Surgical Facial Rejuvenation

A Roadmap to Safe and Reliable Outcomes

Thieme

Surgical Facial Rejuvenation
A Roadmap to Safe and Reliable Outcomes

William H. Truswell IV, MD
Clinical Instructor in Facial Plastic Surgery
Division of Otolaryngology
Department of Surgery
University of Connecticut School of Medicine
Farmington, Connecticut

Thieme
New York · Stuttgart

The progress of this project has been aided by the support and patience of many whom I hold close in both my personal and professional life. To them I owe a debt of gratitude, and to them all I offer this book in dedication.

Thieme Medical Publishers, Inc.
333 Seventh Ave.
New York, NY 10001

Consulting Medical Editor: Esther Gumpert
Managing Editor: J. Owen Zurhellen
Editorial Assistants: Jacquelyn DeSanti, Adriana di Giorgio, Chad Hollingsworth
Vice President, Production and Electronic Publishing: Anne T. Vinnicombe
Production Editor: Heidi Pongratz, Maryland Composition
Vice President, International Sales and Marketing: Cornelia Schulze
Chief Financial Officer: Peter van Woerden
President: Brian D. Scanlan
Medical Illustrator: Joel Herring
Compositor: Thomson Digital
Printer: Everbest Printing Co.

Library of Congress Cataloging-in-Publication Data

Surgical facial rejuvenation : a road map to safe and reliable outcomes / [edited by] William H. Truswell IV.
p. ; cm.
Includes bibliographical references and index.
ISBN 978-1-58890-491-1
1. Surgery, Plastic. 2. Face—Surgery. I. Truswell, William, 1946-
[DNLM: 1. Rhytidoplasty—methods. 2. Face—surgery. 3. Professional Practice. 4. Rejuvenation—physiology. 5. Skin Aging. 6. Surgery, Plastic—methods. WE 705 S96134 2008]
RD119.5.F33S85 2008
617.9'52—dc22

2008014018

Printed in China

5 4 3 2 1

ISBN 978-1-58890-491-1

Contents

Foreword

One can legitimately ask whether another book on facial rejuvenation is needed, given the plethora of texts already available. The answer will be a resounding "Yes" if the question is posed to a resident or fellow aspiring to develop a facial plastic surgery practice or to an established surgeon transitioning their practice to cosmetic facial rejuvenation. These surgeons face an entirely different environment than those of 30, 20, or even 10 years ago. The facial plastic surgeon of yore could provide state-of-the-art facial rejuvenation with a much more limited armamentarium. A reliable facelift, forehead/brow lift, blepharoplasty, rhinoplasty, and skin resurfacing technique allowed one to hang up his or her shingle and successfully build a practice. In most locations, internal marketing was all that was necessary and external marketing was often frowned upon by the medical community. Accreditation of office-based facilities was largely the exception, not the rule.

The amazing growth of public interest in facial rejuvenation has been outpaced only by the number of physicians from multiple specialties now providing these services. The challenge today is further complicated by the emergence of a vastly increased cosmetics industry that turns out a staggering array of products and equipment designed to tap into this growing cosmetic market. Unfortunately, many of these offerings are not outcome-validated, leaving the surgeon at the mercy of slick marketing and product representatives to determine what to incorporate into his or her practice.

To help guide the aspiring facial plastic surgeon through the process of starting or transitioning a practice and the maze of options available for facial rejuvenation, my friend and esteemed colleague Dr. William H. Truswell has assembled a cast of very accomplished facial plastic surgeons, well known as innovators and teachers, to guide the way. I have known Bill for many years through his involvement in the American Academy of Facial Plastic and Reconstructive Surgery and as a teacher and lecturer on facial rejuvenation. Bill is the ideal person to undertake assembling the group of experts who have contributed to this text, as he has intimate knowledge of their areas of expertise. The chapters of this book present safe and reliable techniques and outline solutions for the problems that will inevitably occur with this type of practice.

In addition, Bill Truswell has experienced the transition of his practice to cosmetic facial rejuvenation and understands the necessity of properly setting up the office, credentialing of the facility to accommodate this type of practice, and the internal and external marketing required in these times. Dr. Truswell has always been generous in sharing his time and expertise in teaching facial plastic surgery and he has done so again in undertaking the arduous task of assembling and editing this excellent book. It is a fine guide for the aspiring facial plastic surgeon and a ready reference for any surgeon practicing facial rejuvenation.

Keith A. LaFerriere, MD
Springfield, Missouri

Preface

This book is for you: the facial plastic surgeon wanting a solid reference on rejuvenation surgery; the practitioner developing a practice in cosmetic and rejuvenative facial surgery from within an existing practice in a related field; the resident learning plastic and facial plastic surgery; and the fellow in facial plastic surgery. The chapters of this book are laid out to demonstrate how to establish such a practice from the start and how to evolve an existing practice into a cosmetic one. The use of time, personnel, and space are paramount; credentialing and accreditation are a must. In this field of medicine, perhaps more than any other, marketing is a necessity and will be covered in detail. This text will help you develop techniques to meet these challenges in a practical, efficient, and affordable manner.

The contributors of this text are all accomplished surgeons in facial plastic and reconstructive surgery. They have been in practice many years and are considered experts and masters of their specialty. They are teachers and innovators of techniques and devices employed in facial plastic surgery.

Those of us who have been active in meeting and course presentations over the years receive numerous calls from practitioners asking for advice. They are seeking advice on how to do a part of a procedure, how to avoid a problem, how to handle a complication, how to deal with a difficult patient, how to market and manage their practices, whether to get a new piece of equipment, and many other such issues. The surgical chapters are designed to be a reference and atlas that can be returned to many times for guidance. This text will describe how to achieve reliable, reproducible results safely and efficiently, how to avoid and handle common problems and complications, and how to assess a patient's needs and desires and balance them against realistic expectations on the part of both the surgeon and the patient. The distinctive approach is the stressing of pearls and pitfalls. This is not just a "how to do it" text but rather one that will guide the reader through the penumbra of problems and successes of an accomplished facial rejuvenation surgeon. The accomplished and experienced surgeon may very well routinely perform sophisticated and intricate surgeries. This text will not emphasize those but instead will instruct the practitioner in the safe and reliable surgeries that will help him build his reputation and practice and provide a firm foundation from which to grow.

Acknowledgments

Thank you, Lynn—wife, partner, and friend of infinite patience and understanding—for helping keep this tempest of me somewhat near the ground. And to you, Jason and Jody, my now grown children, you who are the brightness and future.

Thank you Laura, Kathy, Lisa, Cozette, Nancy E., Darci, Jessica, Nancy C., Fawn, and Nancy D., my most wonderful staff, for your loyalty, dedication, hard work, and affection—without you, my practice would be diminished.

I also wish to acknowledge the American Academy of Facial Plastic and Reconstructive Surgery (AAFPRS), the resource for education, guidance, support, and fraternity for facial plastic surgeons throughout the world, and the American Board of Facial Plastic and Reconstructive Surgery (ABFPRS), our certifying body that has raised the bar to the highest and most excellent standard.

Contributors

Peter A. Adamson, MD, FRCS, FACS
Professor of Otolaryngology–Head and Neck Surgery
University of Toronto
Toronto General Hospital
Toronto, Ontario, Canada

Jeffrey M. Ahn, MD
Assistant Professor of Clinical Otolaryngology–Head and Neck Surgery
Director of Facial Plastic and Reconstructive Surgery
Director of Sleep Disorder Surgery
Department of Otolaryngology–Head and Neck Surgery
Columbia University College of Physicians and Surgeons
New York, New York

Richard V. Balikian, MD
Private Practice
Balikian Facial Plastic Surgery
Temecula, California

Anthony E. Brissett, MD
Assistant Professor of Otolaryngology–Head and Neck Surgery
Bobby R. Alford Department of Otolaryngology—Head and Neck Surgery
Baylor College of Medicine
Houston, Texas

Theodore Chen, MD
Surgeon
Department of Head and Neck Surgery
Kaiser Permanente Los Angeles Medical Center
Los Angeles, California

Ted A. Cook, MD, FACS
Professor of Otolaryngology—Head and Neck Surgery
Department of Otolaryngology—Head and Neck Surgery
Oregon Health & Science University
Portland, Oregon

Brian W. Downs, MD
Assistant Professor of Facial Plastic and Reconstructive Surgery
Department of Otolaryngology–Head and Neck Surgery
Oregon Health & Science University
Portland, Oregon

David A. F. Ellis, MD
Professor of Facial Cosmetic Surgery
Department of Otolaryngology–Head and Neck Surgery
University of Toronto
Private Practice
Art of Facial Surgery
Toronto, Ontario, Canada

Kevin H. Ende, MD
Private Practice
The Maas Clinic
San Francisco, California

Mark J. Glasgold, MD
Clinical Associate Professor of Surgery
Department of Surgery
UMDNJ–Robert Wood Johnson Medical School
Highland Park, New Jersey

Robert A. Glasgold, MD
Clinical Assistant Professor of Surgery
Department of Surgery
UMDNJ–Robert Wood Johnson Medical School
Highland Park, New Jersey

Michael S. Godin, MD
Clinical Associate Professor of Otolaryngology–Head and Neck Surgery
Department of Otolaryngology–Head and Neck Surgery
Virginia Commonwealth University
Richmond, Virginia

Jason S. Hamilton, MD
Director of Facial Plastic Surgery
Osborne Head and Neck Institute
Attending Surgeon
Cedars Sinai Medical Center
Los Angeles, California

Mark M. Hamilton, MD
Clinical Assistant Professor of Otolaryngology–Head and Neck Surgery
Department of Otolaryngology–Head and Neck Surgery
Indiana University School of Medicine
Private Practice
Hamilton Facial Plastic Surgery
Indianapolis, Indiana

Robert W. Hutcherson, MD, FACS
Private Practice
Beverly Hills, California

Lisa E. Ishii, MD
Assistant Professor of Otolaryngology–Head and Neck Surgery
Division of Facial Plastic and Reconstructive Surgery
Department of Otolaryngology–Head and Neck Surgery
The Johns Hopkins University
Baltimore, Maryland

Gregory S. Keller, MD
Associate Clinical Professor of Surgery–Head and Neck
Department of Surgery–Head and Neck
University of California Los Angeles
Santa Barbara, California

P. Daniel Knott, MD
Associate Staff
Head and Neck Institute
The Cleveland Clinic
Cleveland, Ohio

Samuel M. Lam, MD, FACS
Private Practice
Lam Facial Plastics
Plano, Texas

Wayne F. Larrabee, MD
Private Practice
The Larrabee Center
Seattle, Washington

Samson J. Lee, MD
Private Practice
Bellevue Ear, Nose, and Throat Clinic
Bellevue, Washington

David A. Lewis, MD
Private Practice
Englewood Ear, Nose, and Throat
Englewood, New Jersey

Corey S. Maas, MD, FACS
Private Practice
The Maas Clinic
San Francisco, California

Jon E. Mendelsohn, MD, FACS
Private Practice
Advanced Cosmetic Surgery and Laser Center
Cincinnati, Ohio

Ira D. Papel, MD, FACS
Associate Professor of Otolaryngology–Head and Neck Surgery
Division of Facial Plastic and Reconstructive Surgery
Department of Otolaryngology–Head and Neck Surgery
The Johns Hopkins University
Baltimore, Maryland

Steven J. Pearlman, MD
Clinical Associate Professor of Facial Plastic Surgery
Columbia University School of Medicine
Private Practice
New York, New York

Stephen W. Perkins, MD
Clinical Associate Professor of Facial Plastic and Reconstructive Surgery
Department of Otolaryngology–Head and Neck Surgery
Indiana University School of Medicine
Private Practice
Meridian Plastic Surgery Center
Indianapolis, Indiana

Adam T. Ross, MD
Assistant Professor of Otolaryngology–Head and Neck Surgery
Department of Otolaryngology–Head and Neck Surgery
Medical University of South Carolina
Charleston, South Carolina

Lorne Segall, MD
Private Practice
Art of Facial Surgery
Toronto, Ontario, Canada

Stephen P. Smith Jr., MD
Director of Facial Plastic and Reconstructive Surgery
Assistant Professor of Otolaryngology–Head and Neck Surgery
Department of Otolaryngology–Head and Neck Surgery
The Ohio State University Medical Center
Dublin, Ohio

Jason P. Sulkowski, MD
Resident of Surgery
Department of Surgery
SUNY Downstate Medical Center
Brooklyn, New York

Jonathan M. Sykes, MD, FACS
Director of Facial Plastic and Reconstructive Surgery
Department of Otolaryngology/Facial Plastic Surgery
UCDavis Health System
Sacramento, California

Monica Tadros, MD
Assistant Professor of Clinical Otolaryngology–Head and Neck Surgery
Director of Facial Plastic Surgery Education
Department of Clinical Otolaryngology–Head and Neck Surgery
Columbia University College of Physicians and Surgeons
New York, New York

William H. Truswell IV, MD
Clinical Instructor in Facial Plastic Surgery
Division of Otolaryngology
Department of Surgery
University of Connecticut School of Medicine
Farmington, Connecticut

Tom D. Wang, MD, FACS
Professor of Facial Plastic, Cosmetic, and Reconstructive Surgery
Department of Otolaryngology–Head and Neck Surgery
Oregon Health & Science University
Portland, Oregon

Edwin F. Williams III, MD, FACS
Private Practice
Williams Center for Facial Plastic Surgery
Latham, New York

Kristina Zakhary, MD, MSc, FRCSC
Private Practice
Calgary, Alberta, Canada

Jose P. Zevallos, MD
Resident of Otolaryngology–Head and Neck Surgery
Bobby R. Alford Department of Otolaryngology–Head and Neck Surgery
Baylor College of Medicine
Houston, Texas

1

Evaluation of the Aging Face

Ira D. Papel and Lisa E. Ishii

Patients who present to a facial plastic surgeon for evaluation of an aging face represent a diverse population with a variety of different concerns. These patients may be male or female, range in age from their twenties to their seventies, and be from different ethnic backgrounds. They may have concerns about specific areas of their faces, or they may want the surgeon to recommend interventions that will improve their general attractiveness. They may have had previous cosmetic procedures or instead be presenting with a cosmetic concern for the very first time. Given the wide spectrum of patients presenting for aging face evaluation for the first time, it is advantageous for the facial plastic surgeon to follow a standard protocol with divergence as appropriate.

The initial consultation should take place in the office or patient evaluation room (**Fig. 1.1**). Lighting should be appropriate for adequate physical examination. A mirror is typically necessary for patients to point out their specific concerns to the physician and for the physician to demonstrate proposed changes to the patient.

It is standard to photograph patients at the time of consultation after obtaining informed consent for photodocumentation. Patient photography should be standardized to enable comparison of preoperative and postoperative photos. Standardization is facilitated by photographing patients in a photo studio using a similar protocol for each photo session. Photographs should be taken in front of a consistent background with lighting that eliminates shadows without flattening the details of the face and skin. The common background color is light blue, which contrasts well with most natural skin tones. The modeling lights are typically umbrellas and or diffusers from a minimum of two directions (**Fig. 1.2**).[1]

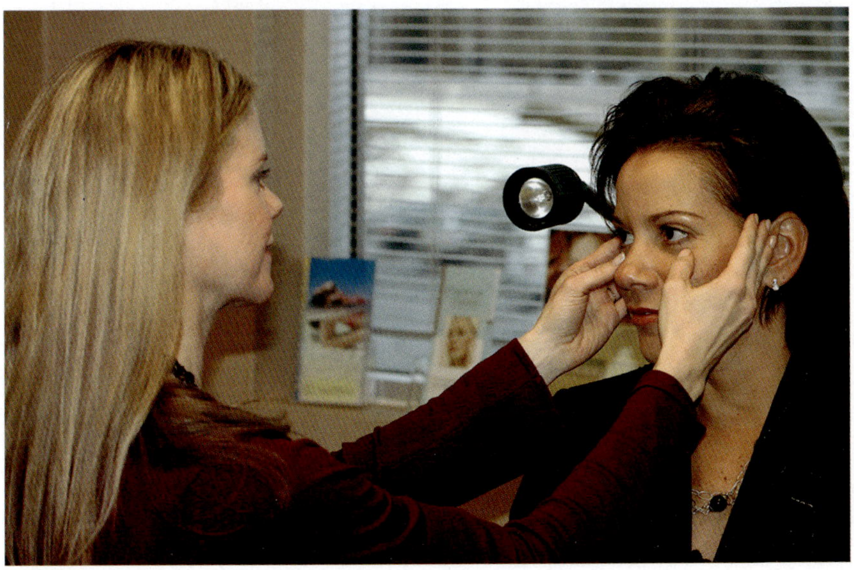

Fig. 1.1 The initial evaluation takes place in an examination room with appropriate lighting.

Fig. 1.2 An appropriate photo studio.

The typical photographic views for patients undergoing rhytidectomy are frontal, left and right profile, and left and right oblique (**Fig. 1.3**). Additional views may be added as appropriate given the procedure. For example, patients scheduled to undergo blepharoplasty should additionally have close-up views of the eyes in the open frontal, lateral, and oblique views (**Fig. 1.4**). The files can be uploaded for computer imaging with commercial systems available in a wide range of prices. Photographs viewed with such software can be altered to demonstrate proposed changes and can help to ensure that the patient and surgeon have similar expectations. In cases of facial rejuvenation surgery, computer imaging is useful for addressing the jawline, neck, and midface.

A

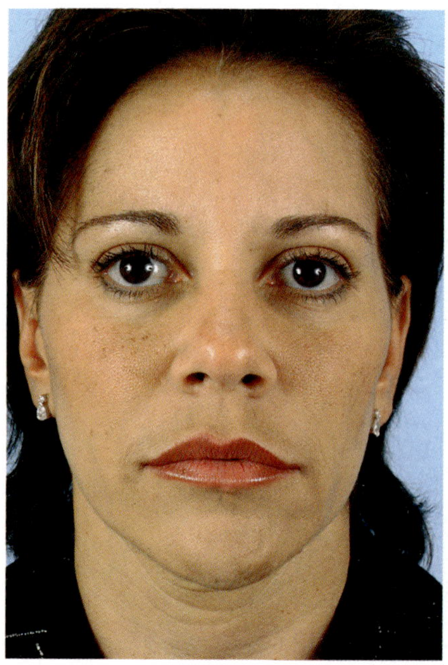

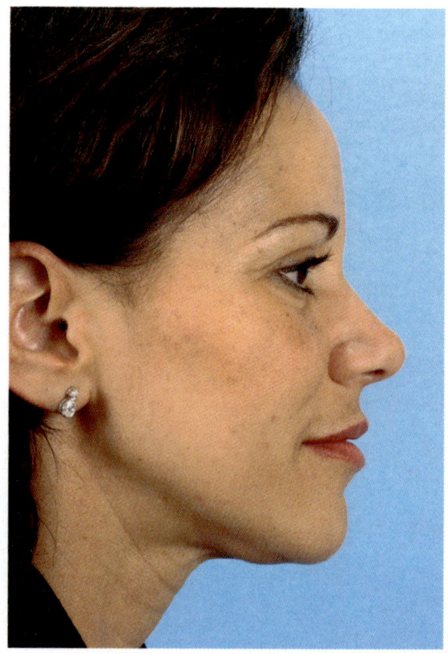

B

Fig. 1.3 Typical photographic views for the rhytidectomy patient: (**A**) frontal and (**B**) right lateral.

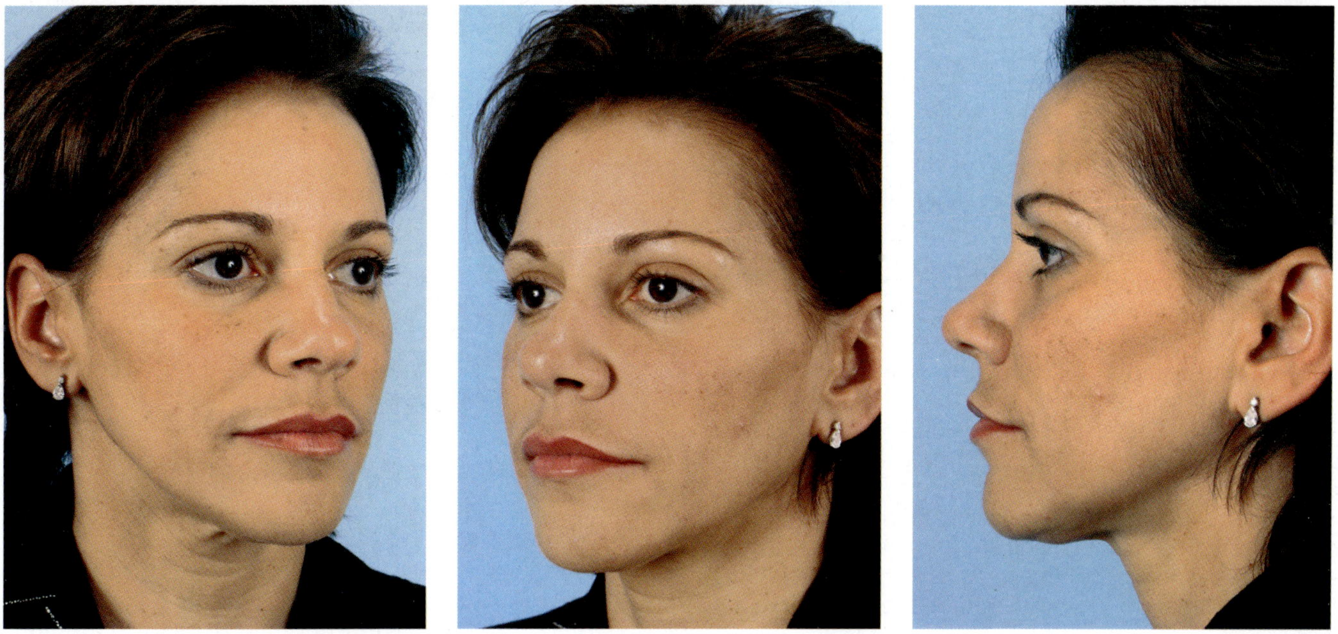

C–E

Fig. 1.3 (*Continued*) (**C**) Right oblique, (**D**) left oblique, and (**E**) left lateral.

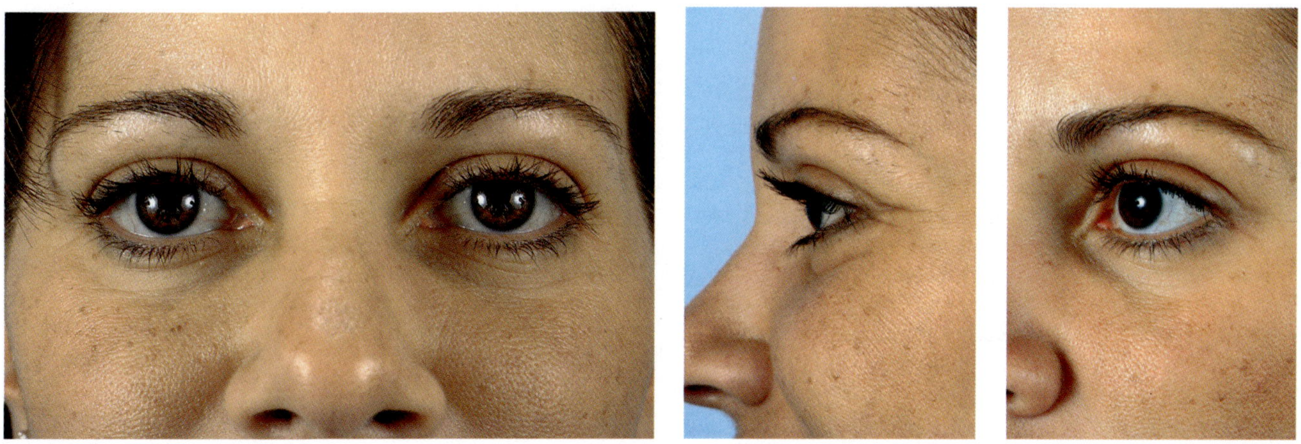

A–C

Fig. 1.4 Typical close-up photographic views for the blepharoplasty patient: (**A**) frontal, (**B**) lateral, (**C**) oblique.

◆ Physical Assessment

The evaluation should begin with a general physical assessment. Each patient should be considered in terms of overall body build and constitution, skin quality, hairline, and bone structure. Additionally, consider whether or not the patient has had prior surgery. Evaluate the face as a whole and in thirds, considering the upper, middle, and lower face and the neck separately.

The initial evaluation should include an appraisal of facial proportions. The symmetric face when evaluated for width can be divided into equal vertical fifths. Each fifth should equal one intercanthal distance, the width of the neck should coincide with a line through the outer canthi on either side, and the lateral-most fifths extend from the lateral canthi to the lateral-most point of the helical rim.[1] Vertical facial height should be measured from the trichion to the menton. Division into equal horizontal thirds should occur at the levels of the glabella and the subnasale. A separate facial height assessment considers only the middle third and lower third of the face. The middle third is delineated superiorly at the nasion with a division to the lower third at the subnasale with its further extension to the menton. In this method, the midfacial height should be 43% of the nasion to menton total distance with the lower facial height comprising the remaining 57%.

Body Build and Constitution

The patient's body mass index (BMI), calculated from height and weight measurements, should be considered prior to treatment planning. Patients with morbid obesity (BMI ≥35) have a three- to fourfold greater risk of respiratory depression from sedative drugs.[2] Additionally, obesity is linked to systemic diseases known to elevate operative risk such as hypertension and diabetes.[3] An increasing number of facial plastic surgical procedures are being performed in outpatient surgery centers as ambulatory surgery. The perioperative cardiopulmonary risk related to obesity or other medical disorders should be considered prior to scheduling outpatient surgery.

Patients who are planning to lose weight should probably delay facial cosmetic surgery until after reaching their target weight. Loss of facial fat associated with overall body weight loss may result in additional skin laxity, particularly in the neck. This increased skin laxity will enable more accurate skin redraping during a facial rejuvenation procedure.

Skin Quality and Hairline

Skin dyschromia, pore size, excess oil or dryness, and hairline position all contribute to the overall appearance of the aging face. Skin quality and hairline must be considered as part of the routine aging face evaluation for optimal treatment planning. Patients experiencing a facial aging appearance due to poor skin quality alone may benefit from a skin care regimen, even in the absence of surgery. For patients with poor skin quality who are planning to undergo a rejuvenating surgical procedure, a skin care regimen in combination with the surgical procedure will provide the greatest improvement in facial appearance. A long-term skin care program, including retinoids, toners, moisturization, and sun block protection, will enhance any surgical result.

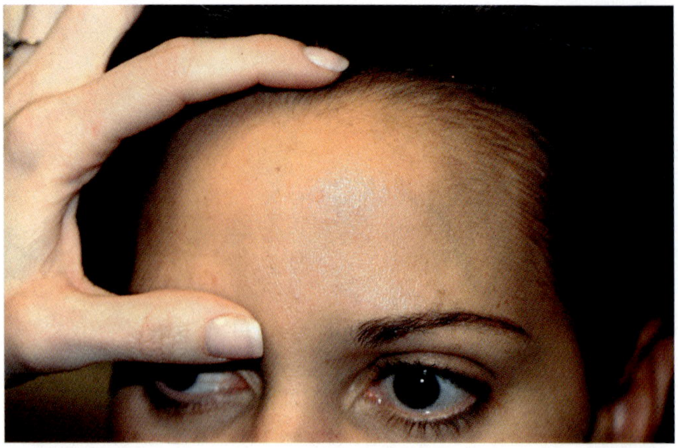

Fig. 1.5 Assessing the position of the anterior hairline.

The position of the hairline must be considered when evaluating patients for surgical procedures and approaches (**Fig. 1.5**). Surgical procedures to rejuvenate the upper third of the face in patients with a high forehead or a receding hairline require careful planning to avoid conspicuous scars or abnormal hairlines postoperatively. For example, the incisions for an endoscopic brow lift may be placed in the hairline for a patient with a normal or low forehead but may need to be placed in a forehead crease for patients with a receding hairline.[4] Frontal and peritemporal trichophytic incisions avoid anterior hairline elevation and maintain preoperative temporal tuft position. These incisions may be particularly useful in patients who have had previous procedures with hairline elevation or unfavorable repositioning of the temporal hair tuft.[5]

Bone Structure

The patient's preexisting bony anatomy can have a significant effect on the outcome of a facial rejuvenation surgical procedure. Hyoid position, chin prominence, and midface vector should all be considered prior to surgical planning. Techniques that address only the soft tissue in patients with unfavorable underlying skeletal anatomy will be unable to restore the desired youthful appearance. The cervicomental angle is the angle created between the horizontal submandibular plane and the vertical portion of the neck. The youthful-appearing neck has an acute cervicomental angle, usually 90 to 100 degrees. Among the factors that can lead to a wide angle, one of the most significant is the position of the hyoid bone. Patients with a low and anteriorly positioned hyoid bone have unfavorable widening of the angle.

Patients with such unfavorable hyoid position may require additional procedures beyond the standard rhytidectomy or submental lipectomy with platysmaplasty to achieve a narrowing of the angle, and they should have realistic expectations about their results.[6]

In addition to hyoid position, chin position affects the cervicomental angle, and retrognathia can cause blunting of the cervicomental angle. The vertex of the angle is at the hyoid bone with the limbs extending through the sternum and the gnathion. The angle is thus affected by the position of the hyoid in relation to the horizontal ramus of the mandible. Patients with a retruded chin have a less distinct transition between the facial and neck aesthetic units, which contributes to the appearance of a heavy, blunted neck.[7] These patients may benefit from placement of a chin or jaw implant in addition to soft tissue procedures to achieve the full desired effect of a smooth neck.

Orbital rim and maxillary hypoplasia may contribute to tear trough deformity, scleral show, and prominent fat pads. Patients with a negative orbital vector are at higher risk for postoperative complications after lower blepharoplasty. The underlying orbital anatomy should be considered prior to performance of a lower blepharoplasty procedure to minimize postoperative complications.[8] For patients with a negative vector, the surgeon should consider a volume enhancement procedure such as temporary injectable fillers, fat transplantation, or permanent implants.

Previous Surgery

Many patients evaluated for facial rejuvenation surgery have undergone previous surgical procedures. This is important to consider as these patients may be at increased risk for complications or may be best served by an alternative surgical approach. For example, patients undergoing revision rhytidectomy may have an increased risk of injury to the marginal mandibular branch of the facial nerve.[9] This results from fibrosis between the subcutaneous tissue and platysma, which increases the difficulty of dissection. Patients who have undergone previous rhytidectomy may have distortion of the temporal hair tuft or unfavorable postauricular hairline realignment. These patients will require special consideration for incision placement and skin flap repositioning. Careful preoperative evaluation with appropriate surgical planning may prevent further distortion and possibly allow for correction of previous complications.

Upper Third of the Face

The evaluation of the upper third of the face takes into consideration the forehead, eyebrows, and eyelids. Patients with aging changes in this region frequently complain of a lingering tired or angry look that is incongruous with their overall disposition. Proper evaluation of this region begins with asking the patient to close his or her eyes for 10 to 15 seconds to relax the muscles. Although they are usually unaware of it, patients with brow ptosis frequently maintain the frontalis muscles in a constant state of contraction to elevate the brows.

The combination of hairline recession and brow drooping typically results in the lengthening of the forehead with aging. Return to a more youthful appearance may be possible with hair restoration procedures to reposition the hairline. This may be particularly beneficial for men. Repeated contraction of the frontalis muscles results in the appearance of horizontal rhytides. Vertical rhytides appear in the glabellar region in response to contraction of the corrugator muscles, and horizontal rhytides in that region result from procerus contraction. The depth of these rhytides should be considered. Patients with minimal to moderate rhytides in this region may respond favorably to Botox® (Allergan Inc., Irvine, CA) injections into the muscles, whereas patients desiring effacement of deeper rhytides may require a surgical procedure.

Brow position changes over time as a result of the pull of gravity. The ideal brow position for the female begins medially at an imaginary vertical line extending through the alar base and medial canthus and ends laterally at an imaginary line from the alar base through the lateral canthus. The medial and lateral ends should be on the same vertical level with a superior arch at its greatest height at the lateral limbus or lateral canthus.[10,11] It should extend ~1 cm above the supraorbital rim. In males, the brow should rest at or just superior to the supraorbital rim with in a more level plane compared with the female arch. Changes in brow position may be achieved with a Botox "chemical brow lift" or with surgical brow lifting techniques such as endoscopic brow lift or transblepharoplasty browpexy.

The eyelids are usually the first facial features to demonstrate signs of aging.[12] The aging appearance of the upper and lower eyelids results from changes in the skin quality, skin excess, and underlying changes in the soft tissue. Effacement of the superior palpebral fold, ideally located one third of the distance between the pupil and the brow, can result from skin laxity and excess.[12] A major blepharoplasty goal is accentuation of this fold. Additionally, excess skin and fat may result in a lack of concavity to the eyelid in the region of the palpebral sulcus. Excision of skin and fat in this region helps restore the more youthful contour.

Evaluation of the lower eyelids should take into consideration the eyelid position, skin quality, lid laxity, and fat pseudoherniation. Additionally, patients should be asked about a history of dry eye symptoms and when there is a concern referred for a formal Schirmer's test. The ideal lower eyelid position is at or slightly superior to the level of the lower limbus. The lower eyelid position may drift inferiorly with age or as the result of scar contracture from prior blepharoplasty. Additionally, in some patients a degree of scleral show is congenital. Patients with crepe-paper eyelid skin and fine wrinkles may enjoy some degree of tightening with a chemical peel or laser treatment, in combination with surgery or alone.[13] The snap test should be performed to evaluate for dermatochalasis of the lower eyelids

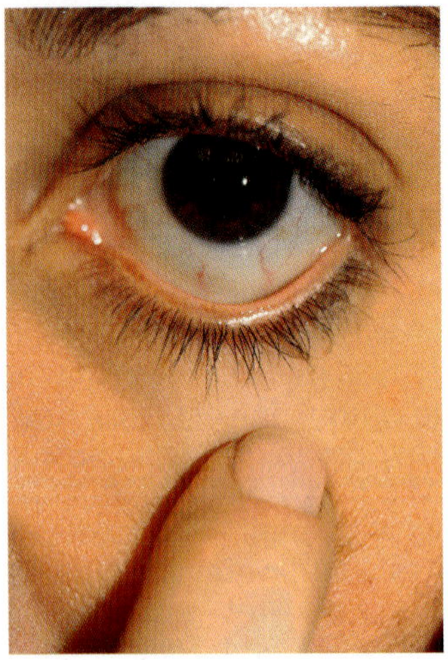

Fig. 1.6 The snap test is performed to assess lid laxity.

(**Fig. 1.6**). Patients with this problem will have a delayed return of the eyelid position after performance of the maneuver. A lateral canthal tightening procedure may be indicated in combination with lower blepharoplasty techniques.

Weakening of the underlying orbital septum can lead to pseudoherniation of fat in the lower eyelid and a *tear trough deformity*. Patients with this problem will complain of dark circles and a chronic tired appearance. The "circles" result from the shadows cast by the protruding fat. It should be noted that some patients may suffer from dark circles due to vascularity or hyperpigmentation. Surgical procedures will not diminish the dark circles for these patients. For patients in whom pseudoherniation is the underlying cause, fat removal or repositioning may improve the circles. For atrophy of soft tissue over the inferior orbital rim, augmentation with injectable fillers or fat transfer will help to obliterate the nasojugal groove and further eliminate the shadow.

Middle Third of the Face

One of the hallmarks of a youthful facial appearance is the convexity of the cheek mounds. The zygoma and overlying soft tissue contribute to this appearance. Over time, the cheek mounds descend and the subcutaneous tissue atrophies such that the youthful convexity is diminished. Additionally, the inferior displacement of the cheek mound results in deepening of the nasolabial fold and nasojugal groove or tear trough deformity. Inferior displacement of the buccal fat pad can lead to effacement of the jawline by jowls.

Identification of underlying bony deficiency such as maxillary hypoplasia may allow for rejuvenation with cheek implants. Alternatively, patients may benefit from temporary effacement of the nasolabial fold and nasojugal groove with injectable fillers such as Restylane® (Medicis Aesthetics, Inc., Scottsdale, AZ) or Radiesse® (BioForm Medical, San Mateo, CA). Long-term midface rejuvenation has historically been challenging. Recent advances in techniques to reposition the cheek mounds with contour threads or Endotine® (Coapt Systems, Inc., Palo Alto, CA) suspension device may contribute to more effective midface rejuvenation.

Lower Third of the Face

Aging changes in the lower third of the face become apparent as skin laxity increases, maxillary and mandibular bone resorbs, and subcutaneous fat thins. In evaluating the patient seeking facial rejuvenation, one should look for the resultant skin excess and soft tissue sagging that leads to blunting of the mandibular line with the appearance of "jowls." As the mandibular line is obscured, the sharp demarcation between the subunits of the lower third of the face and the neck is lost, and this contributes to a less youthful appearance.[14] Submental fat accumulation and submandibular gland ptosis occur as platysma dehiscence occurs anteriorly and contribute to blunting of the cervicomental angle. Aesthetically unfavorable vertical bands running from the chin to the clavicle also appear along the anterior neck with platysma dehiscence and laxity. With aging, the red lip volume diminishes, and perioral radial rhytides become more apparent. Marionette lines may appear as the corners of the mouth begin to droop inferiorly.

◆ Psychological Assessment

The psychological assessment of the patient presenting for facial rejuvenation surgery is just as important as the physical assessment. It is in the best interest of both the patient and the surgeon to invest the time to consider the patient's motives, history, and expectations prior to engaging in a surgical plan. With careful communication and attention to particular problems, physicians may avoid unpleasant surprises after surgery.

Studies have shown that up to 47% of patients seeking cosmetic surgery meet criteria for a mental disorder.[15] It is reasonable to expect that a range of psychiatric illnesses is present in the population presenting for cosmetic surgery just as it is present in the general population. Within that range of illness, the prevalence of disorders involving the individual's appearance such as body dysmorphic disorder (BDD) or narcissistic or histrionic personality disorder may be particularly high.[16] These disorders interfere with rational decision-making, particularly as it relates to one's appearance.[17]

Recognizing patients with these mental disorders can be extremely challenging. Careful attention should be paid to patients who seem excessively needy, anxious, entitled, flirtatious, angry, or depressed, as they may be psychologically impaired. Do they report a history of multiple cosmetic surgery procedures with persistent dissatisfaction with the results? Are they particularly critical of their previous physician(s)? Have they engaged in "doctor shopping" whereby they have sought treatment from multiple cosmetic surgeons?

IRA D. PAPEL, M.D., F.A.C.S. THEDA C. KONTIS, M.D., F.A.C.S

FACIAL PLASTIC & RECONSTRUCTIVE SURGERY
21 CROSSROADS DRIVE • OWINGS MILLS, MD 21117 • 410-356-1100

Pre-Operative Discussions for Face Lifts and Blepharoplasties

1. Problem as the patient perceives it.

a. Forehead
b. Cheeks
c. Nasolabial folds
d. Jowls
e. Midline neck
f. Lateral neck
g. Generalized fine wrinkling
h. Perioral wrinkling
i. Laugh lines
j. Globellar frown lines
k. Upper lid sag
l. Lower lid sag
m. Lower lid bags
n. Nasal deformity
o. Tired appearance

2. Motives, psychological and social status of patient in relation to surgery discussed.

3. Description of problem as I perceive it.

4. Effects of aging on the face are discussed with the patient.

5. Description of operation(s) proposed as to:

a. Anesthesia
b. Location of incisions and resultant scars
c. Probable ancillary procedures
d. Choice of incision as related to hair style and hairline.
e. The goals of improving and unliklihood of perfection stressed
f. Variability of healing from person to person presented
g. Possible complications discussed
 1. Hypertrophic scarring
 2. Hematoma
 3. Infection
 4. Tissue loss
 5. Facial weakness
 6. Loss of sensation of ears and scalp
 7. Loss of hair

6. Weight problem discussed.

7. There is a fairly long period of time for the final exact result of the surgery to be attained.

8. Possibility of secondary procedure discussed.

9. Fees, payment plans, and estimate of hospital costs.

10. Pre-and post-operative instructions read and understood.

Date ____________ Signed ____________

A

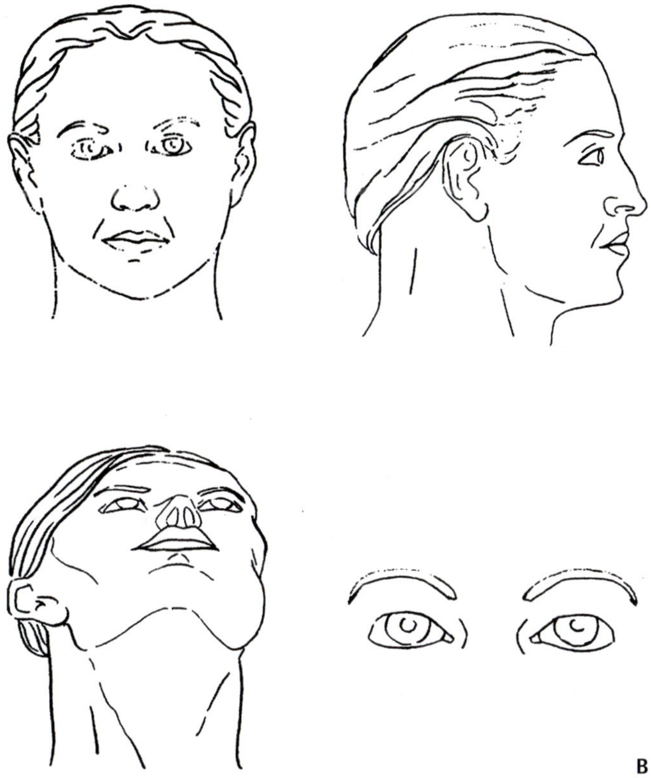

B

Fig. 1.7 Cosmetic evaluation forms: (**A**) front, (**B**) back.

Seven percent to 15% of patients presenting for cosmetic procedures may suffer from BDD, which can be a severely impairing disorder.[16] BDD is characterized by preoccupation with an imagined defect in appearance or an excessive concern over a slight physical anomaly.[17] These concerns may lead to impairment in social and work environments. Patients may engage in excessive checking of the defect or attempts to correct the defect but frequently do so secretly so that the disorder may be underdiagnosed.

The mean age of onset of BDD is in late adolescence and it affects males and females with equal frequency. Rhinoplasty was among the most frequently sought after cosmetic procedures, along with minimally invasive techniques like collagen injection.[16] Because these patients frequently express concern over a relatively minor deformity, they are frequently dissatisfied with the results of an intervention. This may result in frequent and lengthy office visits, phone calls, lawsuits, and even personal threats. Screening questionnaires are available to help identify those patients with BDD.

Patients with narcissistic personality disorder are preoccupied with personal beauty and have a pervasive pattern of grandiosity and a need for admiration.[17] They typically have low self-esteem and react intensely to even minor criticism. They may demonstrate erratic behavior, with outbursts of rage toward the surgeon and the staff followed or preceded by excessive compliments to those same individuals. They should be managed calmly and carefully with extreme attention paid to avoiding critical remarks.

Patients with histrionic personality disorder are excessively emotional and attention-seeking.[17] They use their physical features to attract attention and may be overtly seductive. Patients with histrionic and narcissistic personality disorders may be particularly traumatized by the aging process. Given their inflated views of their appearance, they may be particularly likely to have unrealistic expectations and ultimately dissatisfaction with the results of an intervention.

◆ Checklists

Preprinted forms for the evaluation, informed consent, and posting are helpful to serve as checklists for those portions of the encounter. The evaluation form may include a facial diagram and can be completed during the discussion with the patient. It is a useful aid for describing techniques and anatomy to the patient (**Fig. 1.7**). The preprinted consent and posting forms are useful for increasing efficiency and decreasing errors (**Fig. 1.8**).

Drs. Papel & Kontis
1838 Greene Tree Road, Suite 370
Baltimore, Maryland 21208
Tel: 410-486-3400 • Fax: 410-486-0092

CONSENT FOR SURGICAL TREATMENT

Patient Name: ______________________ Date: ______________

1. I authorize Dr. ______________________ and his/her associates and whomever they may designate as their assistants, to perform the following procedure or operation: ______________________

   and any additional procedure or operation that is considered necessary on the basis of conditions that may be revealed during the course of treatment.

2. I authorize the administration of anesthetics and medications as necessary.

3. Final disposition of any tissues or parts surgically removed is to be handled in accordance with the customary practices of the surgicenter.

4. Indications for surgery: ______________________
   Risks: Bleeding, pain, anesthesia, infection, poor cosmetic or functional result, need for additional surgery, and ______________________

   Alternatives to surgery: ______________________

5. I am aware that the practice of medicine and surgery is not an exact science and I acknowledge that no guarantees have been made to me concerning the results of the procedure.

6. I also give consent for photographs to be taken before, during and after surgery, and give my permission for use of these photographs in scientific presentations and/or medical publications.
   YES NO N/A initials________
   I will allow my photographs to be placed on the internet.
   YES NO initials________

7. I acknowledge that I have read this document and fully understand the planned procedure, indications, potential risks, and alternative modes of treatment.

   Signature: ______________________ Physician: ______________________

   Or:
   Signature: ______________________ Witness: ______________________
   Legal Representative

   ____
   Relationship (if any)

A

FACIAL PLASTIC SURGICENTER, LTD.
1838 Greene Tree Road
Baltimore, MD 21208
410-486-3400

POSTING SHEET

Patient: ______________________ Phone #'s: ______________
Diagnosis: ______________________ Dx Codes: ______________
Procedure: ______________________
______________________ CPT Codes: ______________
Special Equipment: ______________________ Ordered With: ______________
Time Needed: ______________________
Surgical Facility: ❑ FPSC ❑ GBMC ❑ SCOB ❑ SCOP ❑ TENT ❑ MERCY ❑ JHH ❑ Other: ________
❑ OUTPATIENT ❑ INPATIENT (SAME DAY ADMIT)
❑ ELECTIVE ❑ URGENT
Scheduling Preferences: ______________________
ANESTHESIA: ❑ LOCAL ❑ LOCAL / IV SED ❑ GENERAL
Surgeon: ❑ Kontis, M.D. ❑ Papel, M.D. ❑ With Dr. ______________
Preop Consults / Tests: ______________________ Films Needed: ______________

GBMC / Pref. Code # ________ CASE # ________ GOR # ________ ASC # ________

Surgery Scheduled for:

DATE: ______________ ❑ Posted/Date: ______________
LOCATION: ______________ ❑ Called Patient with Date: ______________
TIME: ______________ ❑ Type Up Packet ______________
Arrival Time of Patient: ______________ ❑ Give to: ❑ Dr. Kontis ❑ Papel ❑ Capone
By: (initial) ______________ ❑ Call for Insurance Authorization
Posting Officer: ______________ ❑ FF / NFF
Ins Co. ______________ ❑ Write in Chart
Phone: ______________ ❑ Sign Out Chart to OR
Ins. Authorization #: ______________ ❑ Put in ALL BOOKS / Computer
Auth. Given By: ______________ ❑ Enzymes
❑ Call PCP / NAME / PH # ______________ (For Referral / Surgery)
❑ Waiver

B

Fig. 1.8 (**A**) Informed consent form. (**B**) Posting form.

◆ Conclusion

Both the patient and the surgeon will provide and acquire a significant amount of information during the consultation. Given this large amount of information covered in a typical facial rejuvenation consult, it is useful to conclude the visit with the review of a checklist highlighting the key elements of the visit. The checklist topics may include but are not limited to areas such as realistic expectations, time of healing, and possible complications. Reviewing this checklist with the patient can provide nice closure to the visit and reinforce a mutual understanding of the goals and expectations of the patient and the surgeon.

References

1. Papel ID, ed. Facial Plastic and Reconstructive Surgery. 3rd ed. New York, NY: Thieme Medical Publishers; 2008
2. Chung F, Mezei G, Tong D. Pre-existing medical conditions as predictors of adverse events in day-case surgery. Br J Anaesth 1999;83:262–270
3. Bray GA. Definition, measurement, and classification of the syndromes of obesity. Int J Obes 1978;2:99–112
4. De Cordier BC, de la Torre JI, Al-Hakeem MS, et al. Endoscopic forehead lift: review of technique, cases, and complications. Plast Reconstr Surg 2002;110:1558–1570
5. Holcomb JD, McCollough EG. Trichophytic incisional approaches to upper facial rejuvenation. Arch Facial Plast Surg 2001;3:48–53
6. Prendiville S, Kokoska MS, Hollenbeak CS, et al. A comparative study of surgical techniques on the cervicomental angle in human cadavers. Arch Facial Plast Surg 2002;4:236–242
7. Adamson PA, Litner JA. Surgical management of the aging neck. Facial Plast Surg 2005;21:11–20
8. Jelks GW, Jelks EB. Preoperative evaluation of the blepharoplasty patient. Bypassing the pitfalls. Clin Plast Surg 1993;20:213–224
9. Moyer JS, Baker SR. Complications of rhytidectomy. Facial Plast Surg Clin North Am 2005;13:469–478
10. Ellis DA, Masri H. The effect of facial animation on the aging upper half of the face. Arch Otolaryngol Head Neck Surg 1989;115:710–713
11. Cook TA, Brownrigg PJ, Wang TD, Quatela VC. The versatile midforehead browlift. Arch Otolaryngol Head Neck Surg 1989;115:163–168
12. McCurdy JA Jr. Beautiful eyes: characteristics and application to aesthetic surgery. Facial Plast Surg 2006;22:204–214
13. Halvorson EG, Husni NR, Pandya SN, Seckel BR. Optimal parameters for marking upper blepharoplasty incisions: a 10-year experience. Ann Plast Surg 2006;56:569–572
14. Friedman O. Facelift surgery. Facial Plast Surg 2006;22:120–128
15. Ishigooka J, Iwao M, Suzuki M, et al. Demographic features of patients seeking cosmetic surgery. Psychiatry Clin Neurosci 1998;52:283–287
16. Crerand CE, Franklin ME, Sarwer DB. Body dysmorphic disorder and cosmetic surgery. Plast Reconstr Surg 2006;118:167e–180e
17. Ritvo EC, Melnick I, Marcus GR, Glick ID. Psychiatric conditions in cosmetic surgery patients. Facial Plast Surg 2006;22:194–197

2

Relevant Surgical Anatomy for Rejuvenation of the Aging Face

Wayne F. Larrabee and Samson J. Lee

Surgical techniques for rejuvenation of the aging face have evolved tremendously over the past few decades. This has coincided with a better understanding of the relevant anatomy and the implications of the aging process. Familiarity with the relevant surgical anatomy allows the surgeon freedom in performing surgical dissection in a safe and efficient manner. If a surgeon is hesitant because of uncertainty about important structures, it limits the degree of dissection, ability to manipulate tissue, and may affect results. The first step in evaluating a patient for potential cosmetic surgery is facial analysis.

◆ Facial Analysis

The key to obtaining consistent results in aging face surgery is recognizing the changes associated with aging. Facial analysis should first take into account the sex, race, and age of the individual. Symmetry of the face and any weakness of facial movement should be evaluated and noted. Quality of hair and presence of alopecia should be documented. It is helpful to identify recognizable soft tissue cephalometric points to allow for uniformity in description (**Fig. 2.1**).

The face can be divided into facial aesthetic units.[1] These aesthetic units share similar color, texture, thickness, and mobility of skin. These aesthetic units can be further subdivided for the forehead, nose, and lips (**Fig. 2.2**).[2]

The face is divisible horizontally into thirds and vertically into fifths. The upper horizontal third extends from the trichion to the glabella, the middle third extends to the subnasale, and the lower third extends to the menton. The anterior hairline is usually located 7.5 to 9.5 cm from the glabella. The lower third can itself be further divided into thirds from the subnasale to stomion to mentolabial sulcus to menton (**Fig. 2.3**). The face can also be divided into fifths based on the lateral projection of the helix to the lateral canthus, lateral canthus to medial canthus, intercanthal distance, and so forth (**Fig. 2.4**). Intracanthal distance averages 28 to 30 mm. Faces can come in several aesthetically pleasing shapes, but the oval shape is considered the most pleasing. This corresponds with a 3:4 (height:width) ratio of the face.

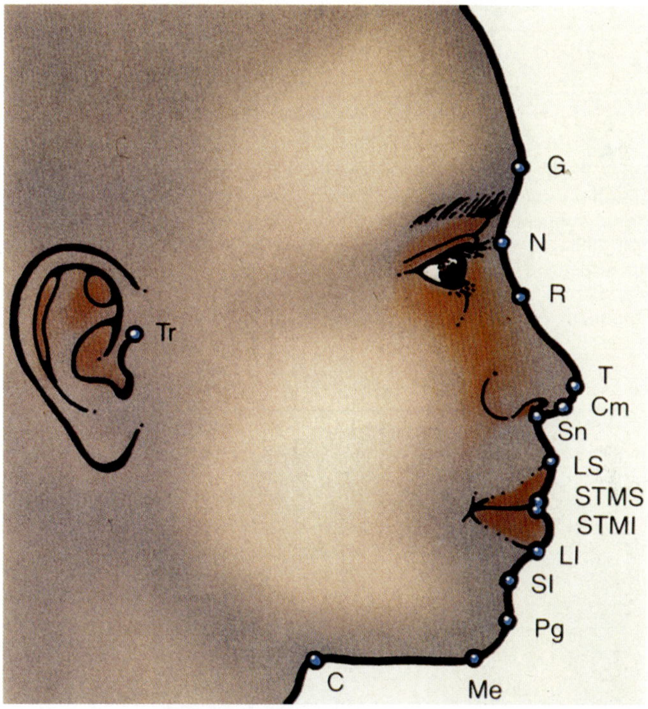

Fig. 2.1 The glabella (G) is the most prominent point in the midsagittal plane of the forehead. The nasion (N) is the deepest depression at the root of the nose in the midsagittal plane. The rhinion (R) represents the junction of the bony and cartilaginous dorsum and is usually the maximum on the nose. The tip (T) is the most anterior projection of the nose. The columella point (Cm) is the most anterior soft-tissue point on the columella. The subnasale (Sn) is the junction of the columella with the upper cutaneous lip. The labrale superius (LS) represents the mucocutaneous junction of the upper lip at the midsagittal plane. Similarly, the stomion superioris (STMS) represents the lower border of the upper lip at the midsagittal plane. The stomion inferioris (STMI) and the labrale inferius (LI) are similarly described for the lower lip. The sulcus inferioris (SI) represents the deepest depression in the concavity between the lip and the chin. The pogonion (Pg) is the most anterior point on the chin. The menton (Me) is the lowest point on the contour of the soft tissue chin. The cervical point (C) represents the junction between the submental area and the neck. The tragion (Tr) is the point at the superior aspect of the tragus. (From Larrabee WF, Makielski KH, Henderson JL. Surgical Anatomy of the Face. 2nd ed. Philadelphia, PA: Lippincott Williams & Wilkins; 2004. Reprinted with permission.)

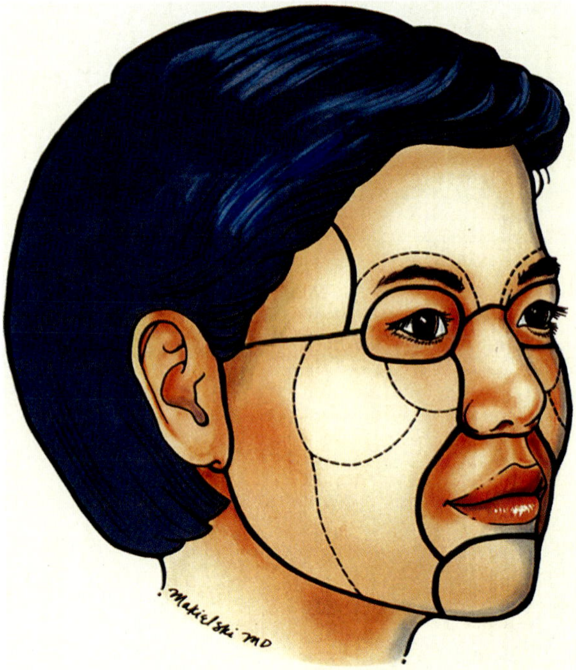

Fig. 2.2 The forehead and the cheek have additional areas of variation in skin thickness (*dotted lines*). The nose is further subdivided into additional subunits (tip, dorsum, sidewall x 2, soft tissue triangle x 2, columella) as well as the lips (philtrum, upper white lip x 2, lower white lip, upper red lip, and lower red lip). (From Larrabee WF, Makielski KH, Henderson JL. Surgical Anatomy of the Face. 2nd ed. Philadelphia, PA: Lippincott Williams & Wilkins; 2004. Reprinted with permission.)

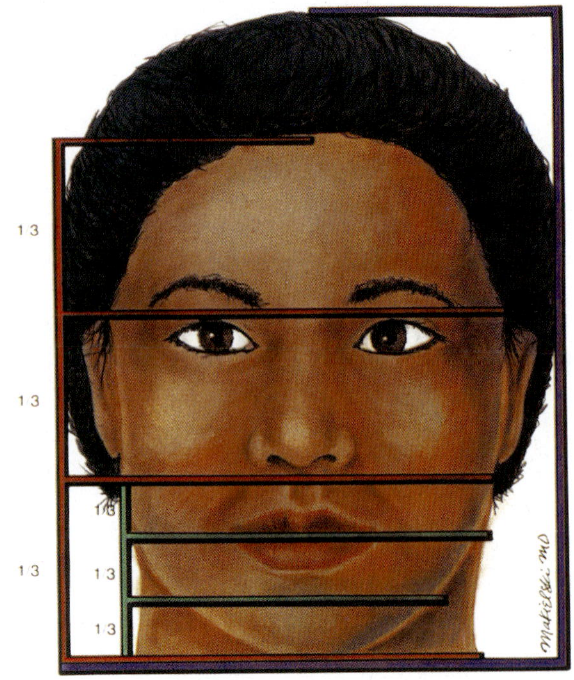

Fig. 2.3 Horizontal facial proportions. (From Larrabee WF, Makielski KH, Henderson JL. Surgical Anatomy of the Face. 2nd ed. Philadelphia, PA: Lippincott Williams & Wilkins; 2004. Reprinted with permission.)

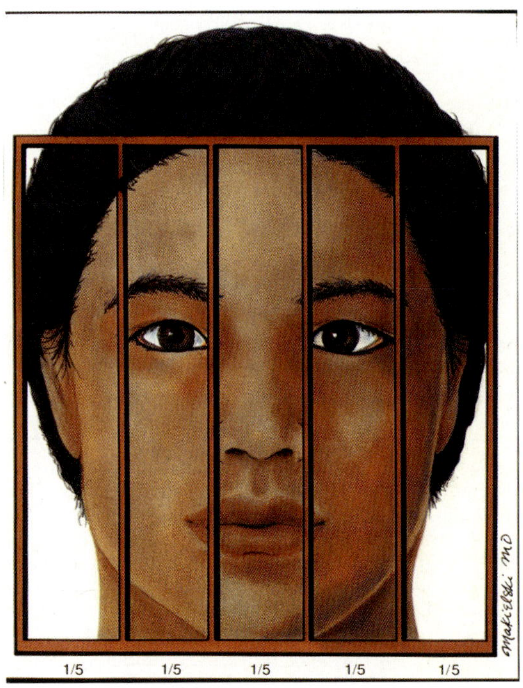

Fig. 2.4 Vertical facial proportions. (From Larrabee WF, Makielski KH, Henderson JL. Surgical Anatomy of the Face. 2nd ed. Philadelphia, PA: Lippincott Williams & Wilkins; 2004. Reprinted with permission.)

A youthful neck contour can be evaluated by the mentocervical angle. This angle is created by a line drawn from the glabella to the pogonion perpendicular to a line from the cervical point to the menton. This angle should be 80 to 95 degrees (**Fig. 2.5**).[3]

Skin

Attention needs to be paid to the quality of the skin. Fitzpatrick skin type should be assessed as well as pigmentary changes. Rhytides, though effaced somewhat by aging face surgery, are better treated by other modalities. This is important to address preoperatively so that the patient has realistic expectations about his or her postoperative outcome. Rhytides can be addressed by resurfacing techniques. As a result of interaction between fixed points, the attenuation in skin, subjacent tissue elasticity, and underlying atrophy of subcutaneous tissue, the accepted younger contours of the face and neck are lost (**Fig. 2.6**). Aging in all parts of the face including the brow, eyelids, face, and neck should be addressed to avoid an unnatural appearance of treating only one area.

Bone Structure

To further assess the overall improvement possible with surgical rejuvenation, the underlying structure of the face must be evaluated critically. Patients who exhibit excellent bony structure of the cheekbones, chin, and jaw during

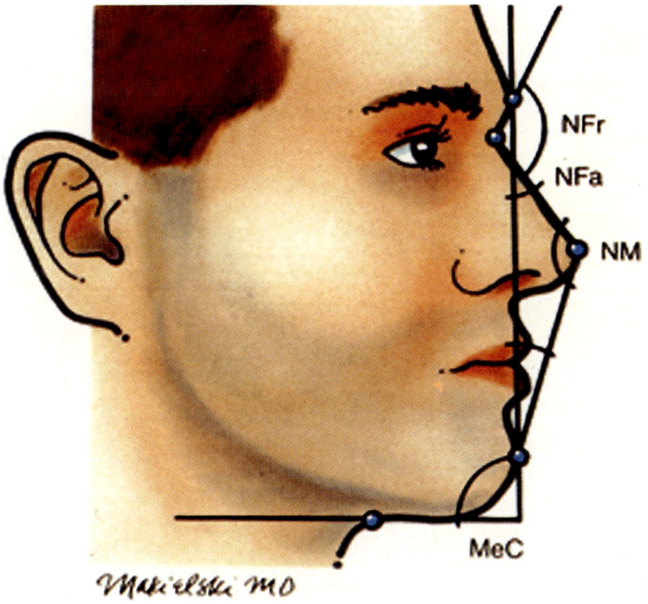

Fig. 2.5 Aesthetic triangle of Powell and Humphreys. A vertical line dropped from the glabella to the pogonion defines the vertical anterior facial plane. A line from the nasal tip is then drawn to the nasion. A line from the glabella to the nasion meets this nasal line and creates the nasofrontal angle (NFr). The nasofacial angle (NFa) is between the anterior facial plane and the line tangent to the dorsum of the nose. The nasomental line drawn from the cervical point to the menton intersects the anterior facial plane and creates the mentocervical angle (MeC). (From Larrabee WF, Makielski KH, Henderson JL. Surgical Anatomy of the Face. 2nd ed. Philadelphia, PA: Lippincott Williams & Wilkins; 2004. Reprinted with permission.)

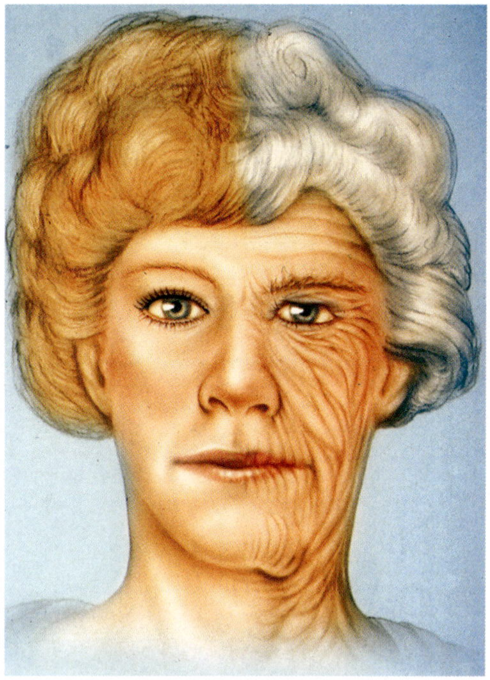

Fig. 2.6 Relaxed skin tension lines depicted on the left side of the face. Notice the changes associated with aging: brow ptosis, upper lid dermatochalasis, lateral canthal laxity and inferior displacement, increased scleral show, cheek ptosis, inferior displacement of the ala, development of the nasolabial and melolabial folds, development of jowling, and downturning of the oral commissure. (From Larrabee WF, Makielski KH, Henderson JL. Surgical Anatomy of the Face. 2nd ed. Philadelphia, PA: Lippincott Williams & Wilkins; 2004. Reprinted with permission.)

their youth have the best results, as the redraping of skin helps to highlight these attractive bony structures. Therefore, patients who have a thinner, angular face and good bony definition are generally much better candidates than are patients with rounder faces, low cheekbones, or short mandibles. With aging there is recession of the mandible and alveolar ridge, particularly evident in edentulous patients, which may limit results without augmentation.

Adjunctive chin and cheek augmentation may be necessary to achieve the desired result. Patients who have a small chin cannot get the desired cervicomental definition without a chin implant or genioplasty. On a lateral view, the line of Gonzales-Ulloa gives an estimate of where the chin or pogonion should lie. This line is dropped perpendicular from the nasion and touches the pogonion. In men, the pogonion should touch this line, and in women, the pogonion should approach this line.[4] If the pogonion does not approach this line, one must address whether there is microgenia (a small chin but normal occlusion), micrognathia (small jaw with possible class II occlusion), or retrognathia (class II occlusion). In addition, the vertical height of the jaw and chin must be addressed. Deficiencies in the vertical dimension are usually better addressed by genioplasty rather than chin augmentation.[5]

Additionally, because the aging process sometimes causes a hollow-cheek deformity due to the atrophy of soft tissue or ptosis of the fat pads, older patients sometimes require submalar augmentation or resupport of the fat pads simultaneously with the facelift. Redraping the skin alone does not replace soft tissue cheek hollowness.

As the underlying structures of the face dictate the aesthetic results possible above the jaw line, those in the neck similarly limit the outcome there. In particular, the position of the hyoid bone relative to the mandible varies from patient to patient. This relationship defines the course of the suprahyoid musculature of the floor of the mouth and delimits the maximum improvement possible in the cervicomental angle. A relatively high and posterior hyoid is ideal, allowing maximum elevation of the submental contour and the greatest definition between the submentum and neck in profile. A relatively low and anterior hyoid limits the possible improvement in the area to a predictable degree. With aging, the hyoid and larynx drop inferiorly causing an aged appearance to the neck in addition to changes in the platysma (**Fig. 2.7**).[6]

Upper Eyelids

The most important part of the preoperative physical examination is the assessment of visual acuity to prevent confusion

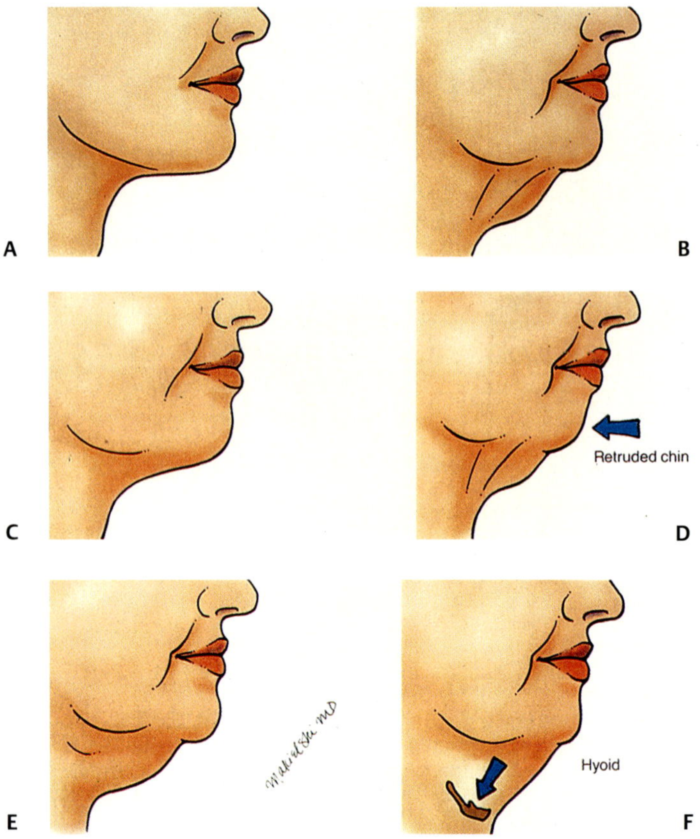

Fig. 2.7 (**A**) A youthful neck with a sharp cervicomental angle and a strong mandibular line. (**B**) Early loss of the cervicomental angle and the mandibular line. (**C**) Chin ptosis, accumulation of submental and submandibular fat, and laxity of submental skin. (**D**) Accentuation of the previous changes plus banding of the anterior platysma. (**E**) Further descent and retrusion of the chin. (**F**) Descent of the hyoid. (From Larrabee WF, Makielski KH, Henderson JL. Surgical Anatomy of the Face. 2nd ed. Philadelphia, PA: Lippincott Williams & Wilkins; 2004. Reprinted with permission.)

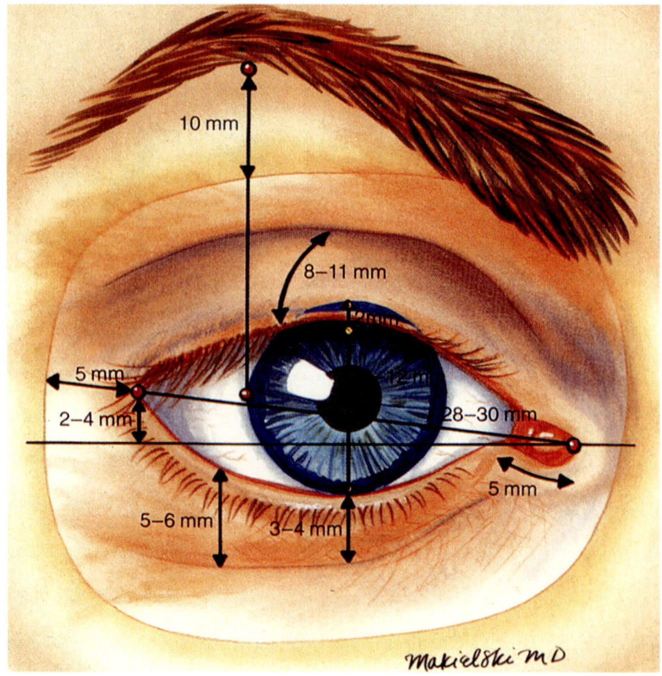

Fig. 2.8 The lateral canthus typically lies 2 to 4 mm superior to the medial canthus. Average palpebral opening is 10 to 12 mm in height and 28 to 30 mm in width. MRD-1 + MRD-2 equals 10 to 12 mm. The distance from the supraorbital rim to the inferior aspect of the brow at the lateral limbus is ~10 mm in Caucasian women. The lower lid crease is ~5 to 6 mm. The high point of the brow is located superiorly somewhere between the lateral limbus and the lateral canthus. (From Larrabee WF, Makielski KH, Henderson JL. Surgical Anatomy of the Face. 2nd ed. Philadelphia, PA: Lippincott Williams & Wilkins; 2004. Reprinted with permission.)

if vision decline occurs in the postoperative period. Ocular movement and function should be tested in addition to asking about symptoms of dry eye.

The upper eyelid is evaluated for the quality of the skin, the quantity of excess skin, pseudoherniation of orbital fat, the position and symmetry of the supratarsal crease, blepharoptosis, retraction of the upper lid, and prolapse of the lacrimal gland. Position of the brow is assessed to prevent pulling the brow inferiorly with upper lid blepharoplasty. Pseudoherniated fat is more commonly found in the nasal compartment of the upper eyelid than in the central compartment. Medial compartmental fat tends to be more whitish and fibrous in texture. Gentle ballottement of the globe can make subtle weakness in the orbital septum evident.

The supratarsal crease is most easily found by lifting the brow and asking the patient to look downward to stretch the eyelid skin, then asking the patient to slowly look upward. The distance from the lash line to the crease at the midpupillary line is 8 to 11 mm in women and 6 to 9 mm in men. If this distance is substantially greater than the reference range, suspect disinsertion of the levator aponeurosis.

Blepharoptosis is determined by measuring the marginal reflex distance (MRD)-1. While the patient remains in neutral gaze, the MRD-1 is measured from the corneal light reflex to the eyelid margin at the midpupillary line. The reference range for MRD-1 is 4.0 to 4.5 mm. Values below the reference range suggest ptosis, whereas values above the reference range suggest upper eyelid retraction (**Fig. 2.8**). In general, the upper lid margin should sit at the upper limbus. Because orbital fat in the temporal compartment is minimal, fullness in this area should alert the surgeon to the possibility of a prolapsed lacrimal gland and the potential need to reposition the gland back into the lacrimal fossa at the time of blepharoplasty.

Lower Eyelids

The lower eyelid is evaluated for the quality of the skin, the quantity of excess skin, pseudoherniation of orbital fat, retraction, and laxity. Pseudoherniated fat in the lower eyelid occurs in three compartments and is most easily assessed by asking the patient to look upward or by gently balloting the globe with gentle pressure on the upper eyelid skin. Hypertrophy of the orbicularis oculi muscle can be assessed by asking the patient to smile and squint. This maneuver highlights redundant or hypertrophied muscle. Another measurement is the MRD-2, which is measured from the corneal light reflex to the margin of the lower eyelid in neutral gaze. The reference range for MRD-2 is 5.0 to 5.5 mm. Evaluation for ectropion or entropion should also be performed. For both the upper and lower lids, fine wrinkling usually cannot be corrected with blepharoplasty alone, and the patient should be counseled about this preoperatively.

Lower eyelid laxity is measured by means of the snap test and the lower lid distraction test. The snap test is performed by pulling the lower lid downward and outward and allowing the lid to snap back to apposition with the globe. The lid should snap back immediately and into full apposition. If it does not, laxity is suggested. The distraction test refers to how much the lower eyelid can be manually pulled or distracted from apposition with the globe. More than 10 mm of distraction is abnormal and suggests laxity. Another important measurement is the relative position of the medial and lateral canthi in the horizontal plane. The lateral canthus is normally positioned 2 to 4 mm superior to the medial canthus with the eyes open. A position inferior to this suggests laxity (**Fig. 2.8**).[6]

Examination of the position of the globe relative to the orbital rim is important. Removing fat from an already retrodisplaced globe or prominent orbital rim can cause a sunken appearance of the eye and should be avoided or prominence of the lateral orbital rim should be addressed. Typically, the distance from the lateral orbital rim to the apex of the cornea is 12 to 16 mm, and the distance from the supraorbital rim to the cornea is 8 to 10 mm (**Fig. 2.9**).[6]

The aesthetics of the lower lid are intimately related to the cheek. Often, to truly address the aging lower lid, the cheek must be addressed in some manner. With ptosis of the cheek fat pad, the vertical length of the lower eyelid increases as the lid-cheek junction becomes more noticeable. To correct this long lower lid and correct the double convexity deformity, the junction between the lid and cheek must be addressed. Often, elevation of the cheek fat pad is not enough, and camouflage of the infraorbital rim is required either by fat augmentation or fat transposition.

Brow

The eyes should be viewed in the context of the entire aging face, especially the forehead and cheeks. The forehead and brows play an important role in the appearance of the eyes. Brow ptosis can account for most of the dermatochalasis in many patients. If blepharoplasty is performed without correcting ptotic brows, the patient is left with a less-than-favorable cosmetic outcome at least and probable worsening of the brow ptosis. For the male patient, brows should be at the level of the orbital rim, whereas the female brow should sit 1 cm above the supraorbital rim. The peak of the brow sits above or just lateral to the lateral limbus in

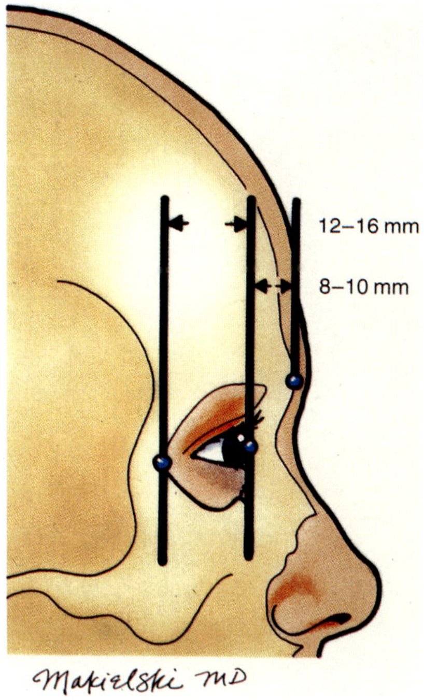

Fig. 2.9 Relationship of corneal apex to lateral orbital rim and supraorbital ridge. (From Larrabee WF, Makielski KH, Henderson JL. Surgical Anatomy of the Face. 2nd ed. Philadelphia, PA: Lippincott Williams & Wilkins; 2004. Reprinted with permission.)

females and is less arched in males. The medial and lateral brow should end at the same horizontal plane. The distal lateral end of the brow should lie at a line tangential to a line adjacent to the ala and lateral canthus.

Cheek

Qualitative analysis of the cheek can be accomplished by two methods. Hinderer's analysis of the malar eminence is performed by drawing a line from the lateral commissure of the lip to the lateral canthus. Another line is drawn from the ala to the superior tragus. The area posterior and superior to the crossing of these lines indicates the location of the most prominent part of the malar eminence (**Fig. 2.10**).

Powell's analysis is performed by a drawing a line from the ala to the lateral canthus; this parallels a line from the tragus to the lateral commissure. Another line is drawn from tragus to tragus. The intersection of the tragal vertical line with the lateral canthal–ala line indicates the vertical position of the malar eminence (**Fig. 2.11**).[6] Settling of the malar fat pad is common after the fourth decade. As the malar fat pad descends, the infraorbital rim becomes more visible as does the delineation between the lower lid and the cheek complex. This results in the double convexity deformity and increased length of the lower lid. This can be corrected by several methods including midface lift, suborbicularis oculi fat pad (SOOF) lift, orbital fat transposition, or fat augmentation.

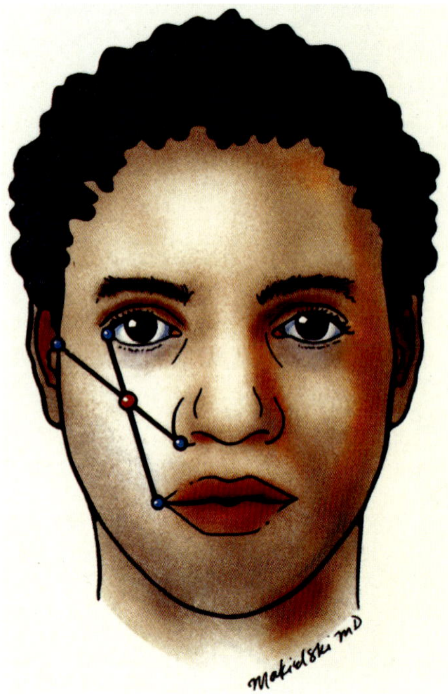

Fig. 2.10 Hinderer's analysis of the malar eminence. (From Larrabee WF, Makielski KH, Henderson JL. Surgical Anatomy of the Face. 2nd ed. Philadelphia, PA: Lippincott Williams & Wilkins; 2004. Reprinted with permission.)

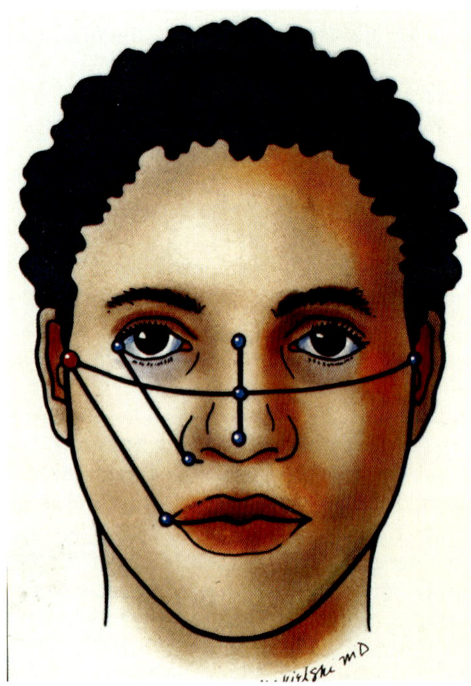

Fig. 2.11 Powell's analysis of the malar eminence. (From Larrabee WF, Makielski KH, Henderson JL. Surgical Anatomy of the Face. 2nd ed. Philadelphia, PA: Lippincott Williams & Wilkins; 2004. Reprinted with permission.)

Lips

As the lips age, several changes occur: increase of upper lip length, blunting of the central defining points, blunting of the philtrum, flattening of the white roll, decrease of vermilion show, downturning of the commissures, and decrease of lip projection.

For assessment of the lips, a line drawn from the subnasale to the pogonion can be used to assess projection. The upper lip should lie 3.5 mm anterior to the line and the lower lip 2.2 mm anterior to the line. Dentition, which can contribute significantly to the projection of the lips, should be evaluated.

◆ Facial Anatomy

Skin

Knowledge of the anatomy of skin is important for all cosmetic procedures involving the face and neck. In particular, knowledge of skin anatomy is important for dermabrasion and skin resurfacing procedures. The integument, or skin, serves as a protective barrier preventing internal tissues from exposure to the outside environment, in sensory perception, immunologic surveillance, thermoregulation, and in control of insensible fluid loss. Beyond this physiologic role, it obviously plays an enormous importance in cosmetic appearance. Skin varies in thickness among anatomic location, sex, and age of the individual. This varying thickness primarily represents a difference in dermal thickness, as epidermal thickness remains rather constant.[7] The thinnest skin is found on the eyelids and in the postauricular region (~0.05 mm thick). Skin on the face in addition to difference in thickness can have varying degrees of dermal appendages and elastin content accounting for differences in elasticity and sebaceous quality. Skin of the forehead, cheek, and lower one third of the nose tends to be more sebaceous and thicker. Male skin is characteristically thicker than female skin in all anatomic locations. Children have relatively thin skin, which progressively thickens until the fourth or fifth decade of life when it begins to thin and lose its youthful elasticity. This gradual thinning occurs primarily in the dermis and represents loss of elastic fibers, epithelial appendages, and ground substance. In addition to thinning of the skin, the subcutaneous tissue thins.

The integument consists of two mutually dependent layers, the thinner epidermis and the thicker dermis, which rest on a fatty subcutaneous layer. Melanocytes are located in the basal layer of the epidermis and primarily function to produce a pigment, melanin, which absorbs radiant energy from the sun and protects the skin from the harmful effects of ultraviolet radiation. With aging, a decline is observed in the number of melanocytes.[7]

The dermis is further subdivided into the papillary dermis and reticular dermis. The pilosebaceous units that control reepithelialization lie in the reticular dermis. These units include sebaceous glands, sweat glands, apocrine glands, and hair follicles. When resurfacing the skin either with lasers, chemical peels, or dermabrasion, care must be taken to avoid too deep an injury to the reticular dermis, which predisposes to scarring secondary to injury to the pilosebaceous units. Underneath the dermis, the subcutaneous layer of fat exists. Nerves, blood vessels, and lymphatics form the subdermal plexus in this layer before supplying the skin.[8] Dissection in this layer traumatizes the subdermal plexus and may lead to hematoma formation.

The papillary dermis is thinner, consisting of loose connective tissue containing capillaries, elastic fibers, reticular fibers, and some collagen. The reticular dermis consists of a thicker layer of dense connective tissue containing larger blood vessels, closely interlaced elastic fibers, dermal appendages, lymphatics, and coarse bundles of collagen fibers arranged in layers parallel to the surface. Although the dominant substance of the dermis is collagen, elastin (which makes up less than 1% of the dermis) has a dominant effect on skin resiliency and elasticity.[7]

The epidermis contains no blood vessels and is entirely dependent on the underlying dermis via diffusion through the dermoepidermal junction. Cutaneous vessels ultimately arise from underlying named source vessels. Each source vessel supplies a three-dimensional vascular territory from bone to skin termed an *angiosome*. Adjacent angiosomes have vascular connections. The cutaneous vessels originate either directly from the source arteries (septocutaneous or fasciocutaneous perforators) or as terminal branches of muscular vessels (musculocutaneous perforators). During their course to the skin, they travel within or adjacent to the connective tissue framework and supply branches to each tissue with which they come into close contact (bone, muscle, fascia, nerve, fat). They emerge from the deep fascia in the vicinity of the intermuscular or intramuscular septa or near tendons and travel toward the skin, where they form extensive subdermal and dermal plexuses. The dermis contains horizontally arranged superficial and deep plexuses, which are interconnected via communicating vessels oriented perpendicular to the skin surface. Cutaneous vessels ultimately anastomose with other cutaneous vessels to form a continuous vascular network within the skin. Clinically, this extensive horizontal network of vessels allows for random skin flap survival.[8]

Skin is anisotropic, meaning that skin's properties vary with direction. Relaxed skin tension lines are lines of minimal tension of the skin. Perpendicular to these lines are the lines of maximum extensibility. When possible, planning incisions parallel to the lines of relaxed skin tension results in less tension and results in a better scar (**Fig. 2.6**).[9]

Hair

Hair follicles have various orientations depending on race. Caucasian hair follicles are oriented obliquely to the skin surface, whereas blacks have follicles oriented almost parallel to the skin surface. Asians have vertically oriented follicles that produce straight hairs. In addition to these racial variations, hair emanates from the scalp in varying orientations depending on the location (**Fig. 2.12**). These anatomic variations are an important consideration in avoiding alopecia when making incisions in the scalp such as brow lifting or correcting alopecia with micrograft transplantation.

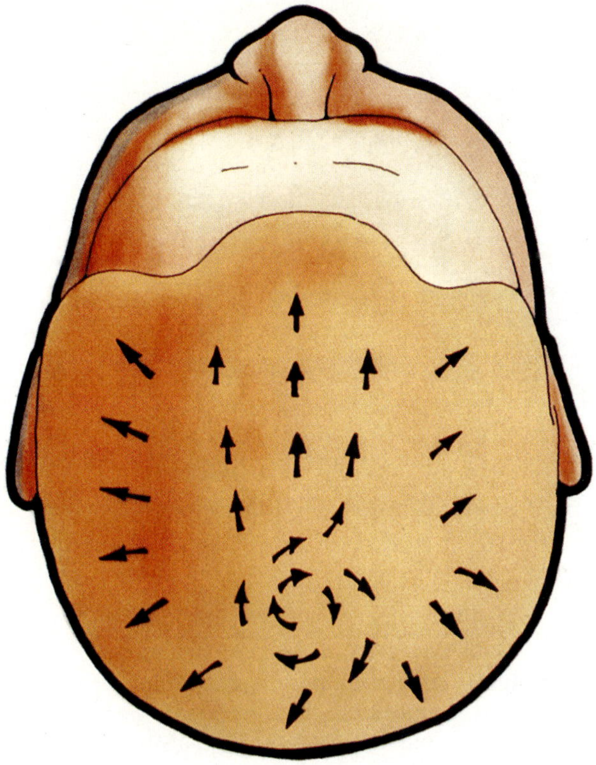

Fig. 2.12 Direction of hair follicles in scalp. (From Larrabee WF, Makielski KH, Henderson JL. Surgical Anatomy of the Face. 2nd ed. Philadelphia, PA: Lippincott Williams & Wilkins; 2004. Reprinted with permission.)

Hair growth exhibits a cyclical pattern. The anagen phase is the growth phase, whereas the telogen phase is the resting state. The transition between anagen and telogen is termed the *catagen phase*. Phases vary in length according to anatomic location, and the length of the anagen phase is proportional to the length of the hair produced. At any one time at an anatomic location, follicles are found in all three phases of hair growth. This is extremely important for laser hair removal because follicles in the anagen phase are susceptible to destruction, whereas resting follicles are more resistant. This explains why multiple treatments of an area may be necessary to ensure adequate hair removal.

Eyelids

Knowledge of the anatomy of the orbit is crucially important to be able to feel comfortable with the myriad of techniques to improve the periorbital complex. The eyelid can be divided into the anterior and posterior lamellae for both the upper and lower eyelids. The anterior lamella is the portion of the lid found anterior to the orbital septum and is composed primarily of the skin and the orbicularis oculi muscle; there is very little subcutaneous fat in this region.

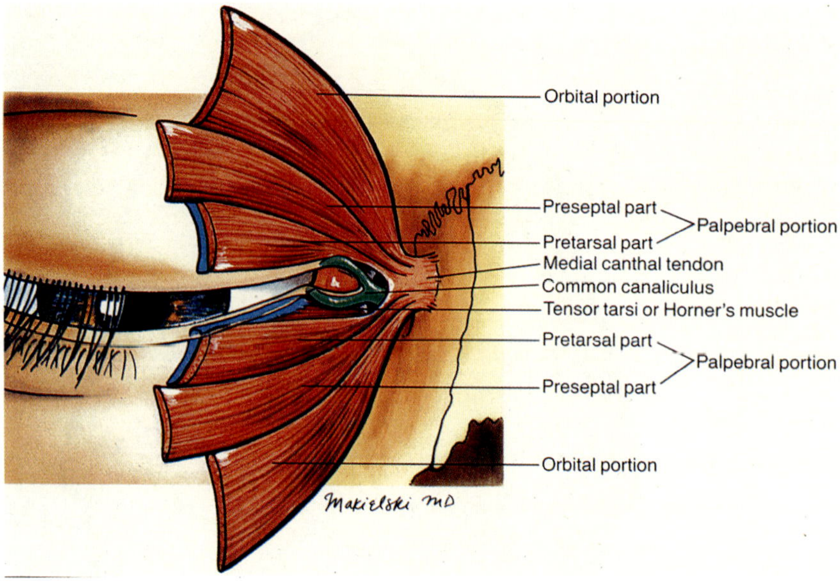

Fig. 2.13 The orbicularis muscle has deep preseptal and pretarsal heads that arise from the posterior lacrimal crest and fossa and a more superficial head from the medial canthal tendon. These heads surround the lacrimal sac and form a pumping mechanism. (From Larrabee WF, Makielski KH, Henderson JL. Surgical Anatomy of the Face. 2nd ed. Philadelphia, PA: Lippincott Williams & Wilkins; 2004. Reprinted with permission.)

The orbicularis oculi muscle is divided into three components: preorbital, preseptal, and pretarsal. The pretarsal orbicularis muscle unites to form the medial and lateral canthal tendons. The medial canthal tendon inserts onto the anterior and posterior lacrimal crests (**Fig. 2.13**). The lateral canthal tendon inserts onto the orbital tubercle of Whitnall.[10]

The orbital septum, which originates from the periosteum at the arcus marginalis at the edge of the orbital rim, fuses with the levator aponeurosis ~3 mm from the upper edge of the tarsus in the upper lid and fuses with the capsulopalpebral fascia in the lower lid. The orbital septum holds back the orbital fat that can be loosely divided into several compartments. In the upper lid, these can be divided into a medial and central fat compartment with the lacrimal gland located laterally. In the lower lid, these compartments are labeled: medial, central, and lateral fat compartments. In the lower lid, the inferior oblique muscle is an important anatomic divider between the medial and central fat compartments. The orbital fat serves as an important anatomic landmark for identification of the levator aponeurosis as it always lies anterior to it in the upper lid. This is particularly important in ptosis surgery. With aging, the orbital septum weakens and allows pseudoherniation of fat to occur.[11]

The posterior lamella is composed of tarsus, levator aponeurosis, Müller muscle, and conjunctiva in the upper lid. In the upper lid, the levator muscle becomes tendinous at approximately the level of the superior rectus muscle insertion and extends anteriorly and then inferiorly to insert into the lower third of the anterior tarsal surface. The Whitnall ligament (superior suspensory ligament of the orbit) is a condensation of connective tissue fibers at the level of the junction of levator muscle and its aponeurosis, which in most instances is anterior to the levator, but it sometimes surrounds the muscle like an envelope. It extends temporally to the lateral orbital rim through the orbital lobe of the lacrimal gland and nasally to the trochlear fascia (**Fig. 2.14**).[6]

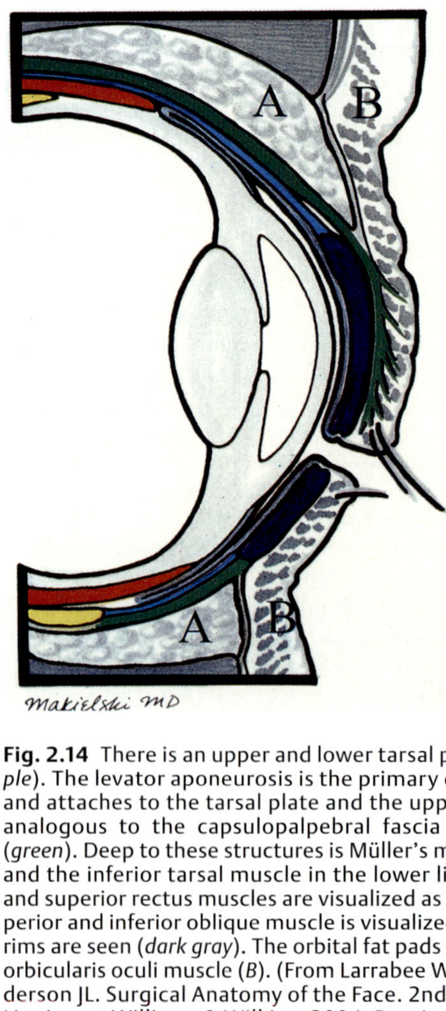

Fig. 2.14 There is an upper and lower tarsal plate in both lids (*purple*). The levator aponeurosis is the primary elevator of the eyelid and attaches to the tarsal plate and the upper eyelid skin. This is analogous to the capsulopalpebral fascia in the lower eyelid (*green*). Deep to these structures is Müller's muscle in the upper lid and the inferior tarsal muscle in the lower lid (*blue*). The inferior and superior rectus muscles are visualized as well (*orange*). The superior and inferior oblique muscle is visualized (*yellow*). The orbital rims are seen (*dark gray*). The orbital fat pads are seen (*A*) as well as orbicularis oculi muscle (*B*). (From Larrabee WF, Makielski KH, Henderson JL. Surgical Anatomy of the Face. 2nd ed. Philadelphia, PA: Lippincott Williams & Wilkins; 2004. Reprinted with permission.)

At about the level of the upper border of the tarsus, aponeurotic fibers arise that extend through the orbicularis muscle to insert into the dermis. These fibers produce the lid crease. In some Asian eyelids, aponeurotic fibers do not insert into the dermis, and this produces the lack of a definable lid crease. In addition, some Asian eyelids possess an epicanthal fold medially (**Fig. 2.15**).[12]

A few aponeurotic fibers also extend to the conjunctiva of the upper cul-de-sac to provide its support and to allow for conjunctival retraction with upward rotation of the eye. The levator tendon is separated from the orbital septum by the preaponeurotic fat, which is an important landmark in the exposure of the tendon during ptosis surgery. The tendon may be somewhat variable in length, usually measuring 14 to 20 mm.[13]

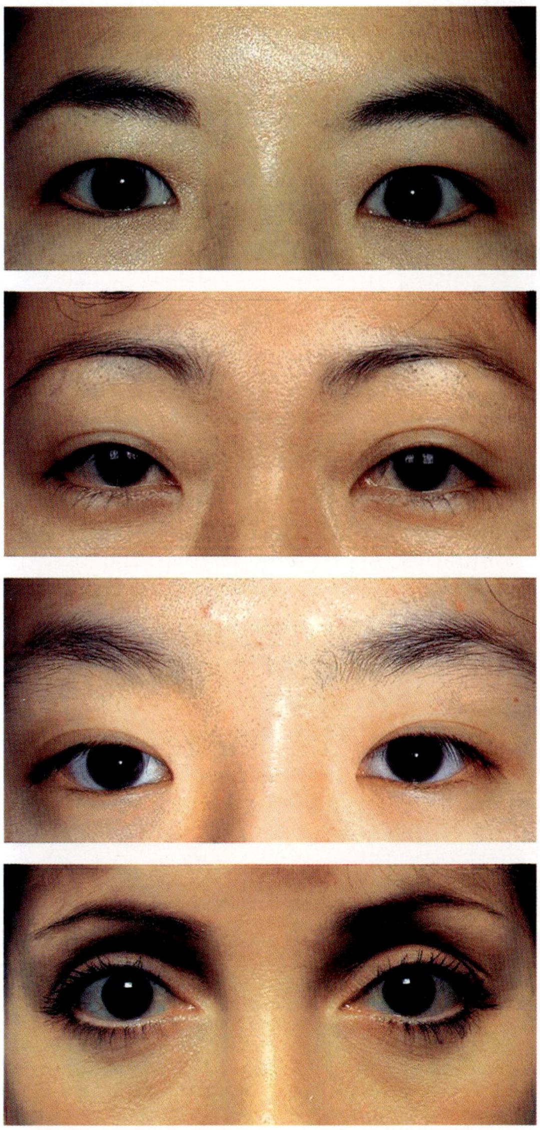

Fig. 2.15 (**A**) Upper eyelid with a crease and epicanthal fold. (**B**) Outer double eyelid. (**C**) Inner double eyelid and epicanthal fold. (**D**) Non-Asian eyelid and no epicanthal fold. (From Larrabee WF, Makielski KH, Henderson JL. Surgical Anatomy of the Face. 2nd ed. Philadelphia, PA: Lippincott Williams & Wilkins; 2004. Reprinted with permission.)

The Müller muscle arises from the inferior surface of the levator originating at the level of the Whitnall ligament and lying between the aponeurosis and the conjunctiva. It passes anteroinferiorly to insert into the upper edge of the tarsus. The Müller muscle is thin and has a slightly darker color than do the levator aponeurosis and levator muscle when seen during surgery. In addition, the peripheral arcade of vessels at the upper edge of the tarsus courses through the Müller muscle and marks its anatomic location. The levator muscle is innervated by a branch of the superior division of the oculomotor nerve (cranial nerve III), which courses through the belly of the superior rectus muscle found beneath it. In congenital ptosis, histologic evidence of muscular dystrophy is present, and fatty tissue and fibrosis replace the levator muscle fibers. As the degree of fibrosis increases, the ptosis becomes more severe. Absence of muscle fibers in patients with congenital ptosis has been documented. The tarsal plate is 10 to 12 mm in vertical height in the upper lid.

In the lower lid, the posterior lamella is composed of tarsus (4 mm in vertical height), conjunctiva, capsulopalpebral fascia, and Lockwood's ligament. The capsulopalpebral head of the inferior rectus is a fibrous connective tissue expansion that attaches ultimately to the tarsal plate allowing for inferior lid retraction during downward gaze. Anteriorly, this capsulopalpebral fascia extends to envelope the inferior oblique muscle and is termed *Lockwood's suspensory ligament*. This ligament attaches to the tarsal plate and contributes to the compartmentalization of the lower lid orbital fat. The orbital septum in the lower lid fuses with the capsulopalpebral fascia 5 mm below the tarsal edge and eventually fuses with the periosteum at the arcus marginalis along the inferior orbital rim (**Fig. 2.14**).[6]

Facial Nerves

Probably the most important relevant surgical anatomy for rhytidectomy is knowledge of the course of the facial nerve. The facial nerve in its initial extratemporal passage lies deep to the superficial lobe of the parotid gland and is not amenable to injury during rhytidectomy in this part of its course. At the superior, anterior, and inferior borders of the gland, the nerve emerges in several branches (temporal, zygomatic, buccal, marginal mandibular, cervical) (**Fig. 2.16**). The superior temporal branches are located within the superficial musculoaponeurotic system (SMAS) or temporoparietal fascia, and the lower branches are located deep to the parotideomasseteric fascia.

As many as three to five temporal branches, which lie anteroinferior to the superficial temporal vessels, may be present. These branches cross the zygomatic arch around 2 cm anterior to the helical attachment of the auricular rim to the face or 2 cm posterior to the anterior-most leading edge of the zygomatic arch. Another simple method is to estimate the distance half-way between the lateral canthus and the helical rim. During endoscopic brow lift and midface

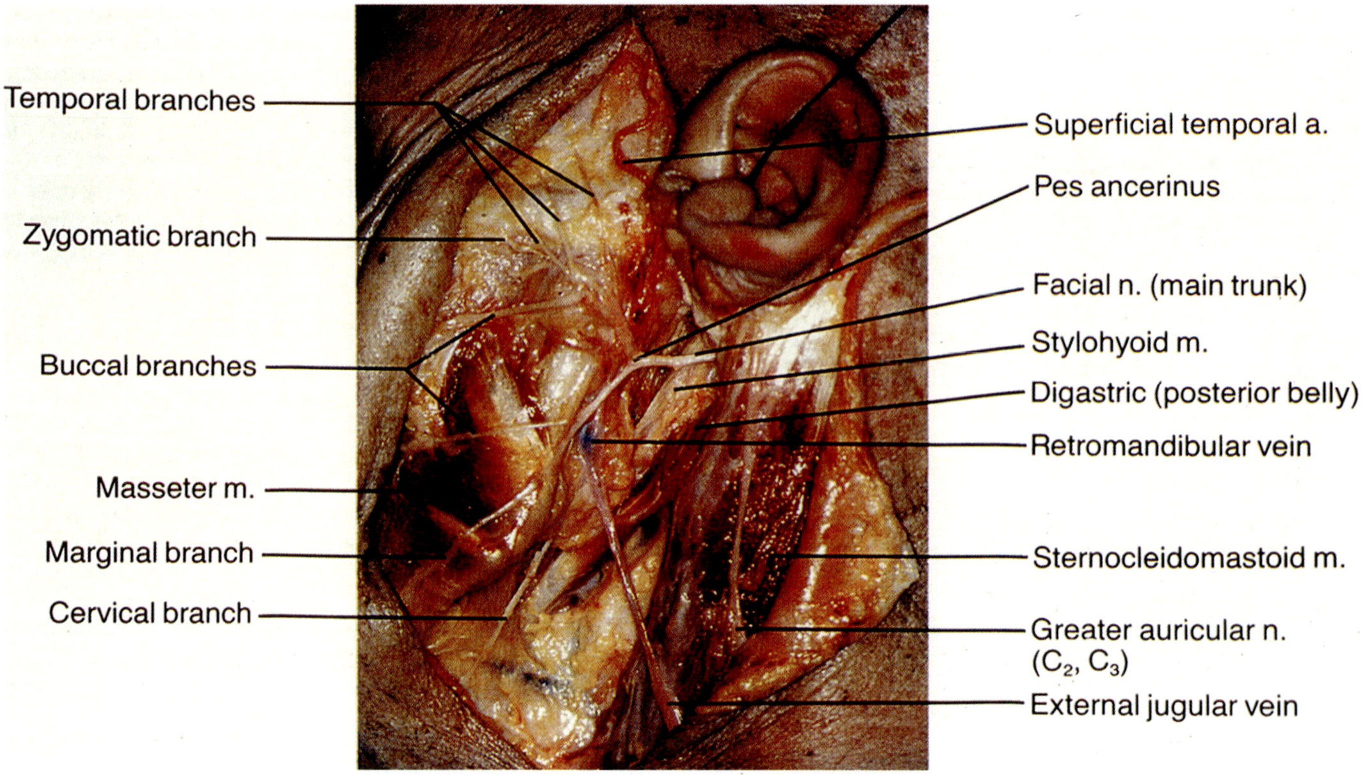

Fig. 2.16 Facial nerve anatomy. (From Larrabee WF, Makielski KH, Henderson JL. Surgical Anatomy of the Face. 2nd ed. Philadelphia, PA: Lippincott Williams & Wilkins; 2004. Reprinted with permission.)

lift, the sentinel (zygomaticotemporal) vein, which is a tributary of the pterygoid plexus, lies lateral to the frontozygomatic suture line. The nerve lies cephalad to the sentinel vein. Caution needs to be exercised around this area to avoid denervation to the frontalis and related muscles. Any cautery in this area should be performed away from the temporoparietal fascia. In addition, the temporal branch of the facial nerve enters the undersurface of the frontalis muscle ~1 to 2 cm above the brow. Care should be taken when taking down the fascial attachments of the temporal line during brow lifting to avoid injury to the nerve as it enters the frontalis muscle (**Fig. 2.17**).[14]

If dissection extends deep to the zygomatic muscles, the zygomatic branches (usually two) are encountered, and risk of trauma occurs. This requires a transition in a deep plane facelift from sub-SMAS to supra-SMAS above the zygomaticus major muscle to avoid injury to these branches. A branch superficial to the zygomaticus major muscle and innervating the orbicularis oculi muscle is described, but the latter muscle is also supplied by frontotemporal branches. Hence, trauma to this branch is largely unnoticed as a result of the dual nerve supply. Occasionally, denervation of this branch can result in problems with the blink reflex. The buccal branches are easily seen lying over the masseter muscle deep to the parotideomasseteric fascia.

The marginal mandibular branch of the facial nerve usually emerges from the parotid gland ~1 cm below the angle of the mandible. It lies deep to the SMAS (platysma muscle) and the parotideomasseteric fascia and posterior to the facial vessels. However, it usually ascends back into the face anterior to these vessels. The mandibular branch may have several tributaries, up to four. The cervical branch lies

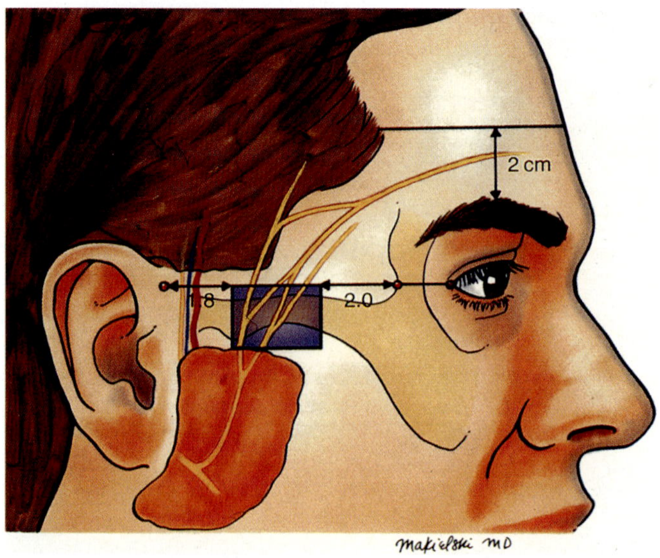

Fig. 2.17 Temporal facial nerve anatomy. (From Larrabee WF, Makielski KH, Henderson JL. Surgical Anatomy of the Face. 2nd ed. Philadelphia, PA: Lippincott Williams & Wilkins; 2004. Reprinted with permission.)

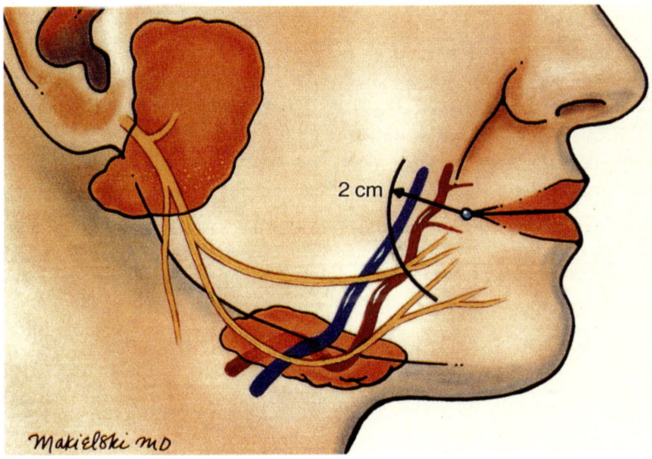

Fig. 2.18 Landmarks for the marginal mandibular branch of the facial nerve. The nerve is deep to the platysma muscle and approaches a point 2 cm lateral to the lateral commissure of the lips. (From Larrabee WF, Makielski KH, Henderson JL. Surgical Anatomy of the Face. 2nd ed. Philadelphia, PA: Lippincott Williams & Wilkins; 2004. Reprinted with permission.)

underneath the platysma muscle and penetrates this muscle ~2 cm below the mandible (**Fig. 2.18**).[15]

The mentalis, levator anguli oris, and buccinator lie deep to the plane of the facial nerve and derive their motor supply on their superficial surface. The facial vessels also adhere to this plane lying superficial to the aforementioned muscles. All other muscles lie superficial to this plane and are supplied on their deep surface.[6]

Other Nerves

The great auricular nerve lies deep to the superficial layer of investing deep fascia as it ascends vertically over the sternocleidomastoid muscle. It lies either in contact or some distance posterior to the external jugular vein, and it divides into anterior and posterior branches to supply the periauricular region. In the posterior cervical and infraaural region overlying the sternocleidomastoid muscle, the skin is adherent to the underlying tissues and may be buttonholed if caution is not exercised. The fibers of the great auricular nerve are in the immediate vicinity. It may be damaged during dissection over the sternocleidomastoid muscle because it is located 6 cm below the tragus at the anterior margin of the muscle to 9.5 cm below the tragus at the posterior margin of the muscle.

The infraorbital nerve deserves attention during subperiosteal lifting in the region of the cheek via an intraoral approach. The nerve emerges from the infraorbital foramen, sandwiched between the superficial surface of the levator anguli oris and the deep surface of the levator labii superioris muscles, to provide sensory innervation to the cheek and upper lip.

The mental nerve emerges from the mental foramen, which lies below the second mandibular premolar. This nerve is vulnerable to injury during chin augmentation or genioplasty.[6] Care must be taken during genioplasty as the nerve in the alveolar tunnel extends 1 cm below the foramen immediately lateral to it.

The supraorbital nerve and vessels usually emerge from the supraorbital notch or canal and continue cephalad in the galea. Occasionally, this neurovascular bundle may exit from a foramen cephalad to the orbital rim, demanding caution with blind dissection within 2 cm of the supraorbital rim.

SMAS and Facial Muscles

Initially, a "skin only" subcutaneous dissection and excision of redundant skin were the first attempts at rhytidectomy. In 1976, the work of Mitz and Peyronie provided a sound anatomic basis by identification and manipulation of the SMAS.[16] Hamra carried facelifting techniques further, involving deeper planes below the SMAS.[17] Further advancements included subperiosteal planes of dissection to achieve facial rejuvenation.[18]

When describing the anatomic dissection planes during facelift, it is helpful to divide the face, temporal regions, and neck into similar units. The layer that corresponds with the facial muscles includes the occipitofrontalis muscle with the intervening galea in the scalp and temporal region and the platysma muscle in the neck. The SMAS layer envelopes and surrounds the facial muscles. The layer that corresponds with the SMAS includes the superficial deep cervical fascia, which envelopes the platysma and sternocleidomastoid muscles in the neck and the temporoparietal fascia in the temporal region. The temporoparietal fascia splits into two layers below the level of the superior orbital margin to enclose the superficial temporal fat pad. In these circumstances, if one proceeds anteriorly under the first layer in a subtemporoparietal fascia dissection, mistaking the deeper layer to be the temporal fascia, trauma to the frontal division of the temporal branch of the facial nerve may occur.

The SMAS is a fibromuscular layer that is thicker and attached to the underlying fascia over the proximal masticatory zone and thinner and more separable from the underlying fascia over the mimetic zone. Hence, proceeding sub-SMAS ~1 to 2 cm anterior to the pretragal crease is advisable. This maneuver also lends skin support to the distal SMAS and skin flap because the SMAS layer may be much thinner and variable in tensile strength further forward. The SMAS has fibrous septae that attach to the overlying dermis, which allows for transferring facial muscle contractions to the skin.[6]

The layers of the temporal region are the skin, subcutaneous fat, temporoparietal fascia (which is the equivalent of the SMAS layer), deep temporal fascia, and the temporalis muscle. The superficial temporal fascia or temporoparietal fascia is separated from the deep temporal fascia by a superficial temporal fat pad. The deep temporal fascia overlying the muscle splits into two layers, enclosing the intermediate fat pad before reuniting ~1 cm above the superior margin of the zygomatic arch and fusing with the parotideomasseteric fascia below. The deep temporal fat pad is an extension of the masticatory fat pad of Bichat under the zygomatic arch and lies deep to the deeper layer of temporal fascia but over the temporalis muscle. The frontal division of the temporal branches of the facial nerve lies in the temporoparietal fascia and is at risk at the level of the zygomatic arch in a subperiosteal facelift operation. Hence, the dissection is carried deep to the superficial temporal fat pad and over the arch. A safer dissection plane is entering deep to the deep temporal fascia 3 cm above the zygomatic arch and under the intermediate temporal fat pad toward the zygomatic arch. At this point, the deeper layer of temporal fascia and zygomatic periosteum is incised anteriorly, and the dissection then proceeds subperiosteally to the superficial surface of the bony zygomatic arch and then over the maxilla (**Fig. 2.19**).

For the forehead region, the frontalis muscle inserts at the medial supraorbital rim into the upper part of the orbicularis oculi muscle and overlying skin. The paired corrugator muscles arising from the periosteum at the superomedial aspect of the orbital rim lie deeper and insert with the frontalis and orbicularis oculi into the skin laterally. The supratrochlear nerves penetrate the corrugator muscle to emerge on the deep surface of the frontalis muscle. Damage to the nerve may occur at this point during corrugator resection. The procerus muscle lies medial and ventral to the corrugator muscles, arising from the nasal bones and

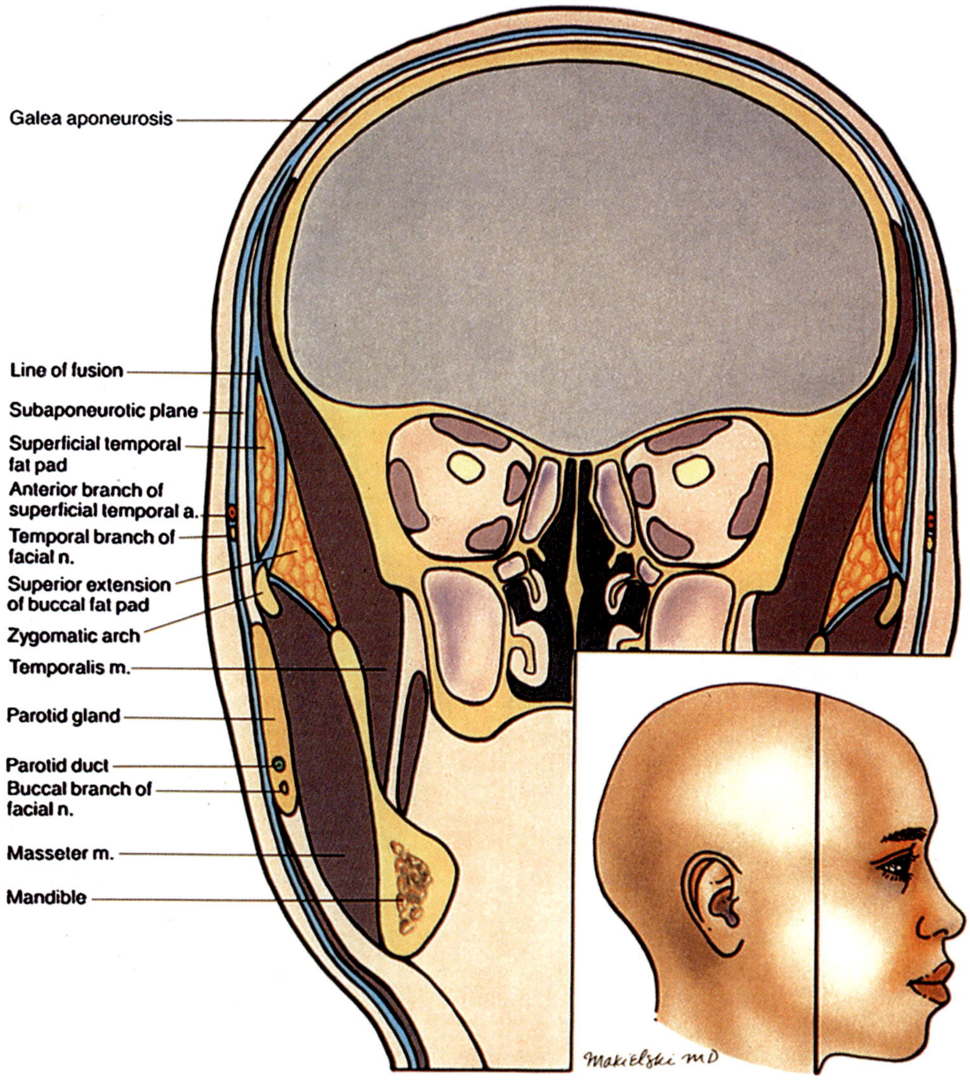

Fig. 2.19 Cross-sectional anatomy of the head depicting the anatomy of the temporal region. Knowledge of this is critical to avoid injury to the temporal branch of the facial nerve. Dissection proceeds under the superficial temporal fascia (temporoparietal fascia) or to be even safer under the intermediate temporal fascia, which overlies the temporal fat pad during subperiosteal midface lifting allowing one to protect the temporal branch of the facial nerve. One should be judicious in preventing too much traumatic injury to the superficial temporal fat pad, which can lead to temporal wasting. Dissection then proceeds just over the zygomatic arch under the periosteum to avoid injury to the temporal branch. (From Larrabee WF, Makielski KH, Henderson JL. Surgical Anatomy of the Face. 2nd ed. Philadelphia, PA: Lippincott Williams & Wilkins; 2004. Reprinted with permission.)

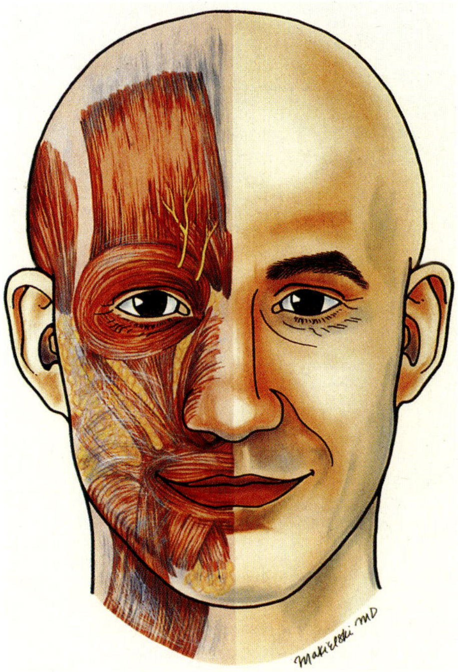

Fig. 2.20 Facial muscle anatomy. Note the position of the supratrochlear and supraorbital neurovascular bundles relative to the position of the corrugator and frontalis muscles. (From Larrabee WF, Makielski KH, Henderson JL. Surgical Anatomy of the Face. 2nd ed. Philadelphia, PA: Lippincott Williams & Wilkins; 2004. Reprinted with permission.)

upper lateral cartilages and inserting into the skin between the eyebrows (**Fig. 2.20**).

Anatomic Planes of Dissection of Rhytidectomy

In a subcutaneous plane, trauma to the facial nerve is not a risk. Dissection proceeds deep to the malar fad pad, which is left attached to the skin, and is advanced superolaterally. A supra-SMAS plane of dissection is similar to the subcutaneous lift; dissection is maintained immediately on the SMAS plane. Again, no trauma to the facial nerve can occur. The sub-SMAS plane in the mimetic zone lies deep to the zygomaticus major, and entrance here definitely jeopardizes its nerve supply. Hence, dissection just lateral to the zygomaticus major muscle needs to shift into the subcutaneous plane. Also, releasing the attachments of the SMAS to the zygomaticus major muscle allows the SMAS layer to be advanced further superolaterally. Leaving the SMAS attached to the skin flap also enhances its viability.

In the temporal region, this plane is the subtemporoparietal fascial layer, and protection to the temporal branch of the facial nerve is thus afforded. In the neck, this layer is subplatysmal, and definite injury to the muscle's nerve supply occurs if dissection is performed in this plane. In the forehead, subgaleal dissection may be permitted up to the supraorbital rim, with identification of the supraorbital nerve and subsequent release of the arcus marginalis to achieve the desired mobility.

A subperiosteal plane of dissection can include the forehead, zygomatic, and maxillary regions. These areas may be approached via an open incision or endoscopically. The bones are denuded of their muscle origins with appropriate caution to preserve the sensory innervation in the region of the supratrochlear, supraorbital, and infraorbital nerves. In this regard, in an endoscopic brow lift, no blind dissection is permissible beyond 2 cm above the orbital rim to allow for the occasional cephalad exit of the supraorbital nerve. Also, careful dissection in the recommended planes in the zygomatic region avoids trauma to branches of the facial nerves. Intraoral dissection in the maxillary and mandibular region must be performed with caution to preserve the infraorbital and mental nerves.

Fat Pads

The malar fat pad lies superficial to the SMAS and overlies the orbicularis oculi, zygomaticus, and levator muscles. It is adherent to the skin, and the zygomatic ligaments traverse it.[6] For efficient placement, dissection must proceed between the muscles and the fat pad so it remains attached to the skin. The inferior extent of the malar fat pad leads to development of the nasolabial fold secondary to the attachments of the SMAS to skin leading to an immobile point of attachment. The superior limit of this cheek fat pad is the orbitomalar ligament, which arises from the arcus marginalis and inserts into the dermis. With descent of the cheek fat pad, this ligament results in a visible separation of the lid-cheek junction ranging from a nasojugal groove to the double convexity deformity.

The ROOF (retroorbicularis fat) pad is located over the superior orbital rim and under the orbicularis muscle. In a patient with brow ptosis, this fat pad can descend and contribute to fullness of the upper lid in addition to the dermatochalasis associated with brow ptosis. This fat pad is routinely visualized during endoscopic brow lift after sectioning of the periosteum.[19]

The buccal fat pad extends laterally over the masseter and buccinator muscles, deep to the plane of the parotid duct and facial nerve branches, and extends anteriorly to the facial vessels. Medially, it may reach into the pterygopalatine space, and an extension lies superficial to the temporalis muscle and its tendon separated from the superficial fat pad by the deeper layer of temporal fascia.[6] (See earlier text for detailed discussion of the temporal fat pads.)

Parotideomasseteric Fascia

This deep layer of fascia splits into two layers to invest the parotid gland. The deeper layer passing deep to the parotid gland is attached superiorly along the base of the skull from the tip of the mastoid process to the lower border of the tympanic plate, as far medially as the carotid foramen. Anteriorly, the fascia may continue deep to the masticatory (buccal) fat pad. The superficial layer over the parotid gland is termed the *parotid fascia*, and it attaches superiorly to the zygomatic process of the temporal bone. The upward continuation is the temporal fascia. With the exception of the temporal branches, the other facial nerve branches lie deep to this layer further anterior in the cheek, in the part known as the parotideomasseteric fascia. This thin layer may be separated from the overlying SMAS between the anterior border of the parotid gland and the anterior border of the masseter muscle. The duct passes forward across the masseter muscle and turns around its anterior border to pierce the buccinator muscle. The duct and facial nerve branches lie superficial to the buccal fat pad.[6]

Retaining Ligaments

The retaining ligaments both may be osteocutaneous or musculocutaneous and may finally insert into the dermis. McGregor first described the zygomatic osteofasciocutaneous ligaments and their role in impairing full mobility of the skin flap. These ligaments anchor the skin to the inferior border of the zygomatic arch contribution from the zygomatic bone. The zygomatic ligaments extend through the malar fat pad, suspending it over the eminence. Accompanying the ligaments are an artery and a sensory nerve. Immediately deep to the ligaments lies a zygomatic branch of the facial nerve. Therefore, care should be exercised to identify these ligaments prior to their incision. With age, these ligaments become lax, leading to inferomedial migration of the malar fat pad and formation of the nasolabial fold. The cutaneous insertion of the zygomatic muscles (i.e., levator labii superioris and levator labii anguli oris) determines the nasolabial crease.

The osseocutaneous mandibular ligament arises from the parasymphysial mandibular body and inserts into the skin inferior to the insertion of the depressor anguli oris, interdigitating with the platysma, which lies deeper to the depressor. If this ligament is left intact and employed as an anchor to allow the jowl lift to pull against it, the perioral area assumes a much more natural look postoperatively. The depressor anguli oris superiorly and the mandibular ligaments inferiorly determine the labiomandibular crease, which similarly is converted into a fold as a result of the laxity of the masseteric ligaments that occurs with age.

The fasciocutaneous masseteric ligaments pass from the region of the anterior border of the masseter muscle toward the dermis. They may represent the points of fusion between the SMAS and the parotideomasseteric fascia layers. With age, laxity of the masseteric ligaments allows the inferomedial descent of the tissues and contributes to the formation of the labiomandibular fold or jowl. The anterior limit of the jowl is the mandibular ligament. The masseteric ligaments need to be freed to achieve skin advancement during facelifting. The masseteric ligament also approximates the midcheek furrow of aging and the posterior boundary of the mimetic muscles (**Fig. 2.21**).[20]

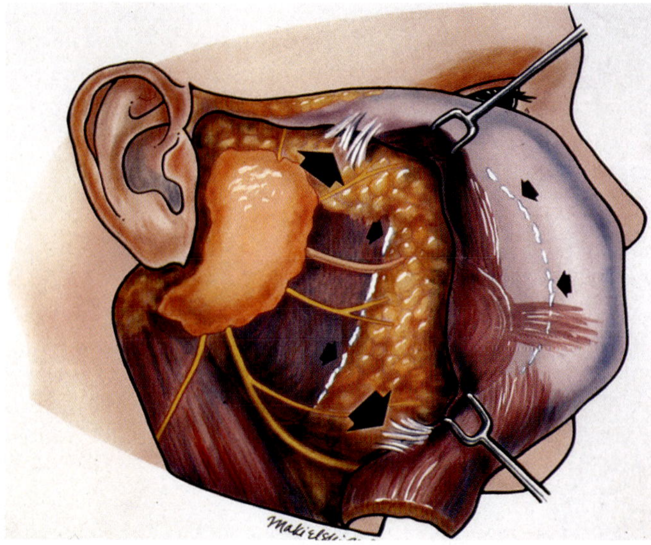

Fig. 2.21 Major retaining ligaments of the face. The SMAS is elevated demonstrating the retaining ligaments of the face. The small arrows delineate the cut SMAS and the large arrows point to the zygomatic cutaneous ligament (superior) and mandibular cutaneous ligament (inferior). A sub-SMAS dissection would proceed under the SMAS but above the facial musculature to protect the facial nerve. Superiorly near the level of McGregor's patch and the zygomatic major muscle, a sub-SMAS dissection should proceed subcutaneously to avoid injury to the nerve that innervates this muscle. (From Larrabee WF, Makielski KH, Henderson JL. Surgical Anatomy of the Face. 2nd ed. Philadelphia, PA: Lippincott Williams & Wilkins; 2004. Reprinted with permission.)

Vascular Supply

The vascular supply to the face is derived from the facial vessels medially and from the superficial temporal vessels laterally. These arteries originate from the external carotid. The facial veins drain into the internal jugular vein, and the superficial temporal veins eventually drain into both the internal and external jugular veins. The supraorbital and supratrochlear branches from the internal carotid system supply the forehead. The generated angular vein joins the facial vein.

Medially, the musculocutaneous branches of the facial artery contribute to the subdermal plexus. Laterally, the fasciocutaneous branches of the superficial temporal artery and the transverse facial artery contribute to the subdermal plexus. These medial and lateral vessels approximate each other lateral to the nasolabial fold. Sub-SMAS dissection transects the lateral perforators, placing supply of the flap solely on the medial musculocutaneous vessels. Subcutaneous dissection transects the subdermal plexus. Both the subcutaneous and sub-SMAS flaps are randomly patterned, based on several vessels with varying patterns of supply dominance.[6]

◆ Conclusion

By understanding relevant surgical facial anatomy, the facial plastic surgeon is empowered to sculpt and manipulate tissue in an efficient manner without fear of damage to underlying structures. The basis of any surgical procedure is critical facial analysis. Facial analysis, in combination with an understanding of how the aging process affects the underlying anatomy, allows the facial plastic surgeon to plan what type of procedure best suits the individual needs of the patient. Though natural selection and evolution are unlikely to significantly change anatomic structures in our lifetimes, surgical techniques will continue to evolve. This evolution of surgical technique will always be dependent on a critical knowledge of the underlying anatomy.

References

1. Gonzales-Ulloa MCA, Stevens E. Preliminary study of the total restoration of the facial skin. Plast Reconstr Surg 1954;13:151–161
2. Burget GCMF. The subunit principle in nasal reconstruction. Plast Reconstr Surg 1985;76:239–247
3. Powell N, Humphreys B. Proportions of the Aesthetic Face. New York, NY: Thieme-Stratton; 1984
4. Gonzales-Ulloa M. Quantitative principles in cosmetic surgery of the face. Plast Reconstr Surg Transplant Bull 1962;29:186–198
5. Sykes J, Tollefson T, Frodel J. Mentoplasty and facial implants. In: Cummings CW, ed. Otolaryngology-Head and Neck Surgery. Vol. 1. New York, NY: Elsevier; 2005
6. Larrabee WF, Makielski KH, Henderson JL. Surgical Anatomy of the Face. 2nd ed. Philadelphia, PA: Lippincott Williams & Wilkins; 2004
7. Moore K, Persuad T. The integumentary system. In: Before We Are Born: Essentials of Embryology and Birth Defects. 5th ed. Philadelphia, PA: W.B. Saunders; 1998:481–496
8. Bennett R. Anatomy and physiology of the skin. In: Papel I, ed. Facial Plastic and Reconstructive Surgery. New York, NY: Thieme; 2002:3–14
9. Larrabee W, Sherris D. Principles of Facial Reconstruction. 1st ed. Philadelphia, NY: Lippincott-Raven; 1995
10. Jones LT. An anatomical approach to problems of the eyelids and lacrimal apparatus. Arch Ophthalmol 1961;66:111–124
11. Neely KA, Ernest JT, Mottier M. Combined superior oblique paresis and Brown's syndrome after blepharoplasty. Am J Ophthalmol 1990;109: 347–349
12. Chen WP. Asian blepharoplasty: update on anatomy and techniques. Ophthal Plast Reconstr Surg 1987;3:135–140
13. Karesh JW. Diagnosis and management of acquired blepharoptosis and dermatochalasis. Facial Plast Surg 1994;10:185–201
14. Bernstein L, Nelson R. Surgical anatomy of the extraparotid distribution of the facial nerve. Arch Otolaryngol 1984;110:177–183
15. Dingman RO, Grabb WC. Surgical anatomy of the mandibular ramus of the facial nerve based on the dissection of 100 facial halves. Plast Reconstr Surg Transplant Bull 1962;29:266–272
16. Mitz V, Peyronie M. The superficial musculoaponeurotic system (SMAS) in the parotid and cheek area. Plast Reconstr Surg 1976;58: 80–88
17. Hamra ST. Composite rhytidectomy. Plast Reconstr Surg 1992;90: 1–13
18. Ramirez OM. The subperiosteal rhytidectomy: the third generation face lift. Ann Plast Surg 1992;28:218–232
19. Most SP, Mobley SR, Larrabee WF Jr. Anatomy of the eyelids. Facial Plast Surg Clin North Am 2005;13:487–492
20. Furnas DW. The retaining ligaments of the cheek. Plast Reconstr Surg 1989;83:11–16

3

The Facelift: A Guide for Safe, Reliable, and Reproducible Results

William H. Truswell IV

The cornerstone of surgical rejuvenation of the aging face is the facelift operation. The method the surgeon uses to perform this procedure will be determined by many factors. The most important consideration is that the surgeon does a procedure with which he or she is comfortable and at which he or she excels. Above all, experience affects outcome. In the beginning of one's practice and experience, a solid approach to sub-superficial musculoaponeurotic system (sub-SMAS) lifting will produce very good results and happy patients. As time passes, the surgeon will gain confidence both mentally and manually with his or her surgical technique and outcomes. This becomes the time to move into more advanced and technical lifting.

Residency and fellowship training, reading texts, listening to lectures, and attending courses certainly provide the scientific and procedural information needed to perform facelifting. Operating over time on the myriad of different facial types, however, imparts the knowledge of what the tissues feel like, how they dissect, how they heal, and how they behave over time after surgery. The emerging facelift surgeon learns through his or her practice how to treat the full spectrum of patients from those with heavy faces and thick, type-III-and-beyond skin, substantial fascia, short necks, and an abundance of fat to those with ultrathin faces and thin, type I skin, tissue paper–like fascia, long necks, and a complete paucity of fat. It is worth repeating that as the surgeon performs more facelifts, his or her confidence grows manually through muscle memory, intellectually as different facial types are encountered and their outcomes studied, and emotionally through both the praise of grateful patients and the problems of the difficult ones.

The first section of this chapter will describe the author's standard for facelift patients from first contact to final farewell and his approach for a sub-SMAS facelift in the uncomplicated face, which over the years has allowed reliable, reproducible results and happy patients. The happy patients make the practice grow.

◆ The Goal: A Happy Patient—The True Measure of Success

First Contact

The goal to which one must strive is more than a satisfied patient; it is a happy patient. This outcome, the happy patient, will be the key that makes one's practice grow and prosper. To achieve this, the surgeon must think beyond the technicalities of surgery. There needs to be a global approach to the cosmetic surgery patient. The process begins with the prospective patient's first contact with the office. The voice, manner, and style of person answering the telephone sets the tone for all that follows. The receptionist must be warm and welcoming, be able to answer questions about the surgeon and his or her experience and qualifications, the practice and its history, and general questions about the procedures done. Clinical questions may be diverted to a nurse or technician, but they too must have these same people skills. A letter is sent out to the patients once they have scheduled a consultation thanking them for making the appointment. The letter tells them what to expect when they arrive at the office and our commitment to patient education. We include a registration form for them to fill out and bring with them. Other enclosures can include a custom practice brochure or brochures from the academy.

The Setting

The office setting will be the first physical impression the patient has of the practice. The reception area and waiting room must be warm and inviting, a place where one will be comfortable and happy to sit for a while. The waiting time should be brief. Information forms should be short, not encyclopedic, or the information could be taken at the patient

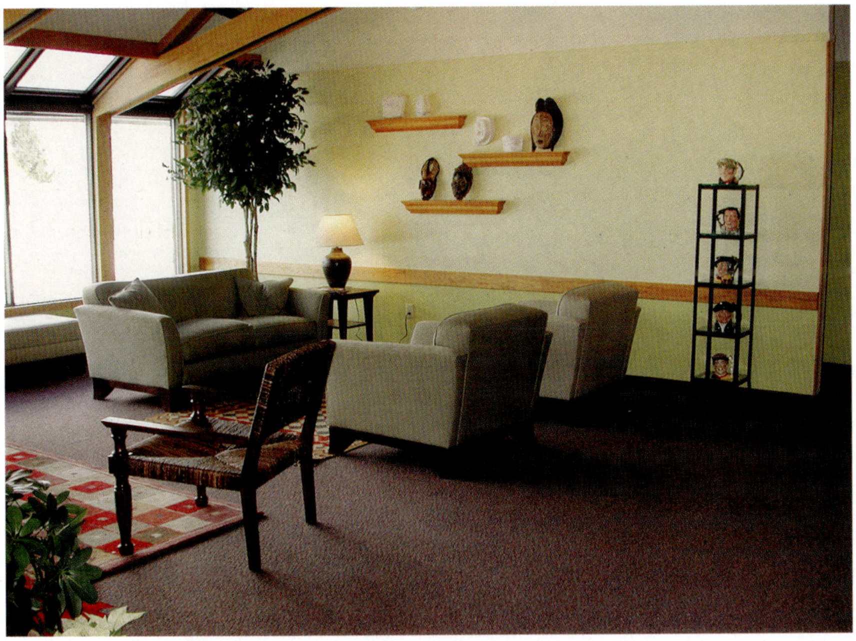

Fig. 3.1 The waiting room should be warm and inviting, a place where one would not mind waiting a while.

coordinator's interview. All that happens before the patient meets the doctor reflects onto the surgeon, and the patient is forming an opinion of the practice and the surgeon starting with the first contact (**Fig. 3.1**).[1]

The Staff

The entire office staff must be friendly and nurturing. They will make the patient feel that she or he will be cared for and cared about. They should dress in a manner that is "upscale" and their grooming must be impeccable. This atmosphere will have the patient feeling that she or he has chosen the best place for his or her needs and desires to be met.

The patient coordinator, nurse, or manager will greet the patient and take digital photographs. The photographs must be standardized for all patients as to position and lighting. This is best done in a dedicated room. The pictures become an integral part of the medical record and should be treated as such. Pictures are taken in frontal, 45 degrees to each side (oblique), and both lateral positions. They are all in the Frankfort horizontal plane. They should also be taken in each position with the patient's hair in its natural style and with the hair up and any high collar rolled down, and earrings and necklaces removed. Standard positions for facelift surgery are full face and neck, right and left oblique, and full lateral right and left. It is important to see the entire ear and all of the neck. This becomes the preliminary step in patient education. At this juncture, a discussion ensues about what the patient's desires are. A skilled coordinator will discern what the patient needs and gently indicate what the doctor may suggest. She will also be able to determine how realistic the patient is and if the patient is a good candidate for the surgery. She will then brief the surgeon about the patient and what he or she may expect.

◆ What Are We Trying to Achieve? The Refeminization of the Female Face

The facelift surgeon should have an understanding of what he or she is trying to achieve. In different parts of the country, patient populations may very well have different ideas about how they wish to look after their surgery. These ideas will also vary within locales.

In western New England, for example, patients have told me for more than 30 years that they do not want to look "done." They want a natural, nonoperative appearance and they often fear being approached by friend or acquaintance with the comment, "You had a facelift." Celebrities they see in the media as well as people they have seen in traveling to more cosmopolitan areas of the country often appear to them as "overtightened" and not looking like themselves. I answer this worry simply by showing them preoperative and postoperative photographs of my patients. It is necessary for the surgeon to understand the style of the demographic where he or she practices.

Unfortunately, as time passes, the soft, lovely, feminine face of youth becomes more masculine (**Fig. 3.2**). Men have low brows, and a woman's eyebrows descend. Men have thin lips, and a woman's lips lose volume. Men have square jaws and heavy necks, and as jowls and wattles appear, the feminine jaw line squares off and the neck tissue falls. Men also have coarser skin, and a woman's skin will coarsen, too. We as surgeons cannot realistically make a 60-year-old face appear to be 40 or even "take 10 years away." I believe the realistic expectations for the surgeon and patient are encompassed by the words *soften, refresh, rejuvenate*, and *refeminize*. This is done by lifting the soft tissues of the face and neck, restoring lost volume, and revitalizing aged, sun-damaged skin to create that more youthful and feminine appearance of youth (**Fig. 3.3**). The patient will know the kind of work the surgeon does from the photographs shown during the consultation. These should not be the most beautiful and successful cases but a collection of faces from those of average appearance to the very attractive, including heavy faces, thin faces, and different skin types. This will present an honest view of what is achieved by the hands of the surgeon.

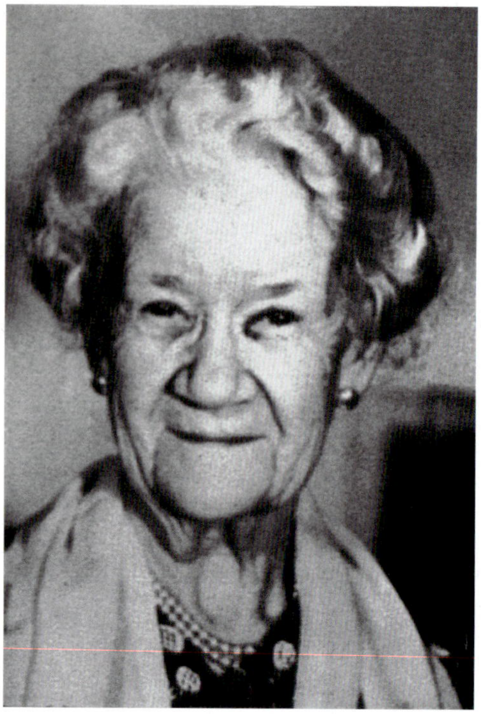

Fig. 3.2 The masculinization of the aging feminine face.

◆ Patient Selection

Patient selection involves the physical, the emotional, and the psychological assessment of the prospective candidate.[1–3] Emotional stability is a must before surgery is undertaken. Recent spousal loss due to separation, divorce, or death causes an emotional wound that must be well healed before a facelift is done. This operation will not fill the void or lift the spirits of the griever. Similarly, psychological disorders such as a bipolar disorder must be in control as well. Lastly, the physiognomy of the person must be well suited to receive reasonable results. The morbidly obese face will not have a pleasing or a lasting result.

Ideally, every patient would be late middle age, normal weight, type I or II skin, with a long elegant neck, good facial

A

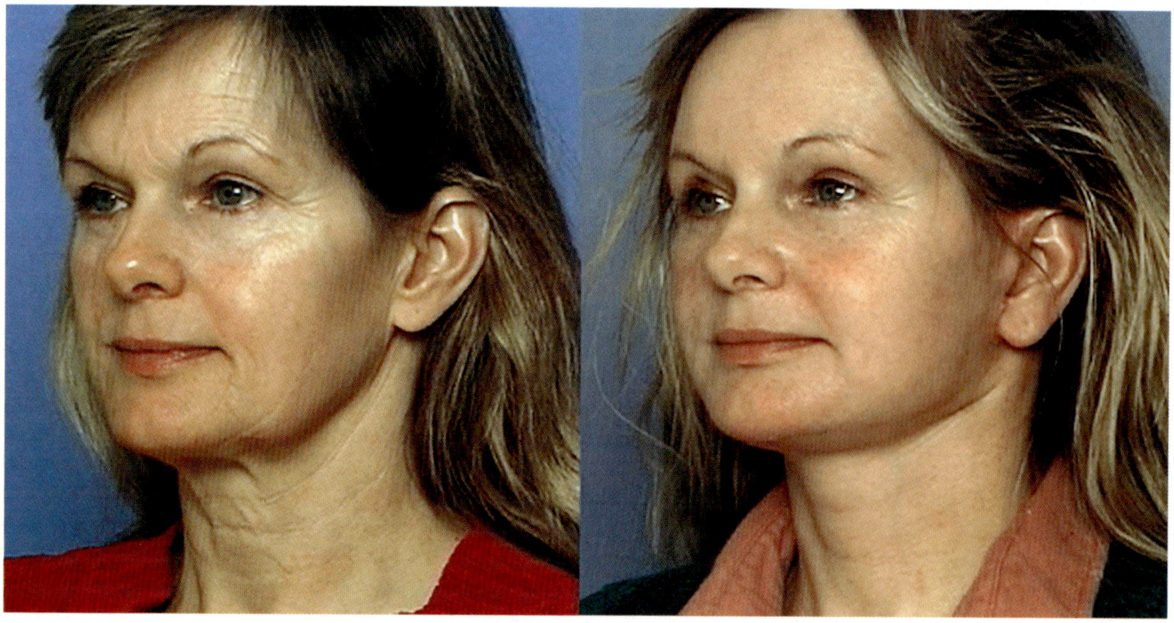

B

Fig. 3.3 (**A**) Before and (**B**) after endoscopic brow and facelifting: restoration of a more youthful and feminine countenance.

bone structure and facial proportion, and in good health. In the majority of cases, however, this is not the situation. The facelift surgeon will sample the whole sea of humanity. It is important, of course, that the patient's health is such that it will not bring risk to the procedure. Medical conditions such as hypertension and diabetes must be stable. Medical clearance should be obtained for the patients preoperatively. The overweight patient should be asked if she is planning to lose weight. Significant weight loss should precede the surgery for optimal results. Facial balance is also important. A recessive chin when corrected will enhance the results of the procedure. Sometimes patients will only want or perhaps can only afford to have the facelift done when in reality they need full facial rejuvenation. It is imperative that they understand and acknowledge the imbalance that will occur between the rejuvenated lower face and the untreated upper face. Both the patient and the doctor must have realistic expectations.

◆ The Consultation

All this attention to detail comes before the patient meets the doctor and should lift her or his expectations. The consultation is the opportunity for the surgeon to convince the patient that there is no reason to look further. It is the start of a very special doctor-patient relationship. It is the time the surgeon will be determining the true motivation of the patient. The attitude, appearance, and personality of the physician will lead to a successful surgery booking. In a relatively short period of time, he or she will listen to the patient's concerns, evaluate the face, explain the options, demonstrate with pictures his or her typical results, perhaps do computer imaging, and enumerate potential problems. Computer imaging is an opportunity for the surgeon to demonstrate the goals of the surgery to the patient by altering the patient's photograph. It must be understood that what is being demonstrated is not an exact representation of the results of any surgery but a simulation of what could be achieved. It is wise to make the imaging somewhat less than the actual results of the surgery.

Preoperative and postoperative photographs of patients who underwent similar surgery are reviewed with the patient. This is an opportunity for the patient to see the kind of results from the hands of her chosen surgeon. The pictures should not be just of the best-looking patients with spectacular results but of faces from all walks of life. Not everyone is beautiful, and the patient should be able to relate personally to some of the pictures. The photographs should be at various intervals after surgery. We show patients at 1 day after, 1 week after, to several years after surgery. The patient should understand the issues of healing and swelling and have a feeling for the natural aging process after facelifting. The patient should come away thinking that there is no reason why this surgeon alone should not take scalpel and scissor to her or his face and change her or his appearance. This task may or may not seem either daunting or arrogant; however, it must be done gently, in a warm and friendly fashion, taking the patient's concerns and fears into consideration.

The consultation is the second and the most important step in patient education. When the patient has a good understanding of what can and cannot be achieved, what the sequelae and possible complications are, and what the operation and postoperative period entail, the entire experience will be smoother with less patient anxiety, more patient compliance with instructions, and realistic patient expectations. The patient should feel that all of their questions and worries are answered, should have no doubt that this surgeon is the best choice, and should never feel rushed.

The surgeon must elicit a medical history from the patient. All previous surgeries including cosmetic procedures need to be explored. It is good to know, in the case of cosmetic surgery, if the patient's expectations were met and if they were happy with their results. This may give an indication of their attitude, goals, and motivation. It should be considered a "red flag" if the patient expresses anger or regret. This would need to be explored thoroughly. The surgeon should be alert for possible personality disorders, the presence of body dysmorphic syndrome,[4] and any unrealistic expectations the patient may have. The existence of significant personality disorder or body dysmorphic syndrome would preclude surgery. If unrealistic expectations cannot be eliminated through patient education, any patient harboring them is not a good candidate for a cosmetic procedure. This is also the time to learn the patient's medical history. It is necessary to know what chronic medical problems the patient may have and what prescription and over-the-counter medications are being taken. Any allergic history to medications and latex must be elicited.

The face, head, and neck should be examined carefully. Assessment of the skin type, solar damage, lesions, rhytides, and elasticity are noted. It is important to note the skin type, the amount of sun damage, and the degree of elasticity in each patient. Skin with severe elastosis and/or significant sun damage may very well benefit from concurrent or sequential resurfacing. In these instances, resurfacing either by laser or peels greatly adds to the result of facelift surgery. The CO_2 laser is uniquely beneficial. Facelifting repositions and recontours the soft tissues of the face and neck, and laser resurfacing, in addition to reducing rhytides, removing lentigines, and improving skin texture, will tighten the skin itself and stimulate the formation of new collagen.

The amount and location of subcutaneous fat needs consideration. The heavier faces, particularly of those patients in need of weight reduction, will have a less than ideal outcome. It is imperative to let the patient know and be certain she understands this limitation. These individuals with heavy skin and subcutaneous tissues will not enjoy a sleek and elegant look from surgery. They will look refreshed, rejuvenated, and, in the case of women, refeminized. They must be taught the realistic outcome of the operation in their individual circumstance. They also must understand that recurrence of aging will be sooner for them than in the thinner, more esthetic face. Using added platysmal support such as the Giampapa suture[5] or securing the elevated platysma with barbed threads to the mastoid fascia may prolong and enhance the effect of the surgery. The surgeon should also assess the use of ancillary procedures such as malar augmentation and a chin implant that could add to the outcome. Again it is best to have a committed weight loss before proceeding with facelifting. If this is not to be, the surgeon needs to have the patient completely understand the likely outcome and maintain realistic expectations.

The position of the hyoid bone is important. A low hyoid will interfere with developing a deep cervicomental angle. Ptotic submandibular glands are visible especially in thinner necks. These attributes must be pointed out to the patient preoperatively. These issues can be demonstrated to the patient with a mirror and imaging. It is important when imaging these patients that the consultant does not demonstrate a deep cervicomental angle where it cannot be achieved nor eliminate the submandibular gland bulge when this cannot occur.

Midface ptosis also must be evaluated and discussed. Many people assume that the standard facelift will also correct this problem. Different approaches to this region include surgical midface lift, malar and/or submalar implants, and barbed thread lifts. These alternatives are covered in other chapters in this text.

Patients often think that facelift means the entire face, the eyelids and forehead included. The entire face should be evaluated and different options discussed. The surgeon must be sensitive to the fact that whereas he or she would like to perform brow lifting, blepharoplasty, chin implant, and facelift, the patient may only be able to afford one procedure. This should be the one that would address her major concern.

Near the end of the consultation, the surgeon will review the probable sequelae and possible complications of the operation. This discussion should be frank but not overwhelming. It is the final part of patient education and an important one. Bruising, swelling, numbness, stiffness, and soreness are all probable. Complications do occur from time to time. It is necessary that patients understand that though unlikely, one could happen. They also must be assured that if one occurs, it will be remedied.[1,6,7]

◆ The Closing and Booking

In this author's opinion, financial and scheduling discussions should be done by a scheduler, patient coordinator, or office manager. This meeting is also very important. It is the third step in patient education. It should be conducted in a comfortable and private setting. When handled correctly, it can in many instances lead a hesitating person into booking the procedure. Financial disclosures can be awkward for some individuals and must be handled in a sensitive manner. Today many patients need to finance their surgery. It is recommended that the physician's practice not extend credit. There are several companies that offer financing for cosmetic surgery. Patients can in most circumstances get better rates with a personal or equity loan from their local bank. The patient should be given the fee in writing and a photocopy retained in the patient's chart.

◆ Preoperative Visit and Instructions

Three to 4 weeks prior to the surgery date, the patient returns to the office for preoperative instructions, the fourth step in patient education. This is also done in a nonclinical, attractive setting by one of the nurses. Patients often express concerns to the nurse that they did not disclose to the doctor. They also listen differently at this meeting than at the initial consultation. The nurse reiterates the nature of their operation and the preoperative and postoperative periods. All of their questions are answered. The discussion should include the nature of dressings and drains, bruising and swelling, what could arise that would necessitate a call to the office, and what they might expect that should not cause a worry. Realistic outcomes are reviewed. It is generally a good idea if the physician is in the office at this time. If there is any misunderstanding on the part of the patient, the surgeon can be available to clarify concerns. Postoperative instructions are delivered verbally and in writing to the patient along with required prescriptions. Consents for surgery and anesthesia are obtained. Preoperative laboratory tests including an EKG and a physical examination are arranged. Fees are collected. Lastly, the nurse records the name of the person who will be staying with the patient on the night of surgery if she will be going home. If necessary or desired, a private duty nurse is arranged for.

◆ The Day of Surgery

On the day of surgery, the patient should be personally greeted at once by the nurse or staff member. She should change clothes in a quiet and private room. The room should be warm with soft lighting and soft music. If the surgeon has his or her own operating suite, there will be more control of the environment than in a hospital. All personnel should behave in an attentive manner designed to calm and reassure the patient that she is the sole object of their concentration and care. Recovery should also be quiet and private with constant attendance and monitoring. If this is a private facility, it must be accredited by an organization like the Accreditation Association of Ambulatory Health Care.

The patient changes into a surgical gown. The surgeon greets the patient in this nonclinical atmosphere and answers any last-minute questions. The face is marked here with the patient in a sitting position. The intravenous line may be started here or in the operating room. After marking is completed, the patient is asked if she needs to use the bathroom one last time and is then brought into the operating room. Here she is helped onto the operating table. A warming blanket is placed over her. The intravenous is started if not already done. She is connected to blood pressure, cardiac, and pulse oximetry monitors. Blood is drawn for the preparation of platelet gel if used. Her hair is put into pigtails around the incision sites. Music is softly playing, she is gently sedated or inducted and prepped and draped. The atmosphere is kept subdued and soothing.

◆ Postoperative Care

If the patient is going home or to a hotel on the night of surgery, she will require a constant companion to stay with her. This person must have the necessary telephone numbers of whom to call for questions or in case of an emergency. Preferably, a private duty nurse will be hired. The evening of surgery, either the doctor or the nurse will call the patient to see how she is doing and to answer any questions. The next day, the patient is seen for dressing change or removal. We remove the dressing and wash out and blow-dry the patient's hair. The patient is given an elastic sling to wear for the ensuing week. Postoperative appointments are made. The patient will return at varying intervals and times depending on what ancillary surgeries were done and how the postoperative course is progressing. Four to 8 weeks later, the patient returns for a cosmetic "make-over" with an esthetician, and postoperative photographs are taken.

◆ Pertinent Anatomy

A keen knowledge of facial anatomy is an obvious prerequisite to performing facial surgery. This topic was covered in depth in Chapter 2. The SMAS is the structure that will be exposed, incised, divided, lifted, and plicated or imbricated in some fashion in facelift surgery. It has intimate and fixed relationships with the motor and sensory nerves of the face as well as with much of the major vasculature. The SMAS encompasses the muscles of facial motion and their investing fascia. This is the layer that is manipulated and repositioned to rejuvenate the aging face. It overlies the parotid fascia, although it is considered by some to incorporate this layer.[8,9] As it extends forward, it becomes clearly associated with the facial muscles first at the zygomaticus major. In the more anterior cheek, it appears thinner and less well defined. In the neck, it is continuous with the platysma muscle. In the scalp, the SMAS is the galea aponeurotica, and as it descends into the temple region it is the superficial temporal fascia (temporoparietal fascia). It becomes entwined and intimately involved with the multiple fascial layers at the zygoma (**Fig. 3.4**).

The SMAS overlies the major vessels and nerves of the face. Smaller branches of these structures extend up to the dermis. Elevating the skin and subsequently the SMAS interrupts these connections. This results in the temporary hypoesthesia all facelift patients experience in the periauricular area after surgery.

There are fibrous connections between the dermis and underlying SMAS known as fasciocutaneous ligaments. These ligaments are significant in that when the SMAS is elevated and repositioned to create a rejuvenated appearance, the skin is drawn along with it. Putting all the tension of lifting

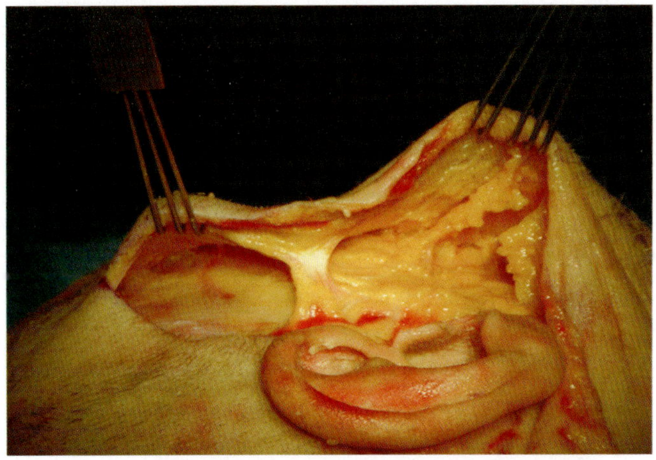

Fig. 3.4 A cadaver specimen demonstrating the transition in dissection from just above the true temporalis fascia in the temple to the sub-SMAS cheek plane at the zygomatic arch. In this confluence lies the temporal branch of the facial nerve. During surgery, this bridge of tissue must be preserved.

on the SMAS and not the skin overcomes the problems encountered in years past when facelifts were essentially done by creating long skin flaps that were lifted and pulled with tension to points before and behind the top of the ear. The viscoelastic properties of skin are such that these skin tension techniques endured short life spans and often resulted in wide scars. There are also two firm attachments of the skin to the underlying bone. These osteocutaneous ligaments are the zygomatic cutaneous ligament, McGregor's patch, and the mandibular cutaneous ligament.[10]

One of the most disastrous complications of facelift surgery is nerve injury, particularly motor nerve injury. The branches of the facial nerve at most risk are the temporal and marginal mandibular. The former rises obliquely from about the attachment of the lobule of the ear. If one were to draw a line from 0.5 cm below the bottom of the external auditory canal to 2 cm above the outer end of the eyebrow and another from this line along the zygoma to the orbital rim, then connect them, a triangle is formed that will contain the temporal branch.[2] In this area, the nerve is within the SMAS over the zygomatic arch just under the skin and on top of the layers of the temporalis fascia. It enters the frontalis muscle from its undersurface. The marginal mandibular nerve runs deep to the platysma muscle in the vicinity of the lower border of the mandible. It has variously been reported to lie above and below the mandibular border.[11,12] Most importantly, it is superficial and at greatest risk in the vicinity of the facial artery and vein. This relationship must be kept in mind when applying cautery to this area.[13,14]

The sensory nerve at greatest risk is the greater auricular nerve. It rises around the posterior edge of the sternocleidomastoid muscle ~9 cm below the external auditory canal and courses upwards across the muscle to divide into anterior and posterior branches below the lobule.[6,10] The nerve lies just under the subcutaneous fat and under the superficial layer of the sternocleidomastoid fascia. It is posterior to the platysma muscle and just behind the external jugular vein,

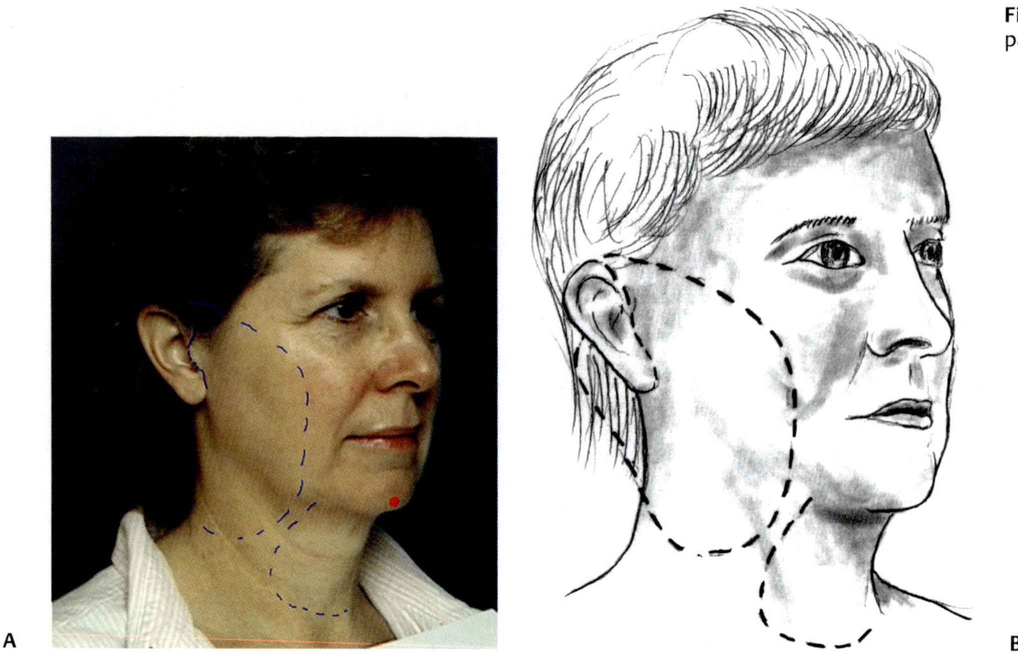

Fig. 3.5 (A, B) Marking the face of a patient.

◆ Marking

The patient is marked in the preoperative room. The surgeon sits on a stool facing the patient who sits upright on a small chair. The anatomic landmarks of the top of the thyroid cartilage, the angle of the mandible, and the midline on the chin are marked. The submental incision is marked in the submental crease from 1 to 3 cm in length. The anterior platysma bands are marked as well as the amount of anterior skin to be elevated. This can vary from a few centimeters below the thyroid notch to the bottom of the neck (**Figs. 3.5 and 3.6**).

The facelift incisions are marked identically on each side. The incision starts either in the temporal hair curving downward to the auricle or through the bottom of the tuft of

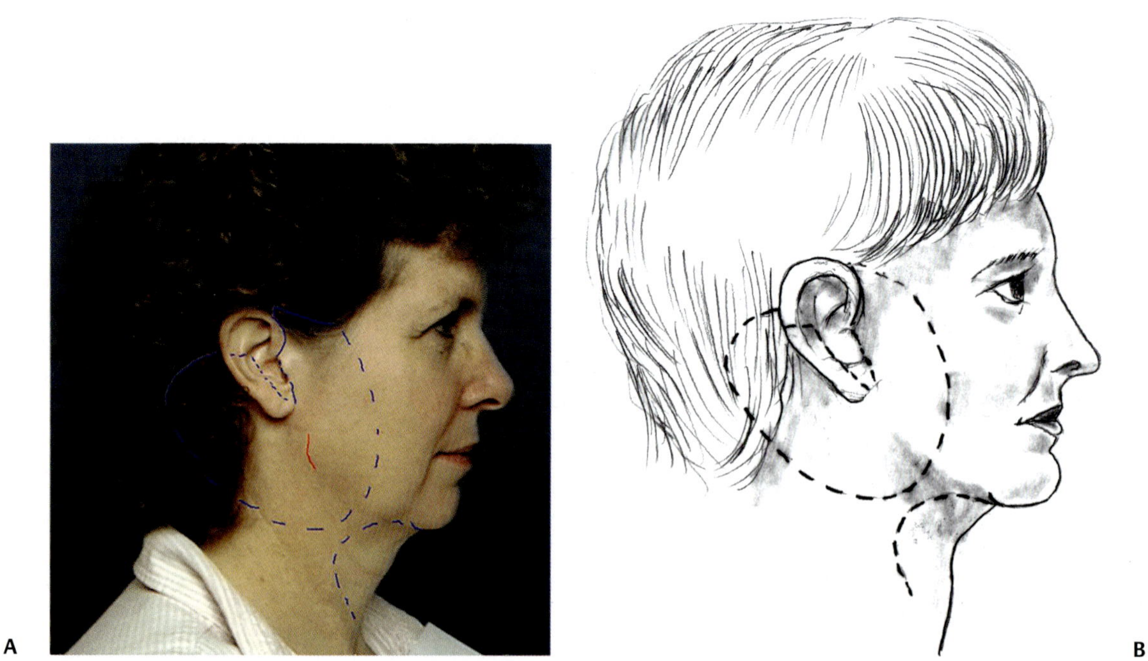

Fig. 3.6 (A, B) Another view of marking the face.

temporal hair backward and upward to the point a few millimeters above the attachment of the auricle. The incision line then drops to the auricular attachment and follows the curve of the anterior helix to the top of the tragus. It then courses along the free edge for 1 to 2 mm behind the tragus and down the prelobular crease. Many surgeons will vary this placement in men. Approximately 1 cm of skin in front of the tragus in men is non–hair bearing. They place the incision in the pretragal skin crease.[12] This reduces the size of the non–hair-bearing skin but keeps it off the tragus. I use the same incision in men as I do in women. Most men in their fifties and older grow an appreciable amount of hair on their traguses that requires trimming every few days. In all patients except those with white hair, laser hair removal can be undertaken in this area. This has never been requested in my experience. I tell my male patients that if this is an issue for them, I can place the incision in front of the tragus but they may have a more visible scar. Men must be informed of the loss or lessening of this non–beard skin in their consultations. A small dart is designed under the lobule to aid in flap trimming and closure. It then rises in the postlobular crease and up onto the posterior conchal surface to a point above the visual junction of the hairline and auricle. Then it traces backward into the postauricular hair, curving slightly downward for approximately 3 or 4 cm and finally downward for 1 cm. This placement will aid in the prevention of postauricular deformities such as a step-off of the hairline. If done in this fashion, the only possibility of visible scar on the face lies at the anterosuperior helix and in the prelobular crease. The approximate extent of the undermining for the cheek and submental flaps are outlined on the face.

◆ Anesthesia

The type of anesthesia used should be the choice of the surgeon. Certainly, the operation can be performed under local anesthesia, local anesthesia with sedation, managed anesthesia care, or general anesthesia. This author's personal preference is managed anesthesia care. In more than 30 years of experience, the patients remain disassociated and comfortable, recover quickly, and have a very low incidence of postoperative nausea. Whatever the choice, the procedure must be performed in an accredited facility.

Various sedative, analgesic, and anesthetic drugs are used in a variety of combinations to maintain a steady state of quiet sedation.[14] The author works either with an anesthesiologist or a certified nurse anesthetist. The typical combination of drugs used includes fentanyl, Versed (midazolam; Roche Pharmaceuticals, Nutley, NJ), and propofol. The patient is sedated most deeply during the lidocaine injection phases of the procedure then allowed to become slightly more responsive to the point of his or her comfort level. One percent lidocaine with 1:100,000 epinephrine is used for the incision sites and 0.5% lidocaine with 1:100,000 epinephrine under the flaps. The flaps are injected in a fan-like pattern. The submental area and right side of the face are injected first. An interval of 10 to 15 minutes is allowed to pass before beginning the procedure. This permits the full vasoconstrictive effect of the epinephrine to occur. It is imperative to not exceed 500 mg of lidocaine within 1 hour to prevent toxicity. This can be avoided by injecting the left side of the face prior to skin closure on the right (**Fig. 3.7**).

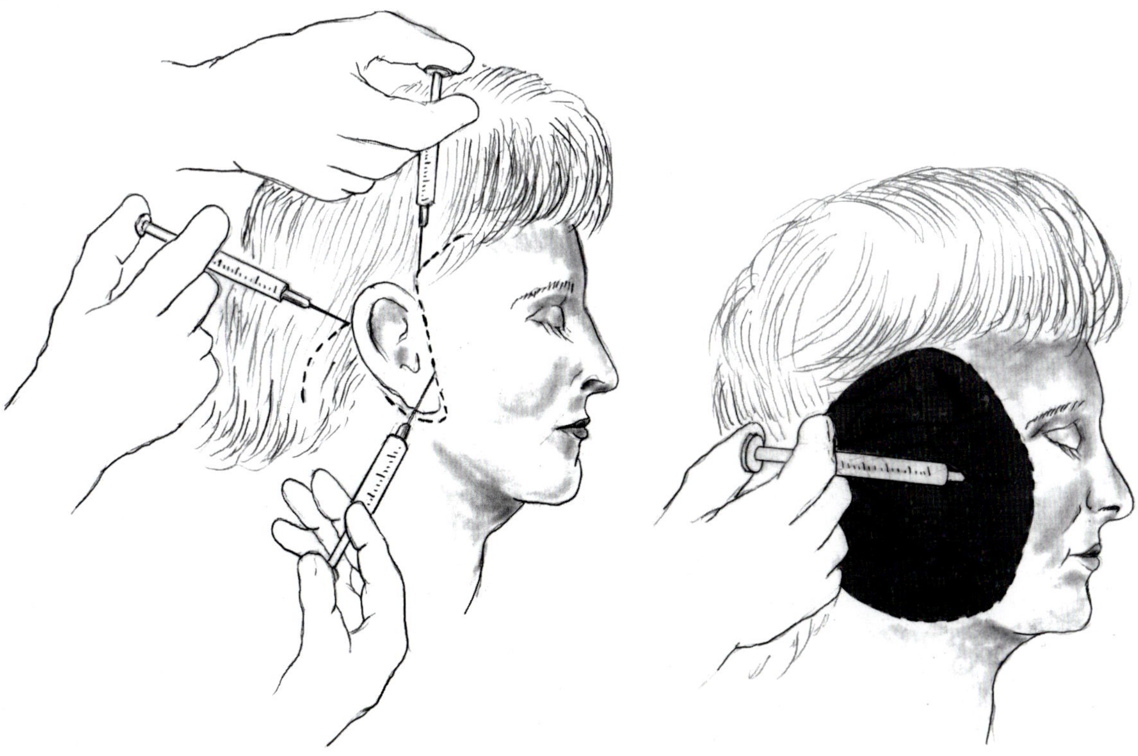

A B

Fig. 3.7 (**A**) Injecting 1% lidocaine with 1:100,000 epinephrine along the lines of incision. (**B**) Injecting 0.5% lidocaine with 1:100,000 epinephrine under the cervico-facial flaps.

◆ A Standardized Approach to Sub-SMAS Facelifting

The Submental Procedure

If liposuction is all that is required in the submental area, a small incision is created in the submental crease just large enough to allow the insertion of a 4-mm liposuction cannula. When work needs to be done on the platysma muscles, a 2- to 4-cm incision is made. The skin flap is elevated with care being taken to leave a layer of fat attached to the dermis. Elevation is done by blunt dissection with scissors, spreading them open to create tunnels. The intervening septa are cauterized with a bipolar cautery and cut for full elevation. The flap is elevated from 3 or 4 cm below the cervicomental angle in the younger, less redundant neck to several more in the older and heavier neck. Lateral elevation extends beyond the area needed for liposuction. In most patients, the platysma bands are dehiscent in the midline. Less redundant, thinner platysmal bands are sutured together with 4-0 Vicryl (Ethicon, Somerville, NJ) from the cervicomental angle to the mentum (**Fig. 3.8**). In the patient with heavy banding, the muscles are elevated from medial to lateral for a few centimeters or more until they are well mobilized. If the bands are particularly thick, a back cut is made for 2 or 3 cm at the cervicomental angle. On rare occasions, when there is great redundancy, the anterior edge of the muscles may be trimmed. The heavy bands are elevated and brought together to assess the amount of redundancy present. Overlapping muscle is trimmed, and the bands sutured with a permanent suture such as 2-0 Ethibond (Ethicon, Somerville, NJ) or a long-lasting absorbable suture such as 2-0 or 3-0 PDS (Ethicon, Somerville, NJ). A running interlocking stitch or horizontal mattress stitches work well. The knots must be buried.

The Cheeks and Neck

The head is rotated to the right. A cotton ball is inserted into the ear canal. The anterosuperior portion of the incision is made through the tuft of hair in front of the ear. The scalpel blade is beveled opposite the direction of the hair follicles and placed low in the tuft so it will not shift the hair upwards and high enough so that with the trimming of the flap a few rows of follicles will remain to grow through and camouflage the scar. The anterior flap is elevated through this incision with progressively longer facelift scissors by advancing and spreading (**Fig. 3.9**). A thin layer of fat should be left attached to the dermis. An unfolded sponge is packed under the flap as a tamponade. The posterior superior incision is made next, beginning at the auricular attachment above the visible junction of hair and ear when the hair is drawn up. It extends backward into the hair for several centimeters as needed for flap elevation and redraping, then downward about 45 degrees for a centimeter to accommodate any dog ear. This flap is elevated and joined with the anterior flap elevation. The greater auricular nerve crosses the anterior border of the sternocleidomastoid muscle in the upper neck. Care must be taken to elevate gently and slowly here to prevent injury. If the nerve is transected it will be easily seen and needs to be reapproximated with a 10-0 suture. This author does not connect the lateral and submental flaps. A band of tissue about 1 cm is left between them. If an expanding hematoma should occur, it will not extend completely across the neck and face but be contained in its original compartment. This flap is also packed

A–C

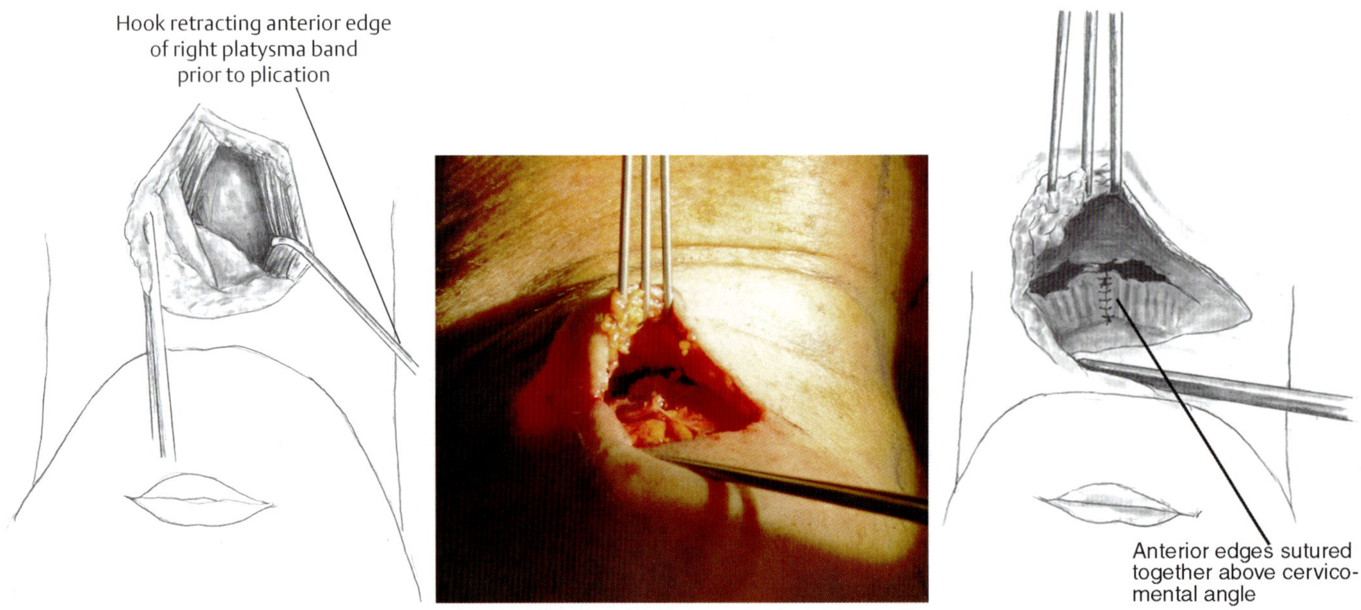

Fig. 3.8 (**A**) Hook retracting the anterior edge of the right platysma band prior to plication. (**B, C**) Plication of the anterior platysma bands.

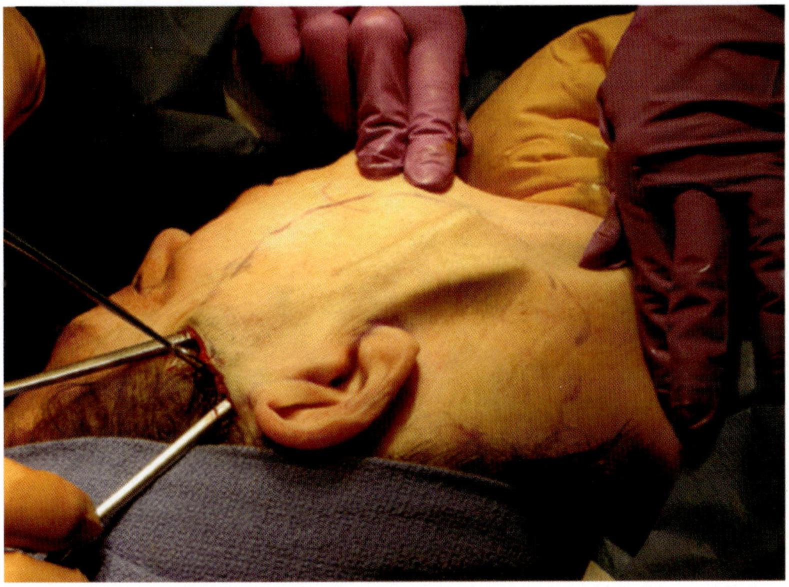

Fig. 3.9 Elevation of the anterior flap.

with a sponge (**Fig. 3.10**). The periauricular portion of the incision is completed with scalpel and scissor. The flaps are raised, and hemostasis is secured. If needed, open liposuction is performed at this time. This can be extended over the jowl if necessary. Care must be taken here to be very conservative to avoid irregularities.

Two incisions are commonly used in the SMAS. One starts at a point 1 cm lateral to and 1 cm down from the lateral canthus and extends inferolaterally to just below the lobule and picks up the platysma's posterior border. The other begins in front of the top of the tragus and below the inferior border of the zygoma. It extends anteriorly for 3 to 4 cm and inferiorly in front of the ear to the lobule then ends at the sternocleidomastoid muscle. The SMAS flap is elevated with care to leave the parotid fascia intact. Elevation proceeds forward to expose the posterior portion of the masseter muscle (**Fig. 3.11**). Elevation is done gently with a small, blunt-tipped scissor. The posterior border of the platysma is elevated as well. It is necessary to be aware of and protect the location of the greater auricular nerve. Once the SMAS elevation is complete, the flap is divided in two, starting just below the lobule and coursing forward along the bottom of the mandible (**Fig. 3.12**). The upper flap is rotated superiorly with tension. This lifts the jowl and helps redefine the jaw line. The excess SMAS tissue is trimmed and discarded. The flap is fixed in place edge to edge with a 2-0 permanent or semipermanent sutures. It is essential to keep the knots buried. If this is not done, the patient will at least feel them, and the thin patient will see them as bumps under the skin. The inferior flap and posterior edge of the platysma muscle

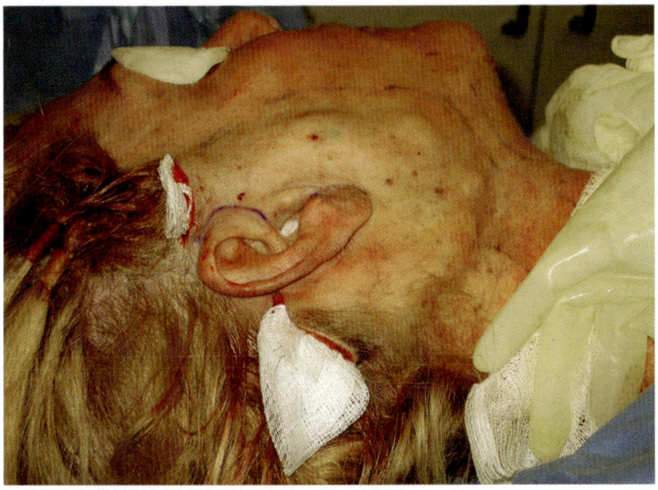

Fig. 3.10 Packing under the flaps.

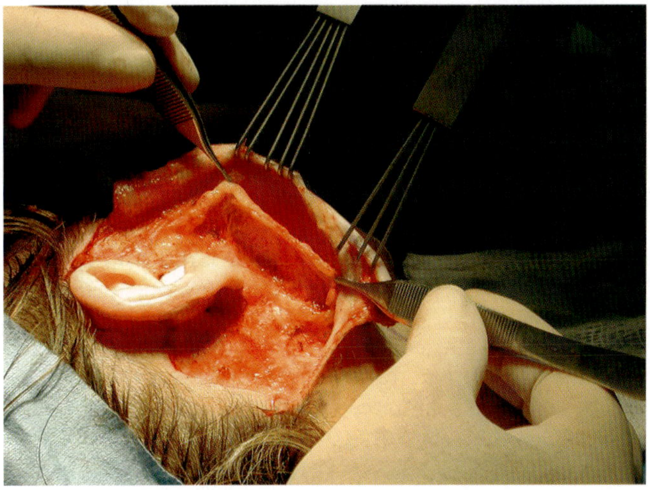

Fig. 3.11 The SMAS flap elevated.

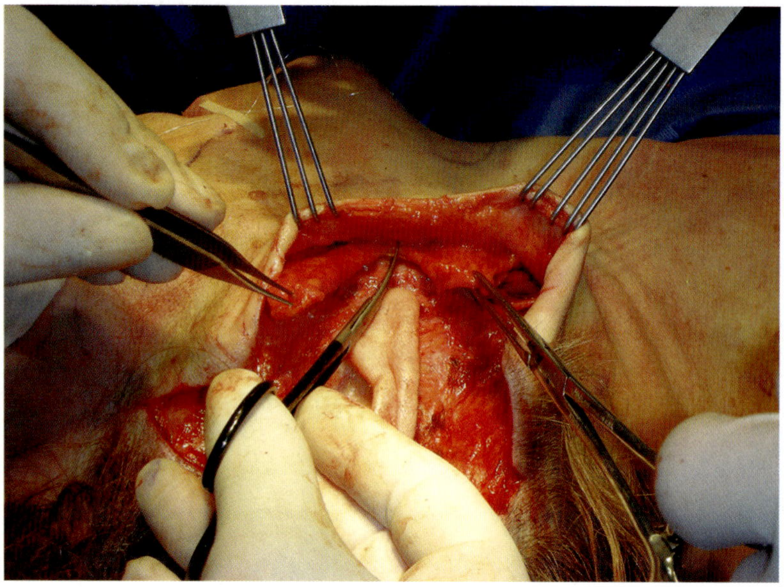

Fig. 3.12 Dividing the SMAS along the mandible.

are elevated posterosuperiorly. The flap is secured with tension to the mastoid fascia. There will be a gap at the lobule between the two flaps. This is closed with 3-point stitch, flap to flap to the fascia below the lobule.

Control of the anterior platysma bands has been a vexing problem in rhytidectomy. This is particularly true in heavy-necked individuals with thick redundant muscles. A variety of techniques of corseting the bands have been described.[15,16] Platysma suspension sutures are used by many surgeons to aid in lengthening the longevity of the cervical portion of the facelift.[5,17,18] This author has been using barbed polypropylene threads to aid in this fashion. Once the SMAS has been lifted, divided, and sutured in place, I pass the double-armed barbed threads through the mastoid fascia then through the platysma with the barbs facing posterior. They are exited through the skin about 1 to 2 cm lateral to the midline. The needles are cut off and the operation is completed. After closure of all the incisions, the free ends of the threads are held with one hand and the skin is pulled back toward the ear anchoring the barbs. The threads are pulled and cut so they drop ~1 cm below the skin level. The incision is closed with 5-0 Vicryl and 6-0 rapid dissolving gut sutures.

The material and technique used for skin trimming and closure can vary greatly from surgeon to surgeon. It is imperative that the skin be under no tension when closed. The following is the author's method. Once imbrication is completed and hemostasis is secured, flap trimming begins. The posterior hairline is positioned first. The skin flap is positioned with two forceps to the point that will remove the redundancy without producing tension on the closure. The posterior flap is rotated superiorly and slightly forward. The junction of the hairline on the flap is lined up with the hairline on the scalp to prevent a step-off deformity. The flap is cut along its hairline until it meets the hairline on the scalp. It is secured here with a skin staple. The posterior-most redundancy is trimmed beveling the cut so the follicles will grow through the scar. Once this point is set, the anterior flap is lifted to its position in a fashion that will produce no wound tension. The rotation of this flap is posterior and slightly superiorly. If too much pull is applied in a posterior direction, the crow's-feet will elongate and a "windswept look" will occur. The first point of fixation is in the incision directly above the superior auricular attachment. In the instance of an incision under the tuft of hair, the excess skin in front of this staple is trimmed ending directly at its anterior extent or using an M-plasty to flatten any bunching. The flap now lies over the lobule. It is incised down the lobule carefully to meet the small dart of skin at that juncture. It is important that the earlobe be slightly pushed upward on closure as it will drift down in healing. This prevents a "pixie ear" deformity. Finally, the remainder of skin behind the auricle is tailored.

The staples are removed and the flaps elevated to check for hemostasis. This author uses platelet-rich plasma, spraying it very lightly on the face and neck tissues and the undersurface of the flap then returning the flap to position securing it with the same two staple placements. Excess platelet gel is rolled out with a gauze and pressure applied for 30 seconds. Others use tissue glue, flat or closed suction drains, or a pressure dressing. The wound is closed with one or two subcuticular 4-0 Vicryl sutures in the anterior and posterior hairline incisions. Prior to closing the cheek incision, the new tragal skin is thinned leaving a very thin skein of fat on the dermis (**Fig. 3.13**). The skin is closed with 5-0 Prolene (Ethicon, Somerville, NJ) in the anterior hairline, at the top and bottom of the tragus, and in the dart beneath the earlobe, 6-0 rapid dissolving gut sutures in front of the ear, 5-0 plain gut behind the ear, and staples in the posterior hairline. The skin closure must be absolutely without tension to minimize the scar (**Fig. 3.14**). To keep the postauricular scar from migrating into view, it is placed on the

A 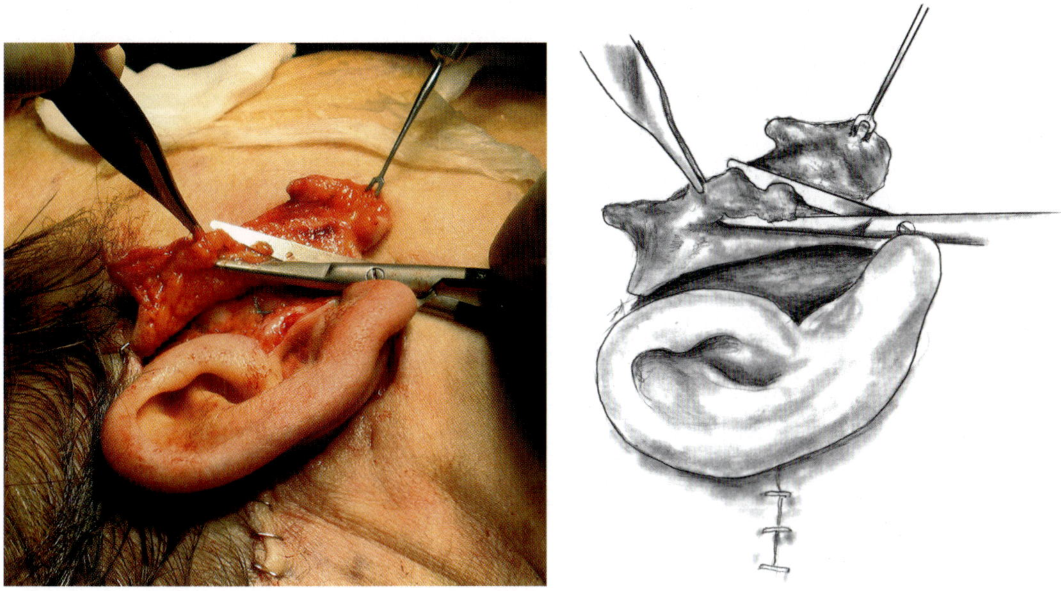 B

Fig. 3.13 (A, B) Thinning the new tragal skin.

back of the ear. The suture is a running locking stitch picking up neck skin, fascia near the postauricular crease, then skin on the auricle (**Fig. 3.15**). The opposite side is done in an identical fashion. With platelet gel or tissue glue, drains are generally not necessary.[19–21]

A dressing of moderate pressure is applied and the patient taken to recovery. The patients are required to have a companion stay with them overnight or to hire a private duty nurse to be with them. We see them the next day. The nurses remove the dressing and wash out and blow-dry the hair. In one of our skin care rooms, we have installed a hair salon type sink and chair for this purpose. This allows the patient to sit semireclined with her hair back into the sink. An elastic sling is applied for continued gentle compression.

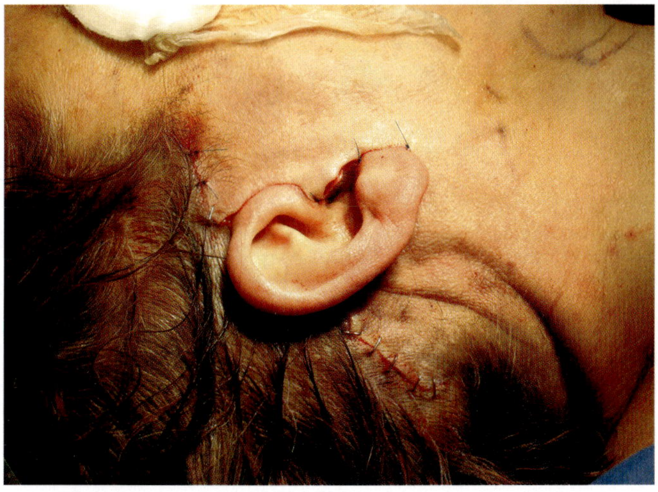

Fig. 3.14 Skin closure with no tension.

Our routine is to have the patient leave it as applied for 1 day. Then she may remove it to shower or eat. She is encouraged to wear it most of the time for the remainder of the week. She takes daily showers and treats the incisions with hydrogen peroxide and an antibiotic ointment. If no care is required for other concurrent procedures, the patient returns on the seventh or eighth postoperative day for suture and staple removal. Most facelift patients will return to work in 10 to 14 days. Vigorous exercise is permitted after 2 weeks have elapsed. The patient returns to our office 5 or 6 weeks later and a complete makeover is done for them by one of our estheticians, and postoperative photographs are taken. Return visits are scheduled at longer intervals throughout the first year after surgery.

Once the facial plastic surgeon has gained an abundance of experience with the standard sub-SMAS lift procedure, he or she may wish to learn more aggressive rhytidectomy techniques. These procedures include the extended SMAS rhytidectomy, deep plane, subperiosteal, and triplane lifts, among other additional aggressive modifications.[22–24] Over the past several decades, the facelift has evolved from subcutaneous surgery. Lipectomy, liposuction, platysma placation, SMAS placation, and SMAS imbrication have all added to the beneficial outcome and longevity of the facelift. As the surgeon contemplates extending his or her technique, he or she must decide if the benefits of more aggressive techniques justify their attendant risks. I would suggest they do not for the young and less experienced surgeon. At the least, they have a higher rate of attendant risks, morbidity, and recovery.[25] The issues of midface results and longevity have long been debated.[26–29] It must be understood that every face is different and will require some individualized modifications of whatever technique is used.

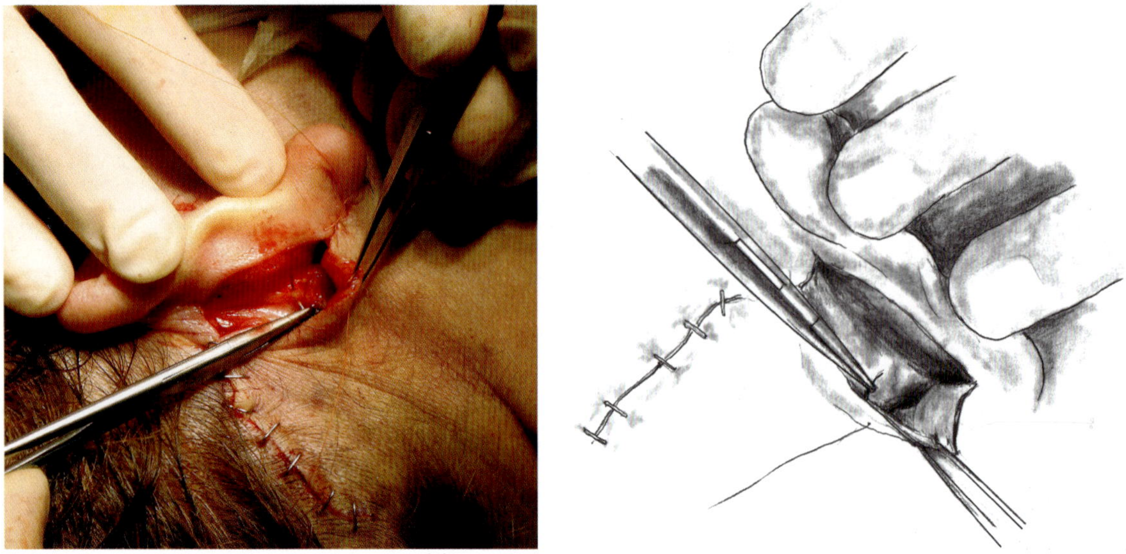

Fig. 3.15 (**A, B**) Posterior auricular closure: skin flap to mastoid fascia to auricular skin.

◆ Complications and Sequelae

Sequelae are what will probably happen, and complications are what we do not want to happen. It is important to educate the patient about what to expect and what to look out for. When the patient fully understands what the postoperative course will be like, that period of time will pass more easily for all involved. Stiffness and soreness will be felt, but patients should not expect pain. I have found that telling patients they will be stiff and sore but that the operation is not particularly painful lessens their expectations of postoperative discomfort. They do feel much better after surgery than those anticipating a painful recovery. Bruising and swelling are to be expected, and they can vary dramatically from one person to another. Different factors affect the degree to which they occur. Older patients bruise and swell more than younger ones. Men bruise more than women. If one surgeon takes twice as long to perform the procedure than another, his patients will tend to bruise and swell more. There will also be some degree of hypoesthesia in the face temporarily. There will be fine scars along the incision lines. I believe scars on the face from cosmetic surgery should be difficult to spot, even without makeup, to the casual observer. The scars that we, as facial plastic surgeons, leave behind are in a sense our signatures. Well-planned and executed incisions will result in fine minimally noticeable incision sites (**Fig. 3.16**).

Complications are things we do not want to happen; however, when one performs enough surgeries, sooner or later a complication will occur. We as surgeons must be prepared to deal with them and with the patient suffering from them. If a complication arises, the physician and staff must deal with it promptly and compassionately. "Handholding" is one of the most important components of a successful outcome in spite of the problem. The patient must be listened to, allowed to vent, seen frequently, and dealt with gently. Sometimes, reassurance can be from a second opinion from a trusted colleague. It is better to send the patient to a peer who is a friend than have the patient go on their own to a less sympathetic competitor. The most common problems in all of surgery are bleeding and infection.

Infection

In facelift surgery, infection rates are low helped in part by the rich vascular supply of the head and neck area. Some

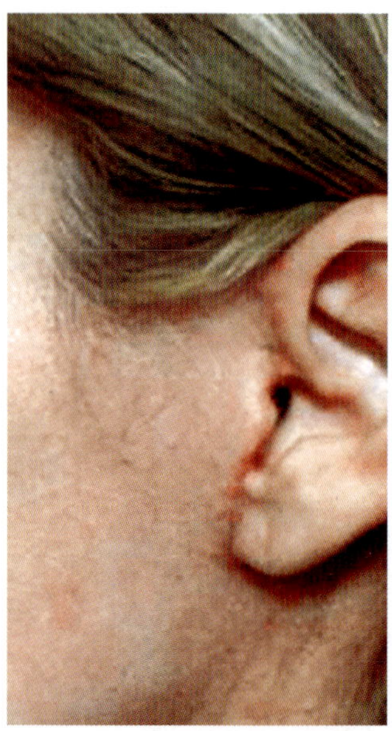

Fig. 3.16 Facial scars should be difficult to spot (scar 2 weeks postoperatively).

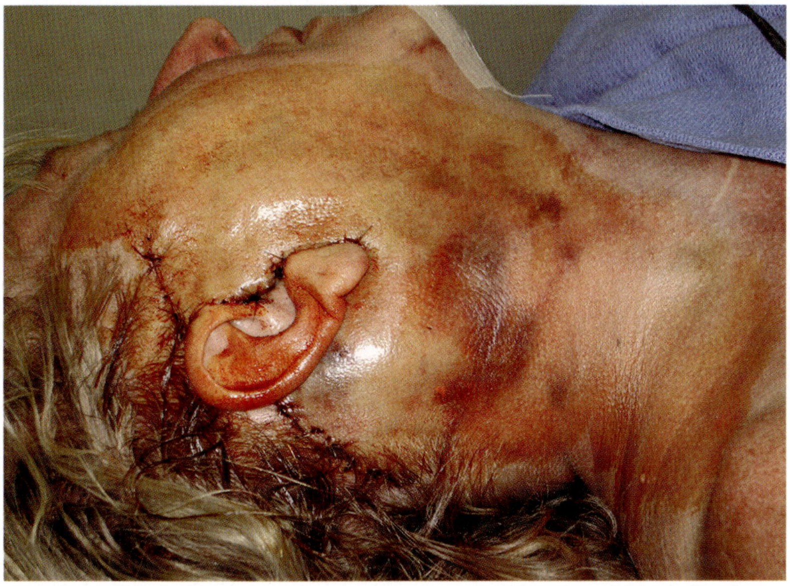

Fig. 3.17 Presentation of expanding hematoma 24 hours postoperatively.

advocate the use of perioperative antibiotics as an additional preventive measure. Increasing redness at the suture line may forewarn of a developing infection. This would be seen in the first postoperative week. If an abscess should occur, sutures in the involved area must be removed and any collection of fluid expressed. Cultures should be taken. Local wound care is instituted with hydrogen peroxide wash and application of a topical antibiotic ointment. Oral antibiotics are started or modified as necessary.

Hematoma

Postoperative bleeding will lead to hematoma formation in as many as 15% of facelift patients[11,30,31] to some degree. Hematomas are more common in men than in women. If a patient complains of localized severe and/or increasing pain, they must be seen as soon as possible. This is strongly indicative of a major or expanding hematoma (**Fig. 3.17**).

One of the reasons I leave the thin bridge of tissue between the central and lateral flaps is that it will contain a hematoma to the space in which it occurs. An expanding hematoma that has free range across the entire neck could compromise the airway. Small ones can be aspirated with a syringe if they are liquefied. Larger yet relatively confined hematomas and those that are clotted are removed by opening a small part of the incision site and milking the blood out. A drain and pressure dressing are applied. The drain is removed the next day and the dressing reapplied for at least one more night. On removal of the dressing, the wound is milked; if there is an appreciable reaccumulation of fluid, the dressing is reapplied until the problem is resolved. Large or expanding hematomas require opening part of the wound to evacuate the hematoma and find and control the source of bleeding (**Fig. 3.18**). Preventive measures include meticulous hemostasis, the use of drains and pressure dressings, and the stopping on the part of the patient of prescription and over-the-counter medications that interfere with blood coagulation. Hypertensive patients must be controlled before undergoing surgery. Strenuous activity begun too early in the postoperative period can cause bleeding under the flaps. The use of platelet gel or tissue glue is advocated by some and may eliminate the need for dressings and drains. I have used platelet gel for several

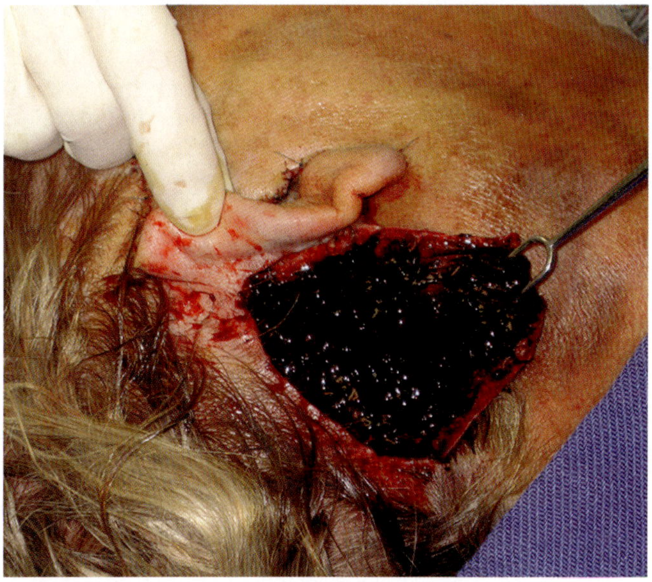

Fig. 3.18 Exposure of hematoma prior to evacuation.

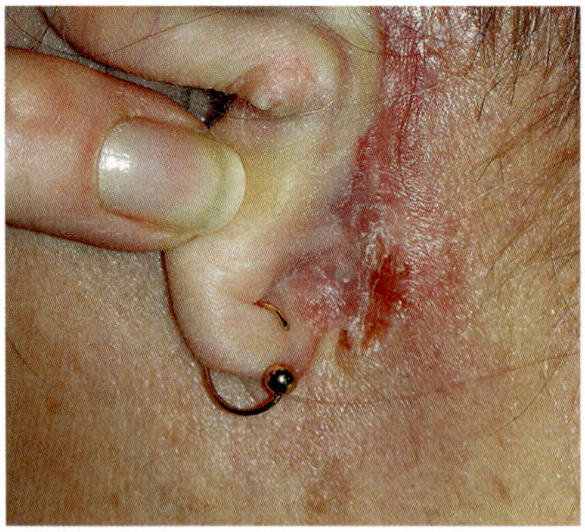
A

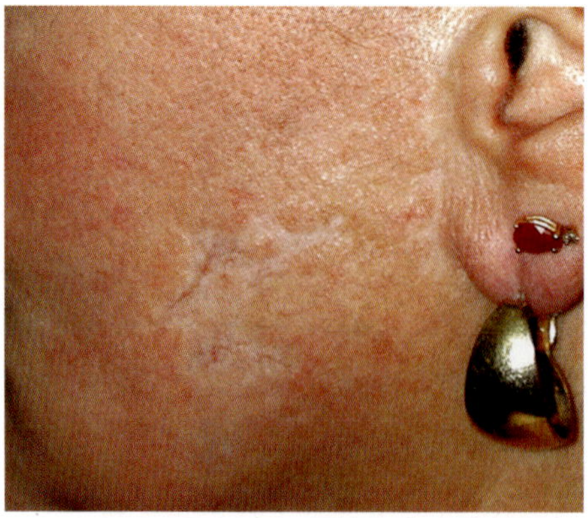
B

Fig. 3.19 (**A**) Necrosis behind ear in a smoker: 2 weeks postoperatively. (**B**) Postnecrosis scar on cheek.

years without drains and have seen less than a 1% incidence of hematomas.

Nerve Damage

The greater auricular is the nerve most frequently injured occurring in up to 7% of procedures.[31] If the nerve is severed, it should be visible. Reapproximation with 10-0 sutures should be done. Reinnervation will diminish the hypoesthesia that occurs. If the nerve is not repaired, a painful neuroma can develop as well as dysesthesia of the affected area of nerve distribution.

Damage to one or more branches of the facial nerve is a devastating occurrence for the patient and for the surgeon. It can leave a lasting and visible disability in its wake. Thorough knowledge of facial anatomy and its variations is paramount to minimize this risk. Surgically induced paralysis of one or more branches of the facial nerve happens in 0.53 to 2.6% of cases.[30,33] The two most vulnerable branches are the marginal mandibular and the temporal nerves. Care in dissection in the vicinity is mandatory. If the temporal branch is injured or interrupted, there will be an inability to raise the eyebrow on the affected side, and the brow depressors will draw it downward. When the marginal mandibular is injured, the lip depressors, the depressor anguli oris and the depressor labii inferioris, are affected. This results in the inability of the lower lip to descend during smiling and talking. The buccal branches can be affected by overzealous dissection in the midface. This will affect the upper lip, angle of the mouth, and nearby cheek area. If paresis should occur, the patient needs to be seen frequently and counseled. Spontaneous recovery will occur in as many as 85% of cases.[30] The recovery comes as swelling resides and cross-innervation takes hold. This may happen from several weeks postoperatively to 6 months or longer. If the temporal branch is affected, Botox Cosmetic (Allergan, Inc., Irvine, CA) can be used on the contralateral side to achieve dynamic symmetry, and a unilateral brow lift may be necessary on the affected side for passive symmetry. Damage to the spinal accessory nerve has been reported resulting in winging of the scapula.[7]

Skin Necrosis

Skin necrosis is an event that will prolong the postoperative course, greatly dismay the patient, and vex the surgeon. It occurs in up to 3% of cases.[4] The most frequently affected area is postauricular (**Fig. 3.19A**). This is where the flap is thinnest, further away from its blood supply, and under the most tension. Scarring can be quite prominent and difficult to remedy if on the cheek (**Fig. 3.19B**). Undetected and untreated hematomas can lead to flap ischemia and, at first, superficial epidermolysis. If they remain untreated, full-thickness necrosis will ensue. Smokers are at a higher degree of risk than are nonsmokers. Common thought is to have them cease smoking or using nicotine gum or patches for 2 to several weeks preoperatively and postoperatively. The exact length of effective time has not been determined. The use of nicotine gum or patches does not lower the risk of skin necrosis; in fact, nicotine itself impairs the healing process by causing vascular compromise. Smokers who continue to smoke up to and through the surgical period have 12.5 times the risk of nonsmokers to develop flap necrosis.[30,33] They should be advised that nicotine patches or gum do not lower the risk. Diabetics are also at risk given their response to wound healing. Care must be taken in flap elevation; if the flap is too thin, damage to the subdermal vascular plexus will occur and necrosis will ensue. If the skin flaps are overly long especially in thin-skinned patients, there is a greater risk of vascular compromise. Too tight a dressing can shut off blood flow to the area and result in necrosis. Cautery must be used judiciously on the undersurface of the flap to prevent damage to the dermis. A bipolar cautery is safer than monopolar in this area. If necrosis should happen, the patient must been seen very frequently for emotional support and wound care. Partial-thickness loss will heal by reepithelialization without a visible scar. If full-thickness necrosis occurs, the wound is kept clean with judicious débridement and the use of hydrogen peroxide and antibiotic ointment. Healing is allowed to occur by secondary intention. Once the eschar is gone, scar revision can be undertaken. If a person continues to smoke or uses nicotine replacements up to the time of surgery, he or she must be allowed to assume the risk and the surgeon must document this discussion.

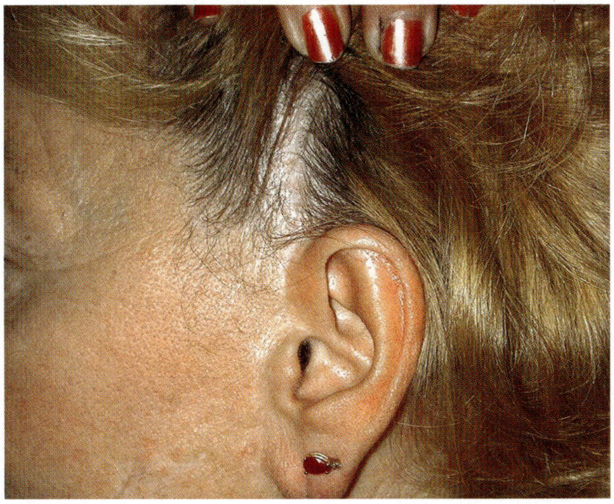

Fig. 3.20 Hair loss.

Hair Loss

Hair loss is the result of surgical manipulation of hair-bearing skin during the surgery. Permanent hair loss is an undesirable and avoidable problem. Common causes that damage the hair follicles include overthinning of the flap, injudicious use of cautery, and too much tension on the wound. If this happens, revision will be necessary. Permanent hair loss has been reported in less than 3% of rhytidectomy procedures.[30,31] Temporary loss of hair can occur. This is sometimes seen in patients with thin growth to begin with. The hair follicles involute and shed leaving an alopecic area. Handholding and reassurance is the only treatment and regrowth will happen over time (**Fig. 3.20**).[32]

Poorly Designed Incisions

Poorly designed incisions are inexcusable. Wound closure in facelift surgery is one of the most important steps. A facial plastic surgeon's calling card is the scar that is left behind. All facial cosmetic surgery should be undertaken with part of the goal being to leave behind inconspicuous, difficult to find scars. Unfortunately, poorly designed incisions are seen all too frequently. The longer one is in practice, the more amazingly poorly done closures he or she will see for second opinions. Care must be taken not to alter the hairline. The preauricular tuft of hair should be left in place. The temporal hairline must not be pulled backward. There must be no step-off in the postauricular hairline (**Fig. 3.21**). If a temple incision is made, it must be within the hairline, never in front of the hair. This would result in a white scar visible whenever the patient pulls her hair back. The ear must not be deformed (**Fig. 3.22**). Closure at the earlobe should push the lobule upward a small amount. Healing with scar tightening and contracture will tend to draw the lobe downwards. Bunching it slightly will avoid the problem known as pixie or satyr or devil's ear deformity

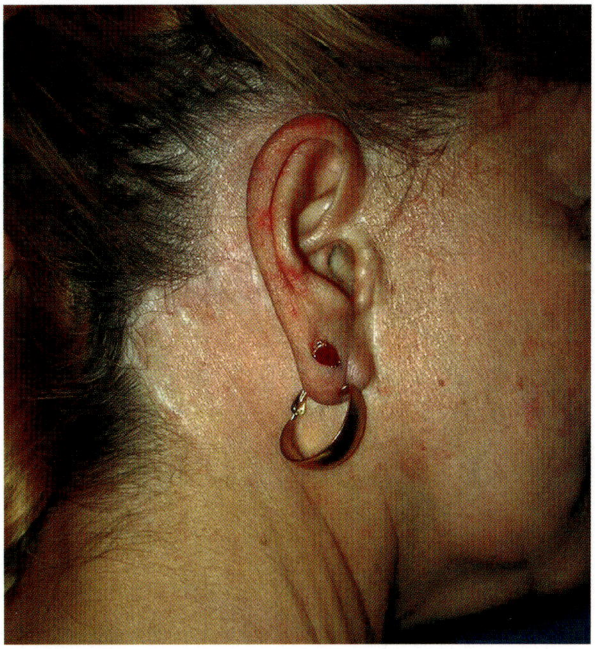

Fig. 3.21 Step-off in hairline.

(**Fig. 3.23**). All of these can be avoided by careful attention to detail.

Hypertrophic Scars

Hypertrophic and keloid scars can happen. The most common site is behind the ear. Sometimes they may be provoked by wound tension. The surgeon needs to inquire if the patient or her family has a history of hypertrophic or keloid scar formation. If the history is positive, the doctor

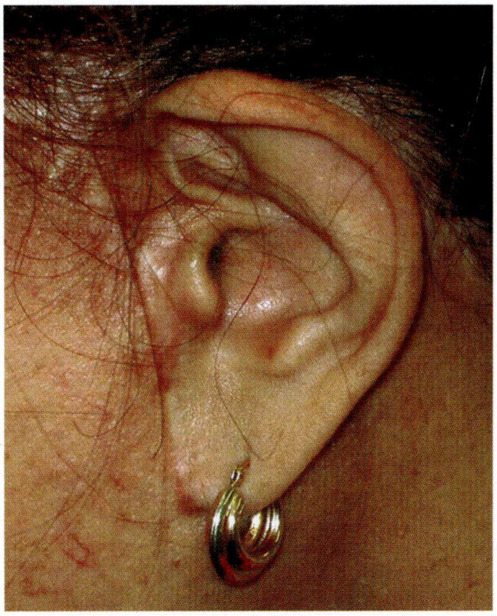

Fig. 3.22 Distortion of auricle.

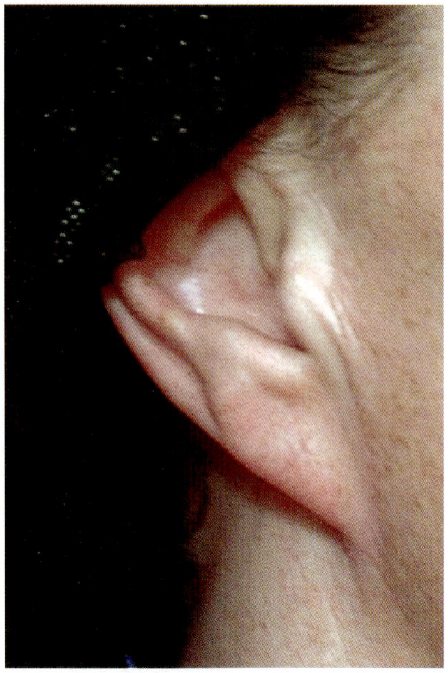

Fig. 3.23 Pixie ear deformity.

needs to discuss it with the patient and let her assume the risk. Reexcision should be delayed for many months. Intralesional steroids, such as triamcinolone 10 or 40 mg per mL concentration, are often helpful and are done at 3- to 4-week intervals. Silicon occlusive dressings can also be used to help ease the problem (**Fig. 3.24**).

Seromas

Seromas may be seen from time to time. They are easily managed by aspiration and a light pressure dressing for 1 or 2 days. They can occur in male patients if they shave early in the postoperative period. Shaving can slide the skin over its underlying bed thus preventing healing. Male patients are instructed not to shave for 7 to 10 days. Seromas will occur if excessive tissue glue or platelet gel is used. With platelet gel, it is important to roll out excess gel after spraying and holding the flaps flat with hand pressure for 30 to 60 seconds. If tissue glue is applied, the flaps should be held for 2 to 3 minutes.

Parotid Fistula

Parotid fistulas or sialomas are rarely seen. They can result with exposure and injury of the gland. If the gland is violated during SMAS elevation, a fistula or sialoma could occur. The use of platelet gel or tissue glue with positioning SMAS tissue over the exposed gland can be preventative. They present as a seroma. If a "seroma" does not respond to aspiration and light pressure dressings in a day or two, a fistula should be suspected. A transdermal scopolamine patch in place for 3 days will often solve this problem.

Erosion of the Sutures through the Skin

Erosion of sutures through the skin is sometimes seen, particularly in thin-skinned individuals with a paucity of subcutaneous fat. They are simply removed if they occur. Avoidance can be achieved by taking care to bury all suture knots. This also prevents palpable or visible bumps under the skin.

Skin Changes

Excessive tension on the wounds can readily cause lightening of the adjacent skin in patients of all skin types (**Fig. 3.25**). Postinflammatory hyperpigmentation of the

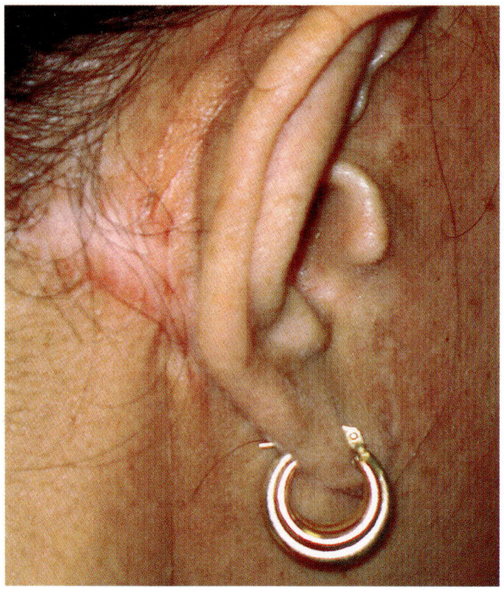

Fig. 3.24 Hypertrophic scar.

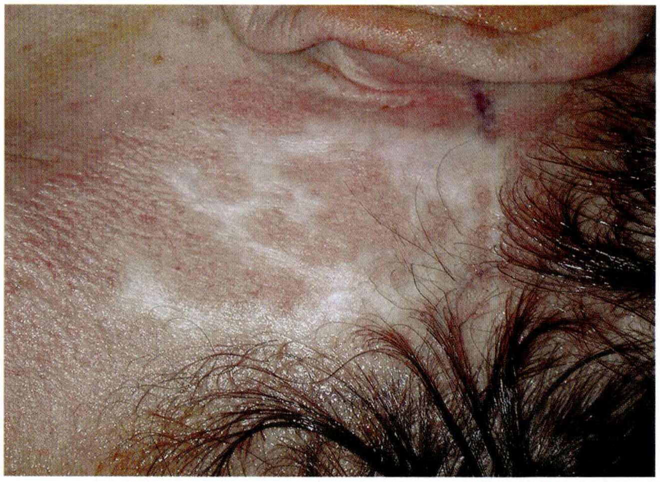

Fig. 3.25 Skin changes from excessive tension on closure.

skin is sometimes seen in individuals with darker complexions. It can be evoked by exposure to ultraviolet light in the postoperative period. Patients should be warned to avoid tanning for several months after surgery. Treatment can include hydroquinones and topical steroids. Patients who have or may be prone to telangiectasias will often experience an increase in these lesions after a facelift. They are best advised of this beforehand. The vessels can be lessened or obliterated with the appropriate vascular laser.

Contour Deformities

Obvious contour irregularities are usually the result of poorly done liposuction. Often, these will soften with massage over time. If they are still unsightly after several months, they will need to be addressed by judicious liposculpture. Overzealous removal of submental fat can lead to a cobra deformity, particularly if the platysma bands are not plicated.

Ptotic Submandibular Glands

Many older people will have ptotic submandibular glands. They may not be visibly evident in a fatty neck, and the surgeon should palpate for them. After a lift procedure, they will become visible or more evident. Procedures such as partial resection and digastric slings have been described. These procedures are quite risky and of arguable benefit. If a patient has ptotic glands, he or she needs to be advised of them and accept their presence (**Fig. 3.26A, B**).

Deep Vein Thrombosis and Pulmonary Embolism

Deep leg and pelvic vein thrombosis and subsequent pulmonary embolism are a very rare but reported event. It is more common in the elderly population and is associated with lengthy surgeries. Although a facelift alone is not a particularly long procedure, it is often one phase of complete facial rejuvenation that may include forehead lifting, blepharoplasty, implants, and even rhinoplasty. The surgeon must remain aware of the risk. If indicated, compression hose and passive or active flexion of the legs during the operation should be considered.

Postoperative Depression

Postoperative depression is not unusual. After a few weeks, if there is lingering swelling or bruising, the patient may "feel the blues" and have some remorse about having gone through "all of this." If symptoms arise, the surgeon and staff need to be gentle and supportive. These feelings are short-lived, and patience and understanding are the best balm. Rarely, counseling will be needed. Prevention is in fact the best armor. Excellent patient education before surgery and cheerful and attentive care afterwards are the best tools for this. Four to 6 weeks after the procedure, we bring the patient back for a makeover and photos. This makes her feel "special" and allows her to see the value of having had the surgery.

The Unhappy Patient

The unhappy patient is one who does not see the improvement she expected. This can occur in a patient who actually has had spectacular results. This phenomenon is different from that of the depressed patient. If patient education and understanding are excellent and the results are what the doctor expected, the unhappy patient may very well have had unrealistic expectations or possibly a personality disorder. It is best of course to recognize these problems during the consultation and not offer surgery. Realistic expectations are paramount. A facelift will not save a marriage, find a sweetheart, or garner a promotion at work. Each one of us gets up in the morning, washes, puts on clothes, maybe makeup and jewelry, fixes the hair, looks into the mirror, and generally feels good about the effort and expects others to like the way we look. Cosmetic surgery should be done for the same end. If there is a fault in a person's appearance and she has the wherewithal and understanding to change it, she will be a good candidate.

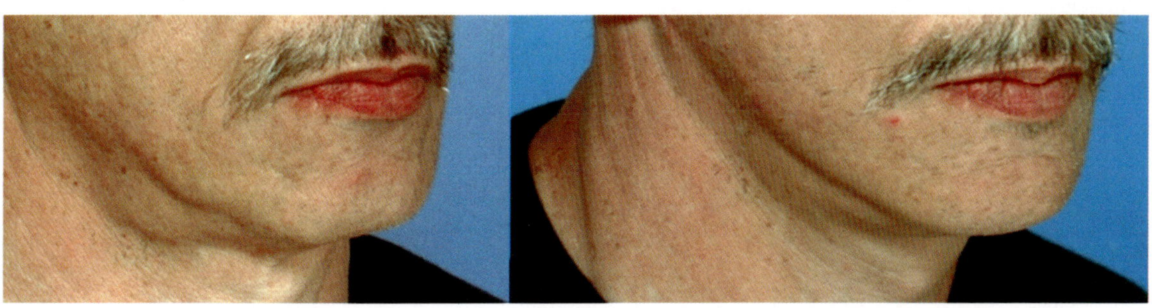

A B

Fig. 3.26 Ptotic submandibular gland (**A**) before and (**B**) after facelift. It is important to identify the presence of a visible, ptotic submandibular gland before performing surgery. This must be brought to the patient's attention so he or she will expect to see it postoperatively.

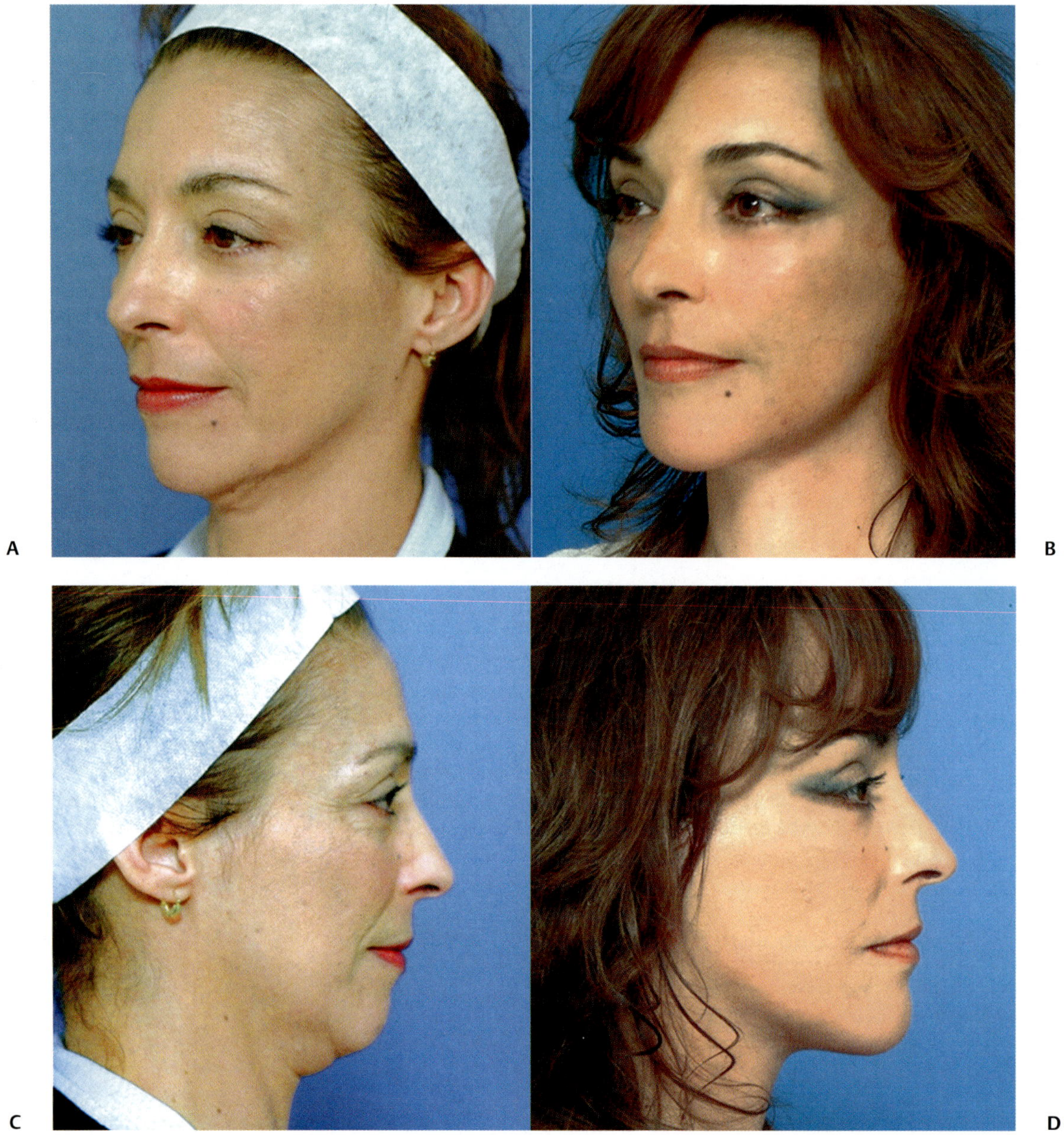

Fig. 3.27 Ptotic submandibular gland (**A**) Preoperative and (**B**) postoperative photographs: 47-year-old woman with facelift, endoscopic brow lift, and chin implant; oblique view. Adding a chin implant brings the features into better alignment and the nose appears less large than in the preoperative picture. (**C**) Preoperative and (**D**) postoperative photographs: 47-year-old woman with facelift, endoscopic brow lift, and chin implant; lateral view. The recessive chin adds to the apparent loss of cervicomental angle. A chin implant restores balance and harmony to the face.

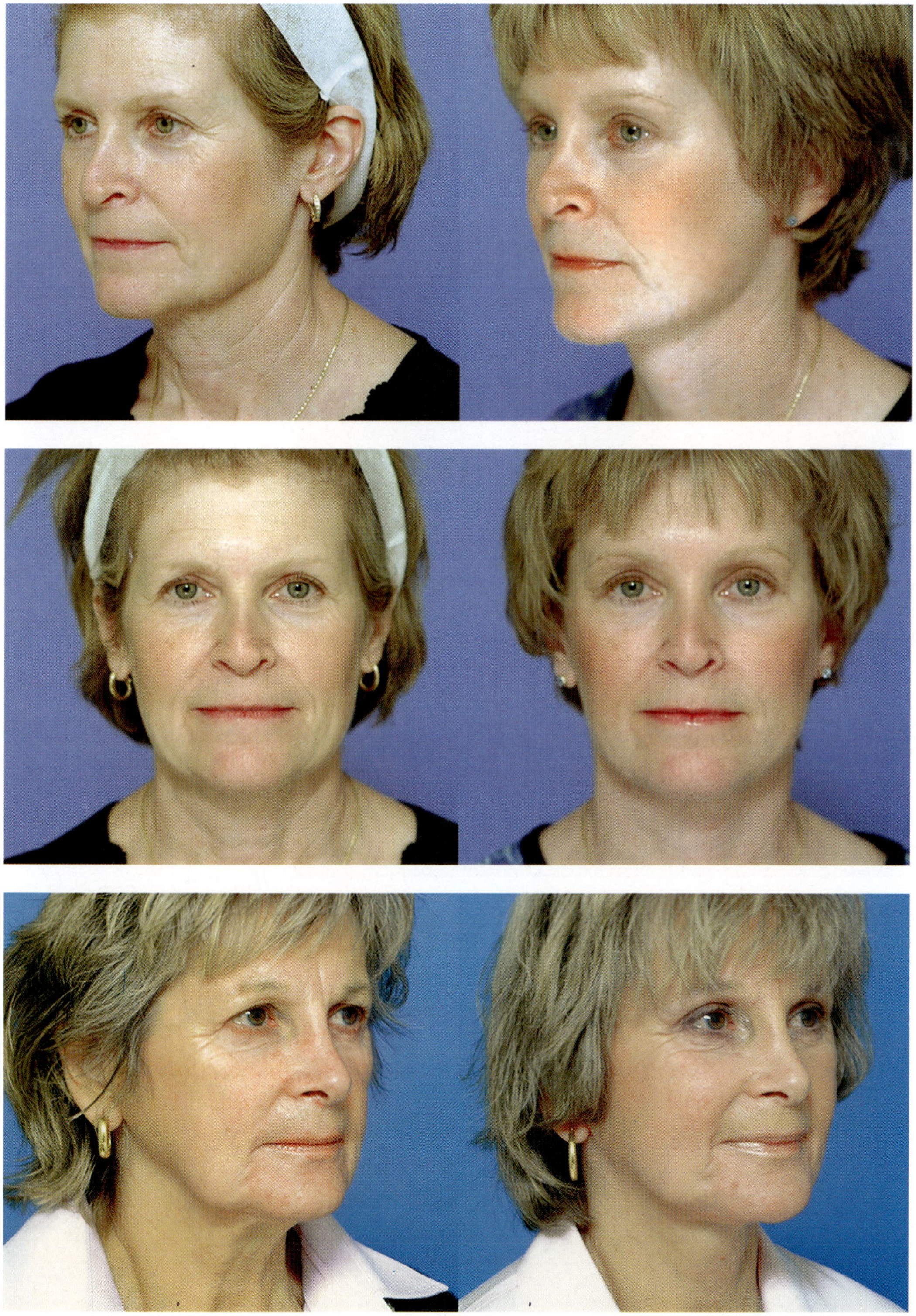

E F
G H
I J

Fig. 3.27 *(Continued)* (**E**) Preoperative and (**F**) postoperative photographs: 55-year-old woman with facelift and endoscopic brow lift; oblique view. Many patients request upper lid surgery when the problem is only a ptotic brow. The lateral hooding in this patient is corrected by the endoscopic brow lift and brightens as well as rejuvenates the eye. (**G**) Preoperative and (**H**) postoperative photographs: 55-year-old woman with facelift and endoscopic brow lift; frontal view. This woman wears little makeup and she looks very natural in the postoperative photograph. It is important to perform rejuvenating surgery without leaving the patient with the stigma of having "been done." (**I**) Preoperative and (**J**) postoperative photographs: 70-year-old woman with facelift and endoscopic brow lift; oblique view. Although the demographic of facelift patients has become younger and younger, we still see many patients in their eighth decade of life. Careful planning and execution of the surgery will result in a more youthful and more feminine face.

(Continued on page 44)

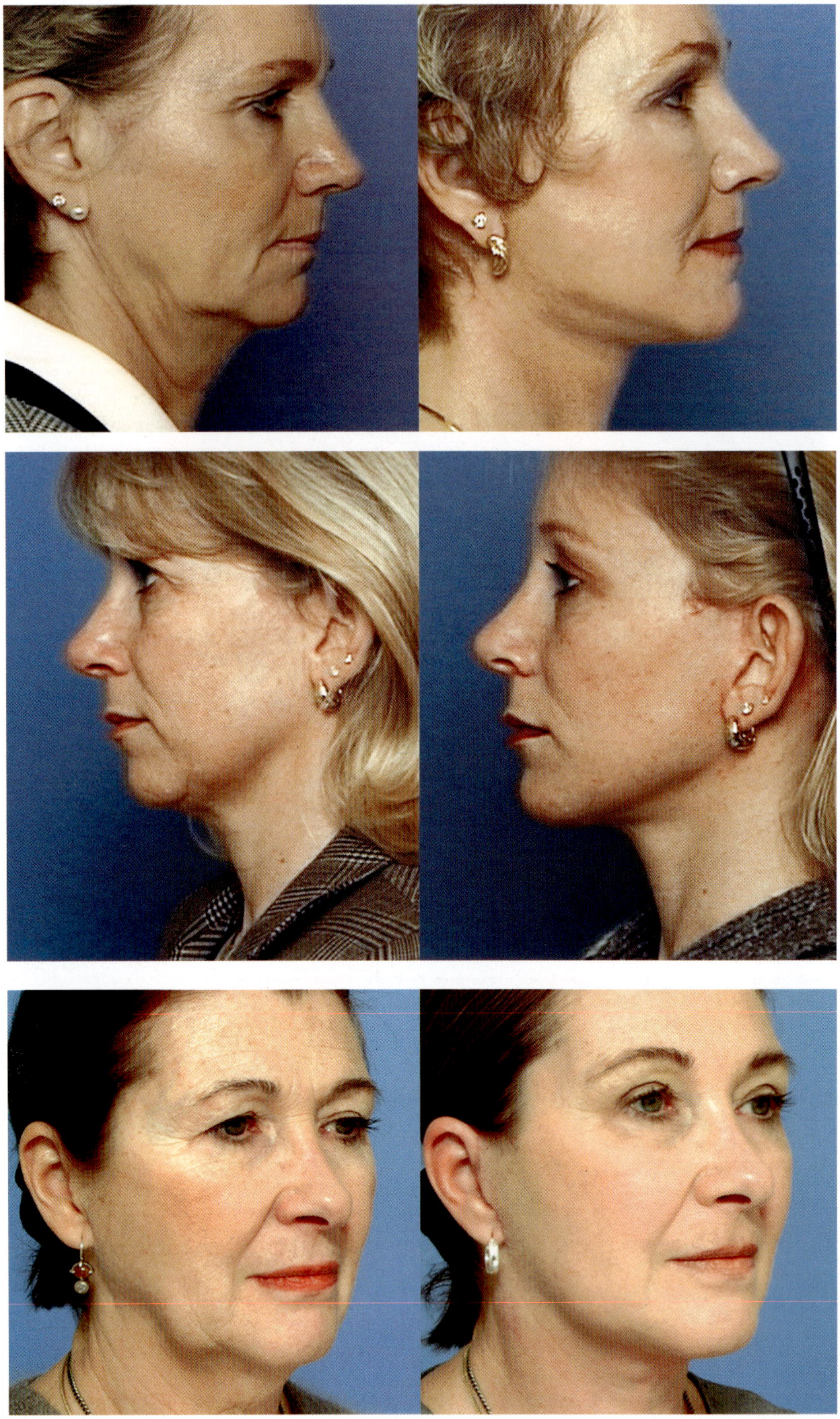

K L M N O P

Fig. 3.27 *(Continued)* Ptotic submandibular gland (**K**) Preoperative and (**L**) postoperative photographs: 60-year-old woman with facelift, endoscopic brow lift, and 4-lid blepharoplasty; lateral view. For many reasons, the surgeon cannot perform all the procedures that he would recommend for a patient. Although this attractive woman would have benefited from upper face rejuvenation, only a facelift was performed. However, she looks refreshed, rejuvenated, and refeminized. The neck is elegant and natural. (**M**) Preoperative and (**N**) postoperative photographs: 44-year-old woman with facelift, endoscopic brow lift, 4-lid blepharoplasty, rhinoplasty, and chin implant; oblique view. As a woman's face ages, it becomes more masculine. Men in general have low brows, thin lips, square jaws, heavy necks, and coarse skin. All these traits can be softened in a woman by carefully planned surgical rejuvenation. (**O**) Preoperative and (**P**) postoperative photographs: 44-year-old woman with facelift, endoscopic brow lift, 4-lid blepharoplasty, rhinoplasty, and chin implant; lateral view. This is a good example of multiple procedures being done to create an elegant and naturally pleasing countenance.

◆ Conclusion

The prepared facelift surgeon will have an understanding of the process of facial aging, a keen knowledge of the pertinent anatomy, and the necessary dexterity to operate efficiently. These attributes are necessary to develop a strong cosmetic surgery practice. Experience in creating reliable and reproducible results in the multitude of different faces that exist will lead to a busy and successful career. Experience, skill, and knowledge are not all that is needed, however. Happy patients will send more and more new referrals to the surgeon who not only does well but treats them well. Kindness, caring, and concern on the part of the doctor and his or her entire staff will be remembered far longer than the results of surgery and will be rewarded many times over with an ever-growing number of patients (**Figs. 3.26 and 3.27**).

References

1. Tardy ME, Thomas JR, Brown RJ. Facial Aesthetic Surgery. St. Louis, MO: Mosby-Yearbook; 1995
2. Cheng ET, Perkins SW. Rhytidectomy analysis: twenty years of experience. Facial Plast Surg Clin North Am 2003;11:359–375
3. Koch RJ, Hanasono MM. Aesthetic facial analysis. In: Papel I, ed. Facial Plastic and Reconstructive Surgery. 2nd ed. New York, NY: Thieme Medical Publishers; 2002:135–144
4. Sarwer DB, Wadden TA, Pertschuck MJ, Whitaker LA. Body image dissatisfaction and body dysmorphic disorder in 100 cosmetic surgery patients. Plast Reconstr Surg 1998;101:1644–1649
5. Giampapa VC, DiBernardo BE. Neck recontouring with suture suspension and liposuction: an alternative for the early rhytidectomy candidate. Aesthetic Plast Surg 1995;19:217–223
6. Perkins SW, Dayan S. Rhytidectomy. In: Papel I, ed. Facial Plastic and Reconstructive Surgery. 2nd ed. New York, NY: Thieme Medical Publishers; 2002:153–170
7. Beeson WH. Selection of "successful" candidates for rhytidectomy surgery. Facial Plast Surg Clin North Am 1993;1:131–134
8. Larabee WF, Makielski KH, Henderson JL. Surgical Anatomy of the Face. 2nd ed. Philadelphia, PA: Lippincott Williams & Wilkins; 2004
9. Jost G, Levet Y. Parotid fascia and facelifting: a critical evaluation of the SMAS concept. Plast Reconstr Surg 1984;74:42–51
10. Ozdemir R, Kilinç H, Unlü E, Uysal AC, Sensöz O, Baran CN. Anatomicrohistologic study of the retaining ligaments of the face and use in face lift: retaining ligament correction and SMAS plication. Plast Reconstr Surg 2002;110:1134–1147
11. Seckel BR. Facial Danger Zones: Avoiding Nerve Injury in Facial Plastic Surgery. St. Louis, MO: Quality Medical Publishing; 1994
12. Wilhelmi BJ, Mowlavi A, Neumeister MW. The safe facelift with bony anatomic landmarks to elevate the SMAS. Plast Reconstr Surg 2003; 111:1723–1726
13. McCollough EG. Facelifting in the male patient. Facial Plast Surg Clin North Am 1993;1:217–229
14. Fletcher M. Anesthesia in facial plastic surgery. In: Papel I, ed. Facial Plastic and Reconstructive Surgery. 2nd ed. New York, NY: Thieme Medical Publishers; 2002:145–152
15. Adamson JE, Horton CE, Crawford H. Surgical correction of the "turkey gobbler" deformity. Plast Reconstr Surg 1964;34:598–605
16. Webster RC, Smith RC, Smith KF. Face lift, 3: plication of the superficial musculoaponeurotic system. Head Neck Surg 1983;6:696–701
17. Connell BF. Cervical lifts: the value of platysma flaps. Ann Plast Surg 1978;1:32–43
18. Henley JL, Lesnik DJ, Terk AR. Contralateral platysma suspension. Arch Facial Plast Surg 2005;7:119–123
19. Powell DM, Chang E, Farrior EH. Recovery from deep plane rhytidectomy following unilateral wound treatment with autologous platelet gel. Arch Facial Plast Surg 2001;3:245–250
20. Hom DB, Maisel RH. Angiogenic growth factors: their effects and potential in soft tissue wound healing. Ann Otol Rhinol Laryngol 1992; 101:349–354
21. Flemming I. Fibrin glue in face lifts. Facial Plast Surg 1992;8:79–88
22. Hamra ST. The deep plane rhytidectomy. Plast Reconstr Surg 1990;86: 53–61
23. Ramirez OM. Three-dimensional endoscopic midface enhancement: a personal quest for the ideal cheek rejuvenation. Plast Reconstr Surg 2002;109:329–349
24. Hamra ST. Composite rhytidectomy. Plast Reconstr Surg 1992;90:1–13
25. Ivy EJ, Lorenc PZ, Aston SJ. Is there a difference? A prospective study comparing lateral and standard SMAS face lifts with extended SMAS and composite rhytidectomies. Plast Reconstr Surg 1996;98:1135–1143
26. Adamson PA, Dahiya R, Litner J. Midface effects of the deep-plane vs the superficial musculoaponeurotic system plication face-lift. Arch Facial Plast Surg 2007;9:9–11
27. Kamer FM, Frankel AS. Rhytidectomy versus deep plane rhytidectomy SMAS: an objective comparison. Plast Reconstr Surg 1998;102: 878–881
28. Kamer FM. One hundred consecutive deep plane face-lifts. Arch Otolaryngol Head Neck Surg 1996;122:17–22
29. Becker FF, Bassichis BA. Deep-plane face-lift vs. superficial musculoaponeurotic system plication face-lift. Arch Facial Plast Surg 2004;6:8–13
30. Adamson PA, Moran ML. Complications of cervicofacial rhytidectomy. Facial Plast Surg Clin North Am 1993;1:257–271
31. Moyer JS, Baker SR. Complications of rhytidectomy. Facial Plast Surg Clin North Am 2005;13:469–478
32. Parkes ML, Kamer FM, Bassilios MI. Treatment of alopecia in temporal region following rhytidectomy procedures. Laryngoscope 1977;87: 1011–1014
33. Rees TD, Liverett DM, Guy CI. The effect of cigarette smoking on skin flap survival in the face lift patient. Plast Reconstr Surg 1984;73: 911–915

4

Extended Superficial Musculoaponeurotic System (SMAS) Facelift

Stephen W. Perkins and Richard V. Balikian

With the recent advances in surgical technique, a variety of anatomically sound techniques are available to the rhytidectomy surgeon. No one operation has been created that is best for treating the aging face. The astute surgeon will understand the importance of each patient's individual needs and offer techniques most appropriate to each individual patient. One such technique that leads to a natural result is the superficial musculoaponeurotic system (SMAS) flap rhytidectomy.

◆ Preoperative Planning

Proper incision planning and marking are crucial for creating long-term patient satisfaction. Avoiding changes in hairline and visible scars is critical to a successful outcome. Patients with well-hidden scars and unchanged hairlines will have more freedom with which to style their hair, leading to greater satisfaction. Often, the surgeon who takes care in incision planning will garner referrals by hairdressers and cosmeticians, who will recognize superior results.[1]

In considering the placement of incisions, three points must be considered: first, maintaining the preauricular tuft of hair, including the sideburn. Each patient is different in terms of the location of the lower portion of the sideburn and the width at which it extends anteriorly from the insertion of the helical curvature. If the preauricular tuft is 1 or 2 cm below the insertion of the superior portion of the helical insertion, it may be appropriate to design an incision that curves up into the temporal hair and allows some posterior superior lifting of the hairline. The curved hairline incision rather than a straight vertical incision is required to interrupt forces of contracture, maintain a minimally wide scar, and to avoid alopecia. As long as the hairline is not lifted higher than the insertion of the superior helical insertion, the patient will have no cosmetic disturbance of the area. If the sideburn is at the helical insertion preoperatively, an inferior sideburn incision is required. At no time should the incision be carried anteriorly around the sideburn tuft and along the pretemporal hairline. All scars in this area will be visible and cannot be camouflaged by the fine, severely sloped hair as it exits the skin naturally in a posterior direction. All incisions should be beveled to allow hair regrowth through scars created during incision.[2]

Second, preauricularly, the incision starts at the helical insertion and follows the apparent curvatures of the auricle itself to the helical root. The incision then goes behind the tragus ~1 to 2 mm, then exits at the junction of the earlobe with the face. In male patients, a pretragal incision is used to avoid lifting and placing hair-bearing skin over the tragus (**Fig. 4.1**).

Third, postauricularly, the incision must be directed up onto the posterior aspect of the auricle, above the sulcus so that when the ear settles posteriorly and the scar heals with some contracture of the skin, the scar falls into the sulcus. At the level of the helical insertion or eminence of the concha, the incisions curve gently toward the hairline. Depending on the amount of skin laxity needed to be removed from the neckline, the incision will be directed horizontally through the hairline (for minimal skin laxity) or down along the hairline (for greater skin laxity). When advancing the postauricular skin posteriorly and superiorly, the posterior hairline can then be approximated with no step-off or other deformity (**Fig. 4.2**).[3]

◆ Surgical Technique

The beginning of the facelift operation requires treatment of the neck first prior to posterior shortening and suspension of the platysma muscle. In addition, treating the fatty tissues of the jowl, submentum, submandibular region, and neck sets the stage for proper contouring of the neck and jaw line with treatment of the SMAS tissues. The procedure is started by making a 2- to 3-cm incision in the submental crease, followed by 0.5-cm elevation of the skin to expose the subcutaneous tissue. After hemostasis is achieved, a small, 3-mm, round liposuction cannula with three rectangular holes on one side is used to preelevate tunnels into the jowl in a radial, fanlike fashion from the left submandibular area completely to the submandibular area on

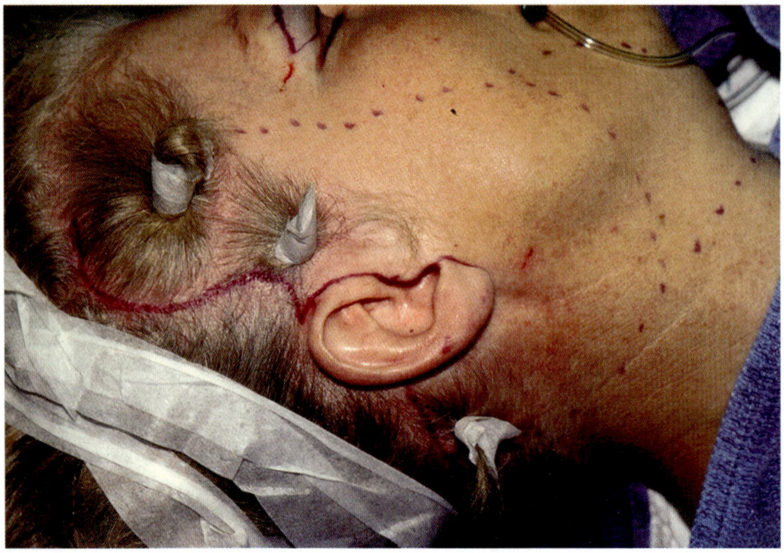

Fig. 4.1 Preauricular incision designed to prevent pretragal scarring and protection of the preauricular hair tuft.

the right. Once pretunneling has been accomplished, a judicious liposuction at 1 atm pressure of each jowl is performed to avoid dimpling. Symmetric and adequate liposuctioning can be accomplished by using the nondominant hand to palpate the jowls, then lifting the tissues and excess fat into the cannula. Care should be taken to avoid turning the holes of the cannula toward the dermis to avoid dimpling. For patients with significant lipoptosis, a 5-mm spatula liposuction cannula can be used in addition to the 3-mm cannula in the central neck compartment. Liposuction adds a tremendous amount to the overall initial and long-term results in facelifting with the caveat that one should underreduce the fat in any compartment rather than overremove it. Overzealous suctioning may make the ptotic submandibular gland more visible, thus a more difficult aesthetic issue for the patient.[4]

In most types of facelifting, further work is required to tighten the ptotic anterior platysma muscle as well as remove

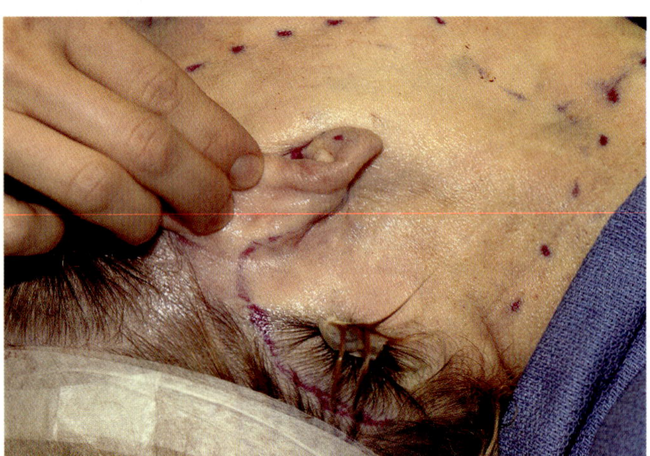

Fig. 4.2 Postauricular incision just above sulcus and across the hairline.

some subplatysmal fat in the anterior midline area. The Kelly clamp technique for submental platysmaplasty can be used for safe, reliable results. To accomplish the Kelly clamp platysmaplasty, complete undermining of the neck skin is required. This is done with Kahn beveled facelift dissection scissors. From the submental incision, the elevation is continued to the anterior part of the sternocleidomastoid bilaterally and across the cervicomental angle. Direct visualization of the remaining ptotic tissues is easily done. The forceps is used to pick up the loose anterior platysmal bands, as well as the subplatysmal fat that is redundant in the midline. A large curved Kelly clamp is then used to tighten these tissues in the anterior midline. Once tightened, creating firmness to the anterior tissues, sequential cauterization, excision, and suturing together with mattressing buried 3-0 Vicryl sutures (Ethicon, Somerville, NJ) is performed (**Fig. 4.3**). This sequential excision and suturing is done from the submental crease down to and sometimes across the cervicomental angle. Excision of digastric muscle and/or repositioning the hyoid muscle may be more surgical intervention than is indicated for the cosmetic surgical patient. In the patient with a very heavy neck, 3-0 Tevdek suture is used in a figure-of-eight fashion to oversew the anterior platysmal plication. Thus, at this point a firm anterior corset has been created setting the stage for bilateral posterior suspension and imbrication of the platysma.[5]

The degree of undermining of the neck skin is directly related to the amount of redundancy of skin in the neck and whether or not excisional plication of the platysma is required. The neck skin is undermined completely to redrape these tissues in a posterior superior fashion. The degree of laxity in the midface and concerns over viability of skin flap often dictate a lesser degree of undermining in the midcheek tissues and more attention to the underlying structures via the deep plane approach. By employing sub-SMAS and deep plane techniques in the midface, much less undermining of the facial skin is required, thereby decreasing the risk of vascular compromise, particularly in smokers. The number

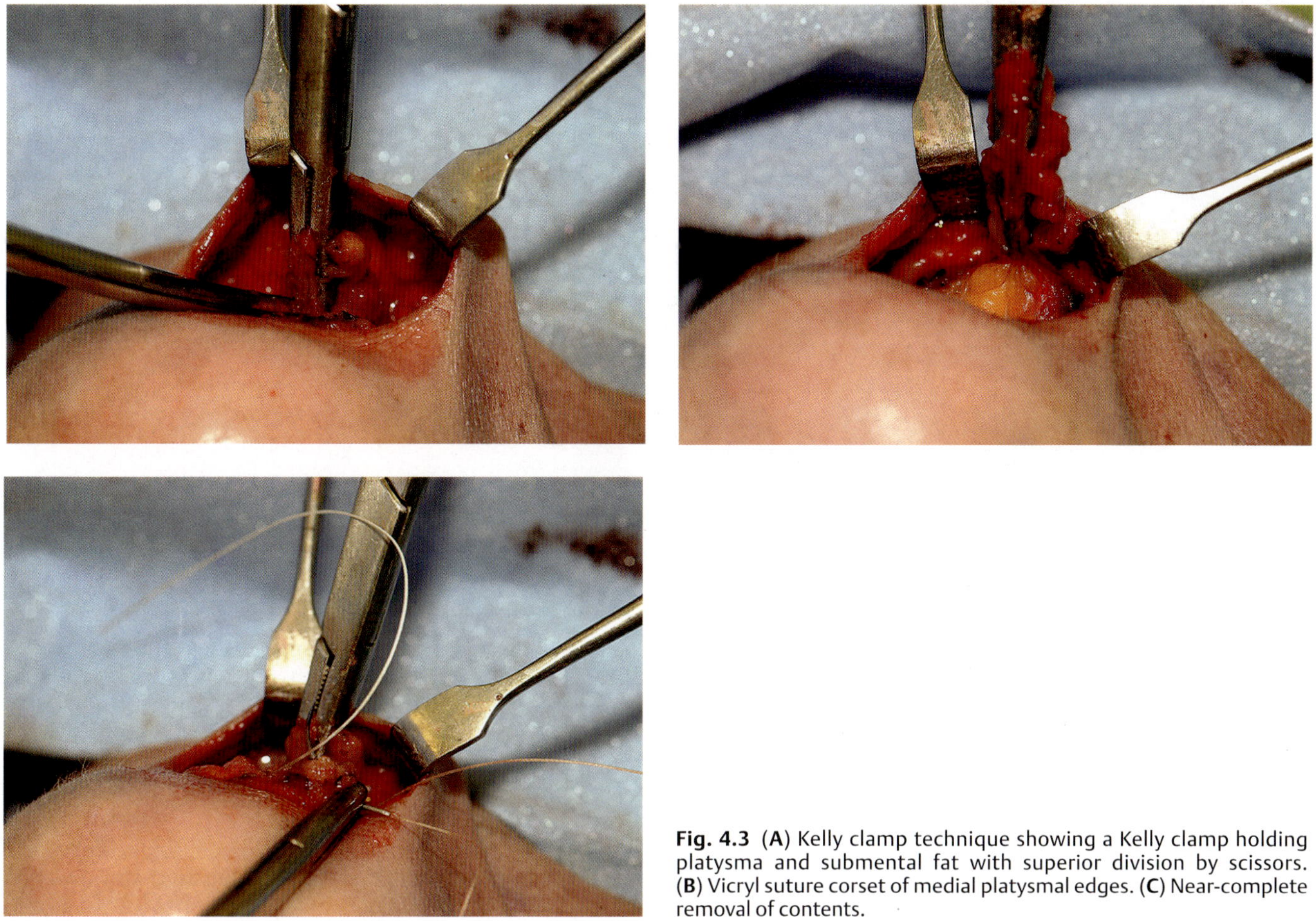

A C B

Fig. 4.3 (**A**) Kelly clamp technique showing a Kelly clamp holding platysma and submental fat with superior division by scissors. (**B**) Vicryl suture corset of medial platysmal edges. (**C**) Near-complete removal of contents.

of seromas, hematomas, and other irregularities in this area are also effectively reduced as well.

After temporal, preauricular, and postauricular incisions have been fashioned and beveled appropriately, skin flap elevation can be performed. Elevation of postauricular skin flap is performed first. Dissection begins deep to the hair follicles and superficial to the fascia of the sternocleidomastoid muscle, then turns more superficial until it is in the immediate subcutaneous plane. This dissection can be carried to connect to the previously elevated neck skin flaps if necessary. Using Kahn beveled facelift scissors in an advanced spread technique with the tips up assures the surgeon that he or she is in the proper plane.

Next, attention is directed to the temporal region, where elevation is performed in the subgaleal supratemporalis fascia plane all the way to the lateral orbital rim. Dissection is continued down near the upper border of the zygomatic arch in this plane. In the event that an inferior sideburn incision has been made, a disconnected temporal incision is made to accomplish this temporal lift.

Preauricular skin elevation is then begun at the level of the helical insertion and in the subcutaneous plane. Initial dissection begins beneath the hair follicles of the sideburn and then extends out in the subcutaneous plane to the lateral orbital crow's-feet region. This can be done safely in the subcutaneous plane without risk of injury to the frontal branch of the facial nerve coursing just beneath this level of dissection. As long as one preserves the layer within the temporalis fascia in a subcutaneous plane, there is no risk to the frontal branch of the facial nerve from direct dissection. Elevation is continued ~3 to 4 cm in the preauricular region connecting down to the elevated neck and postauricular flaps.

Once hemostasis is obtained, one can visualize all the way down below the mandibular margin into the neck (**Fig. 4.4**). An incision is then made in the SMAS extending from the inferior border of the zygomatic arch at the malar eminence diagonally down to the level of the earlobe and then continuing inferiorly 1 cm in front of the anterior border of the sternocleidomastoid. One then uses a horizontal scissor dissection for the first centimeter of SMAS elevation. Further elevation of the SMAS is then performed by spreading the scissors in a more vertical fashion, directly visualizing tunnels and bridges as the dissection is carried anteriorly. Dissection is carried underneath the platysma muscle ~3 to 4 cm. Just above the mandibular margin, dissection is continued superficial to the masseter muscle over the premasseteric fascia. The marginal mandibular nerve is often easily visualized. Dissection is then begun in the malar region just above the zygomatic buttress in the subcutaneous plane

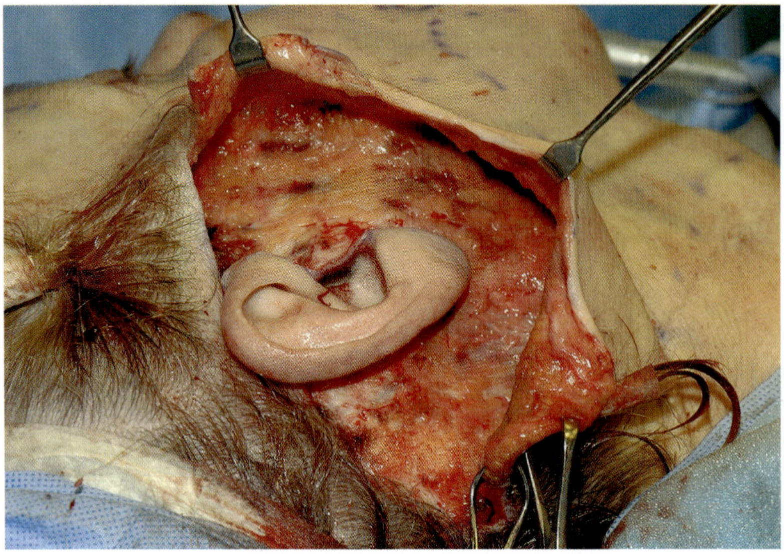

Fig. 4.4 Skin flap after elevation and connection of cheek and neck flaps.

extending just inferior to the orbicularis muscle. This dissection requires release of strong dermal attachments to the malar eminence. Some control of bleeding is often required here. Elevation is then easily extended superficial to the level of the zygomaticus muscle into the midcheek region if necessary. Individualization of the extent of midcheek SMAS undermining is important. Not all patients require full SMAS elevation of the midcheek, as has been reported for the standard deep plane facelift. Once good mobilization of the jowl has been accomplished as well as freeing and mobilization of the malar eminence, a complete elevation transition from deep to superficial to the zygomaticus muscle is not generally required. Increased safety is the result of modifying the deep plane technique, which leaves the zygomatic and buccal branches of the facial nerve in less danger of being injured.

The other modification of this technique that differs from a standard deep plane is that there is a 4-cm amount of skin elevated in addition to the SMAS, creating two separate flaps for later biplane vector suspension. At this stage, the suspension of the midface and jowl tissues is accomplished by advancing the SMAS–subcutaneous skin unit in a posterior superior fashion. There is a tremendous lift and improvement of the lower and midface with the mobilization of the SMAS. This is because there are significant skin-dermal-adipose-SMAS fibrous connections. In addition, the soft tissues of the midface are elevated in continuity with this compound unit. The superior triangular portion of the SMAS is advanced, and Metzenbaum scissors are used to incise the redundant preauricular portion of the SMAS. The superior slip of this SMAS is left intact and suspended to the dense preauricular temporalis fascia at the level of the helical insertion with a deep buried 0 Vicryl suture. Occasionally, a secondary support of one 3-0 Tevdek suture is used in the patient with heavy cheeks. Attention is then directed toward the overlapping platysma-SMAS at the level of the earlobe. Metzenbaum scissors are used to incise this so a posterior-inferior slip of platysma-SMAS can be suspended intact to the mastoid fascia with a 0 Vicryl suture (**Fig. 4.5**). This is literally hanging the platysma to the mastoid, creating a firm corset across the midline to the opposite side. Some redundancy of fatty tissue and SMAS overlapping the lower portions of the sternocleidomastoid are trimmed to avoid extra lumpiness in this area. Next, 3-0 PDS (Ethicon, Somerville, NJ) sutures are then used to reinforce the platysma-SMAS unit to the posterior mastoid-sternocleidomastoid fascia. The preauricular area is also trimmed and sutured end to end with 3-0 PDS sutures to complete the SMAS imbrication. If only a small amount of jowl repositioning and posterior repositioning of the platysma muscle is required, plication of the SMAS may be the only maneuver necessary.

At this stage, the skin is easily advanced up and redraped over the auricle in a different, more posterior vector. There remain only 2 to 3 cm of undermined skin in the preauricular region. The skin from the neck is advanced to the posterior mastoid hairline region posteriorly, and then it is rotated superiorly. These three different lifting vectors achieve a similar effect as described by Baker with the triplane rhytidectomy. This is to ensure the re-creation and maintenance of the postauricular hairline and avoid step-off deformity. A single suspension in the high postauricular region is performed, the hair-bearing portions are reapproximated with staples, and the skin is suture with 5-0 plain interlocking catgut suture. The preauricular skin is moved in a much more posterior direction rather than superior to avoid any undue movement of the temporal hairline. The skin is trimmed judiciously in the preauricular area, ensuring that the earlobe is cradled in a superior fashion to avoid *satyr's ear deformity* and a migrating scar in this region.[6]

The tragal flap is designed to be extremely redundant and is pie-crust sutured in a running interlocking fashion with a 5-0 plain catgut suture. No tension is left on the tragal

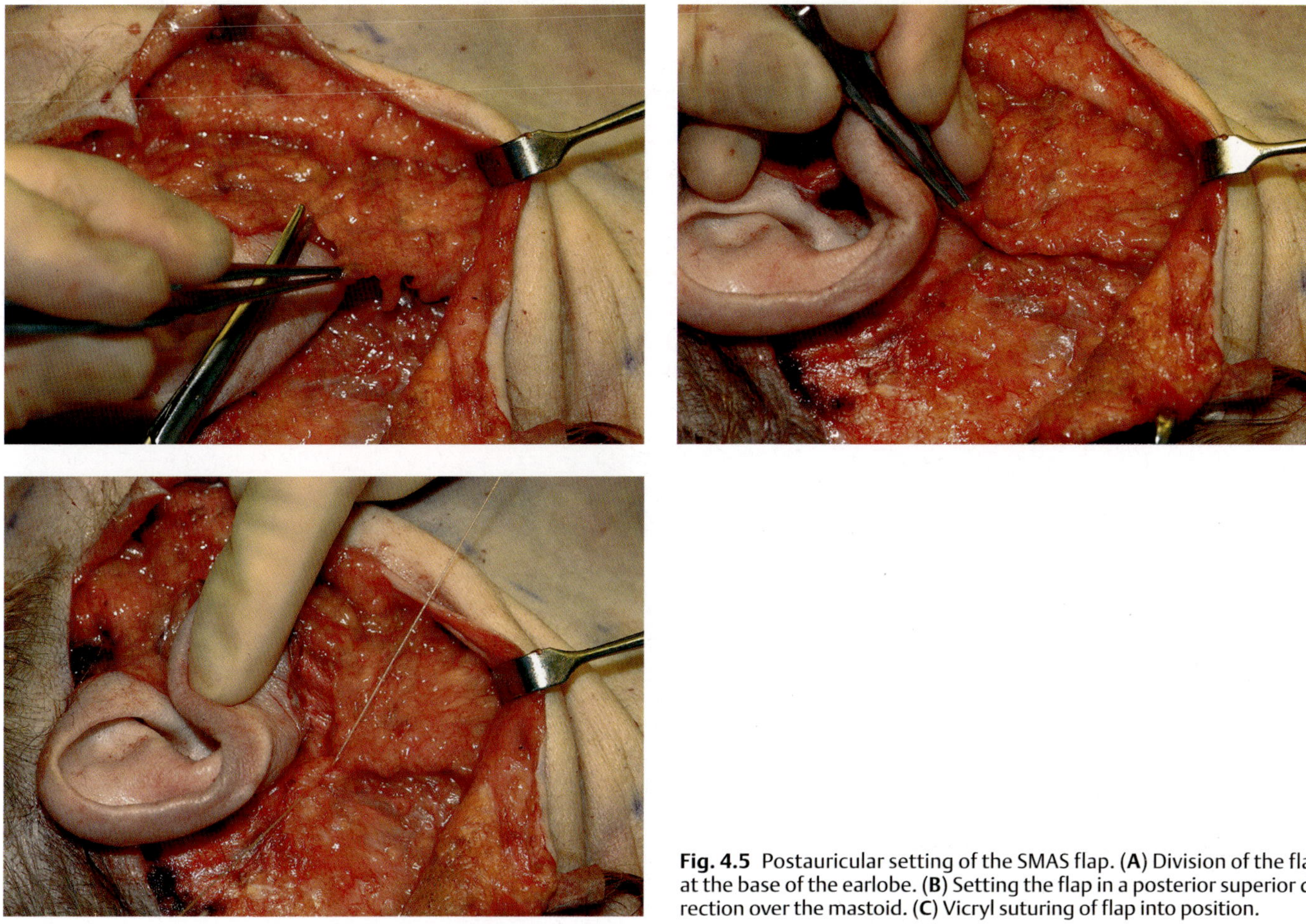

Fig. 4.5 Postauricular setting of the SMAS flap. (**A**) Division of the flap at the base of the earlobe. (**B**) Setting the flap in a posterior superior direction over the mastoid. (**C**) Vicryl suturing of flap into position.

skin, and it is thinned judiciously to avoid overthinning and loss of viability. The closure in the temporal hair-bearing portion of the skin is performed by incrementally excising the redundancy and placing one buried 3-0 Vicryl suture holding the galeal suspension to the temporalis fascia. The scalp is then approximated with interrupted staples. Just prior to the conclusion of the closure, a drain is placed into the neck portion of the wound on either side to assist in the overall reduction of seromas and small hematomas. This has been demonstrated to reduce the hematoma/seroma rate significantly. A permanent 6-0 nylon suture is placed at the earlobe and left in for 10 days, and the remainder of the catgut sutures either dissolve or are removed at 1 week. Placement of the drain also reduces the need for any kind of compressive dressing, but a light compression dressing using an abdominal dressing/combine dressing and elastic chin strap is used for patient and family convenience. Mild compression is used in the preauricular area to prevent any fluid collection in this region.[7] Significant compression dressings used in the past without suction drainage resulted in increased incidence of skin viability problems. Pressure dressings can create poor venous outflow and skin necrosis, which can occur from venous congestion even when arterial vascular perfusion is adequate. Slow venous flow within the flap creates an increased chance of infection further inflaming the flap and creating loss of perfusion and ultimate potential loss of viability.[8]

After the appropriate initial follow-up to ensure proper healing, all patients are followed for at least 1 year, when postoperative results are assessed and photos are taken. Most patients continue to return for follow-up for years to monitor the lasting results of their facelifts (**Fig. 4.6**).

◆ Complications

Although it has been reported that facial nerve injury can occur in 0.5 to 6.0% of all facelift patients, it really should not ever occur even with the deep plane techniques available today.[9] In nearly 2000 patients, the only facial nerve occurrences were two cases of temporal frontal branch paresis, caused by stretching the nerve while elevating the temporal portion of the skin flap. These both resolved within 2 to 4 months. With meticulous dissection techniques in the midface region, use of this modified SMAS elevation should prevent any injury to the facial nerve.

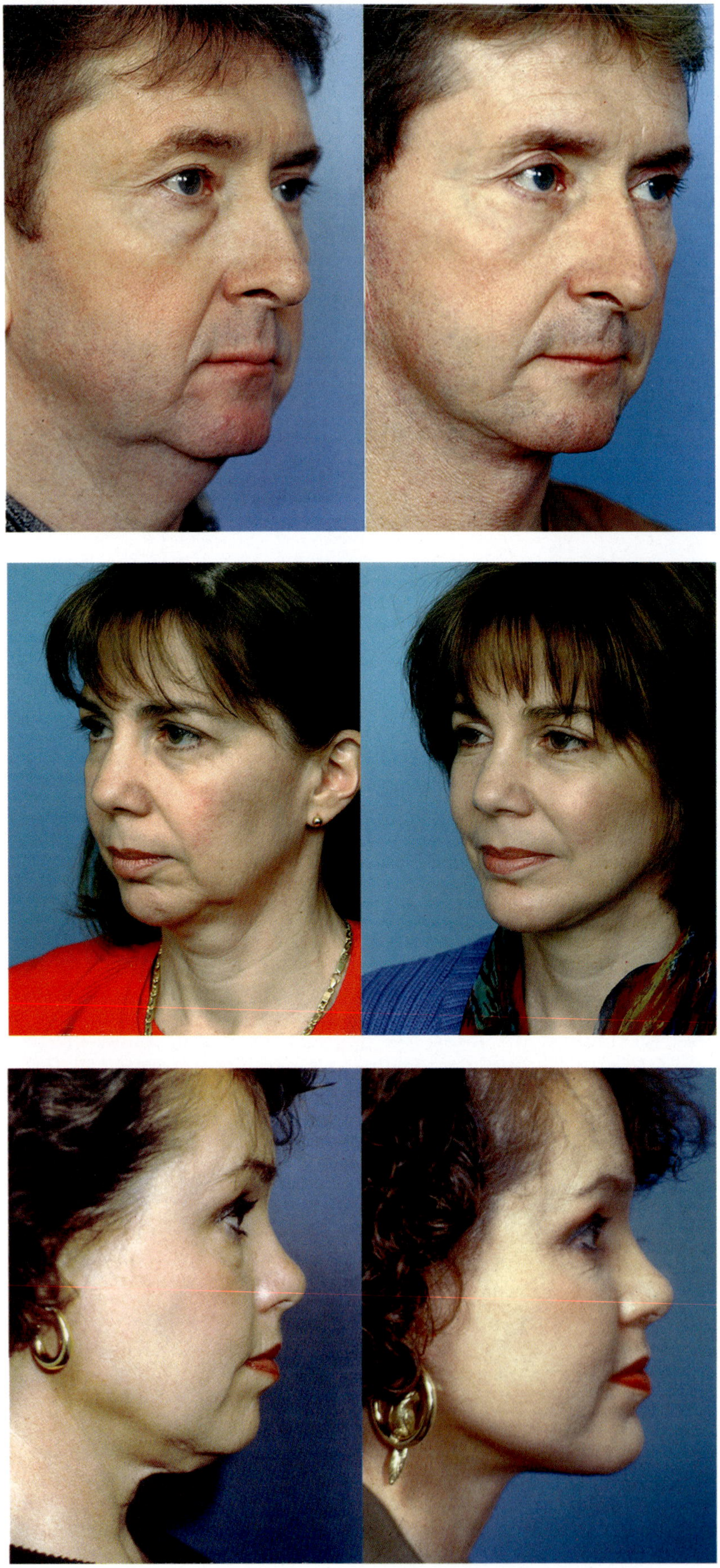

A–B

C–D

E–F

Fig. 4.6 (**A, C, E**) Preoperative and (**B, D, F**) postoperative photographs of three patients showing natural, long-lasting results.

Injury to the facial nerve is the most feared complication of rhytidectomy. Having a patient with paralysis could be detrimental to your long-term successful practice. Choosing a facelift technique that is safe, without the risk of facial nerve injury, is highly recommended rather than being more aggressive surgically, which may risk a facial nerve injury for a small extra potential benefit in the result.

◆ Conclusion

As more and more rhytidectomy techniques are developed, many options exist for the rhytidectomy surgeon. The extended SMAS flap rhytidectomy provides the surgeon with a proven method of achieving a natural, long-lasting result. Care must be taken to tailor planning and surgical technique for the patient's individual needs to achieve maximal results.

References

1. Hamra ST. The deep plane rhytidectomy. Plast Reconstr Surg 1990;86: 53–61
2. Kamer FM. One hundred consecutive deep plane face lifts. Arch Otolaryngol Head Neck Surg 1996;122:17–22
3. Baker SR. Tri-plane rhytidectomy. Arch Otolaryngol Head Neck Surg 1997;123:1167–1172
4. Ramirez OM. The subperiosteal rhytidectomy: the third generation face lift. Ann Plast Surg 1992;28:218–232
5. Koch BB, Perkins SW. Simultaneous rhytidectomy and full-face carbon dioxide laser resurfacing: a case series and meta-analysis. Arch Facial Plast Surg 2002;4:227–233
6. Ashbell TS. Photographic simulation: an express warranty. Plastic Surgery Products; April 2002.
7. Perkins SW, Williams JD, MacDonald K, et al. Prevention of seromas and hematomas following facelift surgery with the use of postoperative vacuum drains. Arch Otolaryngol Head Neck Surg 1997;123: 743–745
8. Straith RE, Raju D, Hipps C. The study of hematomas in 500 consecutive face lifts. Plast Reconstr Surg 1977;59:694–698
9. Castanares S. Facial nerve paralyses coincident with or subsequent to rhytidectomy. Plast Reconstr Surg 1974;54:637–643

5

Periorbital Rejuvenation

Tom D. Wang and Adam T. Ross

Rejuvenation of the periorbital region provides a more youthful appearance to one of the focal points of the face. As the average age of our population increases, these procedures are likely to become increasingly more common. Accurate preoperative examination, assessment, and counseling are imperative to achieve an excellent result. Also, careful selection from the spectrum of available techniques, combined with meticulous surgical precision, will assist the surgeon in rejuvenating the individual patient. Although no one ideal surgical procedure exists, many safe and effective strategies have been developed as we have learned more about the effects of aging. This chapter provides a history of techniques used in eyelid rejuvenation, as well as an overview of the evaluation process.

Rejuvenation of the periorbital region can be one of the most rewarding procedures for both patient and surgeon. Many believe that the "eyes are the window to the soul," and as such they significantly contribute to the general appearance of the patient as perceived by an observer. As time passes, a youthful appearance fades as tissues stretch, adipose tissue settles and atrophies, and skin becomes redundant. Thus, procedures to rejuvenate the periorbital region are designed to counteract these changes related to aging.

A thorough review of the literature written on rejuvenation of the periorbital region can be somewhat perplexing for the young facial surgeon. The myriad of techniques offered for each orbital finding encountered in the aging patient illustrate that, to date, there is no perfect technique to reliably rejuvenate this area. Compounding the complexity of choosing a course of action is the common admission that different techniques work better in the hands of different surgeons.

Clearly, the search for the ideal technique continues, and to the credit of modern-day, evidence-based surgeons, more emphasis has turned to defining the etiology of the signs of aging rather than simply offering techniques used to camouflage appearance. Many techniques, even those most commonly performed, have the limitation that they further alter anatomy in a nonanatomic fashion, but often will produce excellent results. We predict that the time will eventually come that prevention of the changes related to aging will be more successful, leading to a reduced need for rejuvenation procedures. As the population ages, attention will likely be turned to procedures that more closely replace the anatomy found in youth. Until that time comes, however, we are left to use one or many of the excellent, safe, and successful techniques that are well described in the literature.

Obviously, an exhaustive discussion of orbital anatomy, its changes, and those techniques available to correct the aging eye are beyond the scope (and length) of this chapter. However, a brief overview of anatomic changes and available techniques will provide a base from which those interested can pursue further study.

◆ History of Eyelid Surgery

Although exact dates are somewhat ambiguous, the documented history of eyelid surgery finds its beginnings in the writings of Susruta, a legendary Indian surgeon who is thought to have lived more than 2000 years ago. Although the practice of surgery became less popular after early interest (and clear technological disadvantages), it experienced a rebirth in the 10th and 11th centuries. At that time, Arabian surgeons were noted to remove excess skin folds to improve vision—our first documentation of functional blepharoplasty. It was not until 1792 that Beer, an Austrian ophthalmologist, provided the first illustration of this upper eyelid deformity in his textbook, and in 1818 Von Graefe coined the term *blepharoplasty* to describe reconstructive procedures of acquired eyelid defects.[1] Shortly thereafter, European surgeons began to focus on upper lid reduction, and in 1844, Sichel first described the lower lid pseudoherniation of fat found with aging.

In the early 20th century, advances in anatomic description of the periorbita were reported, as were early attempts at cosmetic blepharoplasty. Bourquet, in 1929, was the first to describe the presence of two separate fat compartments of the upper eyelids and procedures to remove them. Claoue and Passot, in 1931, went on to describe the transconjunctival approach to remove these fat pads. Castañares, in 1951, was the first to provide detailed anatomy of the orbital fat compartments and popularized skin and fat resection of the aging lower lid.[1] In 1952, Fox suggested *dermachalasis* as a term to describe the relaxation and redundancy of eyelid skin over time. We continue even today to more accurately describe eyelid anatomy with respect to aging, facilitating new surgical techniques to reverse or obscure these changes.

◆ Eyelid Anatomy

An accurate understanding of periorbital anatomy and function is clearly a prerequisite for any surgeon performing cosmetic or reconstructive surgery in or around the orbit. Excellent texts currently exist with more detail than space permits in this chapter.

Upper Eyelid

The current discussion of upper eyelid anatomy will focus on the Western eyelid, although ethnic variation is well described in the literature and an understanding thereof is clearly important before proceeding with any surgical intervention, especially with regard to the Asian eyelid. As well, the contribution of the upper third of the face, specifically the eyebrow subunit, to the upper eyelid must be evaluated correctly, and often intervention involves modification of both regions.

The skin of the eyelid is the thinnest in the body (1 mm) and therefore heals extremely well without hypertrophy or contraction. However, the skin thickens as it extends to the brow and lateral orbital rim, where it is more susceptible to unpredictable scarring. The upper eyelid skin has very little subcutaneous tissue but is firmly connected to the underlying orbicularis oculi muscle through fine connective tissue attachments.

The orbicularis muscle is divided into pretarsal, preseptal, and orbital components, with the orbital component responsible for voluntary closure of the eye and the remaining regions responsible for involuntary and reflexive closure. The medial canthal tendon is formed as the superficial and deep heads of the pretarsal orbicularis insert onto the anterior and posterior lacrimal crest, respectively. Likewise, the lateral canthal tendon is formed from the coalescence of orbicularis laterally into the orbital tubercle of Whitnall.

Just deep to the orbicularis is the orbital septum, a thin fibrous sheet that originates at the orbital rim from the arcus marginalis and is continuous with orbital periosteum. The septum fuses with the levator aponeurosis 2 to 5 mm above the superior tarsal border. The tarsal plate and conjunctiva lie deep to the orbital septum.

A preaponeurotic fat pad lies, divided into central and medial components, posterior to the orbital septum and anterior to the levator aponeurosis. These fat pads are separated by the trochlea. The lacrimal gland occupies the lateral aspect of the orbit.

The levator palpebrae superioris muscle and Müller's muscle are the retractors of the upper lids. The levator palpebrae superioris muscle originates at the lesser wing of the sphenoid and inserts onto the anterior, inferior one third of the tarsus and into the orbicularis muscle and skin. This insertion into the skin and muscle of the upper eyelid forms the upper eyelid crease, which falls 10 to 11 mm above the Western eyelid margin.[2]

Lower Eyelid

Unlike the upper eyelid, there are no significant racial differences in lower eyelid anatomy, which is similar in many ways to the upper lid, with skin, orbicularis, and septum encountered similarly.[2] The presence of the lid retractors differentiates the lower lid anatomically. The capsulopalpebral fascia of the inferior rectus muscle encompasses the inferior oblique muscle, and these fascial layers reunite anteriorly to contribute to the formation of Lockwood's suspensory ligament. In addition, the capsulopalpebral fascia also fuses separately with the orbital septum ~4 to 5 mm below the inferior tarsal border, and this structure along with the inferior tarsal muscle allows retraction of the lower lid.

The medial and lateral canthal tendons, with the overlying pretarsal orbicularis muscle, form a tarsoligamentous sling to maintain normal lower lid tone. The medial canthal tendon attaches anteriorly to the frontal process of the maxillary bone and posterior to the posterior lacrimal crest. The lateral canthal tendon attaches to the lateral orbital tubercle of Whitnall.

Between the orbital septum and lower lid retractors lies adipose tissue divided into lateral, central, and medial compartments. The inferior oblique muscle separates the medial and central fat pads. The central and lateral fat pads are separated by the arcuate expansion of the inferior oblique muscle. The medial fat pad has a characteristic lighter color than that of the central or lateral pads. The size of these fat pads is not related to body habitus and they do not appear to regenerate once removed.[3]

The midface plays an equally important role with respect to the lower eyelid as the brow does with respect to the upper eyelid. Inferior to the orbital rim and posterior to the orbicularis oculi muscle is a fat pad called the suborbicularis oculi fat (SOOF) pad. Along with the malar fat pad, changes in position of these midface structures contribute to lower eyelid appearance and clearly need to be addressed simultaneously.

◆ Age-Related Changes of the Eyelids

Upper Eyelid

The appearance of the upper eyelid may be affected by changes in eyebrow position that are well described. Specifically, lateral ptosis of the eyebrow may add fullness to the upper eyelid, adding to skin redundancy and functional visual field loss. Combined with the loss of frontal volume and the reabsorption of retroorbicularis oculi fat (ROOF), eyebrow changes may accentuate aging changes inherent to the eyelid.[4] The ROOF fat pad, which rests on the lateral portion of the superior orbital rim between periosteum and eyebrow, may descend and exacerbate lateral bulging of the eyelid.[5]

The orbicularis may hypertrophy over time presumably due to the necessary blinking that one does throughout life. This causes the preseptal portion of the orbicularis to become redundant and may roll over the firmly attached pretarsal orbicularis.[2] The descent of the eyebrow, and therefore the orbital portion of orbicularis, compounds this redundancy. Gravity and constant repetitive motion conspire to cause the skin to lose its natural elasticity.

Although usually less significant an issue in the upper eyelid than in the lower eyelid, a weakened septum may permit pseudoherniation of the orbital fat. Fullness in the lateral aspect of the upper eyelid may also result from ptosis of the lacrimal gland. Weakening of the suspensory ligaments of the globe with aging also causes the eye to descend inferiorly into the orbit. This manifests as a superior sulcus deformity, which is accentuated by gradual age-related loss of intraorbital fat.[6]

Lower Eyelid

It is now recognized that a youthful, cherubic appearance is associated with a single convexity evident on lateral view that begins at the inferior margin of the lower eyelid tarsus and extends down to the cheek, lateral oral commissure, and angle of the mandible. Contributions to this convexity include all of the structures previously described, as well as their natural blend into a well-supported midface, and changes in position and volume of these structures are the culprits of lower eyelid and midfacial aging (**Fig. 5.1**).

Baggy eyelids, one of the tell-tale signs of lower lid aging, are caused by pseudoherniation of lower eyelid fat under a weakened orbital septum. This is exacerbated by attenuation of the orbicularis muscle, as well as by the previously described descent of the globe pushing on orbital fat. The orbital septum bows but prevents this fat from descending below the orbital rim at its attachment at the arcus marginalis.

Concurrently, the malar fat pad and SOOF descend, separating the eyelid and midface subunits from each other, skeletonizing the orbital rim, and creating a tear trough deformity medially. Crucial to the formation of these sulci and deformities is the presence of cutaneous insertions of the orbicularis retaining ligament and zygomatico-cutaneous ligaments well described by Mendelson et al.[7] With this separation, a double convexity is formed, and aging is evident. Progressive ptosis of the skin and the orbicularis oculi muscle also contribute to the skeletonizing effect of the orbital rim seen in the aging face.

The lower eyelid loses its support as the malar fat pad and the SOOF descend, and as a result, the lower eyelid (especially laterally) is pulled with it, causing senile ectropion.[8] The snap test and careful photographic documentation and review are important to correctly identify this deformity.

The effects of gravity in an aging face manifest in a double convexity contour on profile. An understanding of the changes that cause this double convexity contour in the aging face are essential to resorting the youthful single convexity contour and rejuvenating the periorbital region.

◆ Patient Evaluation

Standardized photographic views are a crucial component of the preoperative evaluation. Particular views with respect to blepharoplasty are also obtained, most importantly of the eye region with the head neutral but the eyes looking straight ahead and then superiorly. This allows for identification of lower eyelid pseudoherniation, as well as quantifying the contribution of each compartment to lower lid fullness. Medical factors that might predispose patients to poor outcomes need to be addressed and particular attention taken to discontinue medications or herbal therapies that might affect

A–C

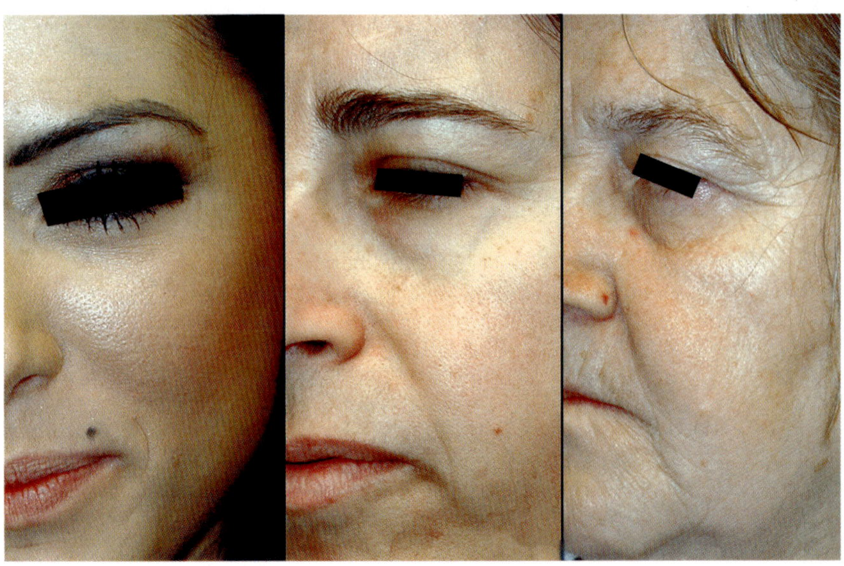

Fig. 5.1 Age-related changes in the periorbital region: (**A**) 22-year-old, (**B**) 48-year-old, and (**C**) 75-year-old women. Note the progression of lateral upper eyebrow ptosis, progressive lateral upper lid redundancy, lower lid pseudoherniation of fat, infraorbital hollowing, and descent of the midface over time.

platelet function. A history of dry eyes or irritation must be assessed, and presence of asymmetry or lower eyelid laxity identified and appropriately evaluated. Preparation for eyelid surgery is well described in the literature.[9,10]

A useful tool when assessing patients is a review of pictures from an earlier age. Once enough of these pictures are studied, surgeons will recognize that sagging is not the only culprit but rather is present in combination with volume loss. Recent techniques appropriately focus on restoring volume as well as altering anatomy.

◆ Eyelid Rejuvenation Techniques

With the previous description of the aging process in the periorbital region, there are a multitude of techniques in the literature that address each of these age-related findings. Whereas individual procedures will be discussed, most patients require a combination of techniques to achieve the most aesthetically pleasing result. The surgeon must recognize what works well in his or her hands and must correctly apply techniques to each individual patient. Whereas general patterns of aging are useful descriptively, patients may vary in their individual components.

Techniques have evolved that allow a myriad of approaches to address the aging periorbital unit, most often in combination with adjacent facial subunits. Although many observed that patients do not lose fat with age, many techniques served to treat the appearance rather than the underlying cause of the deformity. The removal of periorbital fat is one such prime example. Although there is no clear ideal method to perfectly rejuvenate the eyelid, preservation and augmentation seem to be the modalities of the future.

Upper Eyelid

The descent of the eyebrow and orbicularis oculi muscle must be addressed first. In fact, it is not infrequent for brow lifting procedures to obviate the need for further eyelid procedures. This is especially true laterally, as the unopposed orbicularis depression of the eyebrow combines with gravity to cause lateral hooding. Preoperative manipulation of the eyebrow while the patient is sitting often will indicate whether eyelid procedures will be necessary. It is quite easy to illustrate this effect to the patient, and most patients will recognize that brow descent has occurred. Techniques for brow lifting are not discussed in this chapter.

Recent techniques have also focused on volume augmentation of the frontal region.[4,6] Injection of fat, hyaluronic acid, and other fillers may be effective in creating a more full eyebrow and may even reposition the eyebrow superiorly. Volume augmentation can aid in the reversal of the superior sulcus deformity, although clearly this effect is not anatomically correct as the globe continues to be lowset, and periorbital fat remains lost. The correct plane of injection is suborbicularis, which serves to reduce irregularities that are visible or palpable. When performing volume augmentation, one should not violate the orbicularis to improve graft or injection survival, and preservation of structures goes hand in hand with augmentation.[4]

The use of botulinum toxin, although only approved by the U.S. Food and Drug Administration for glabellar rhytides, may also be useful to sculpt the eyebrow. This is performed through injections laterally in the vertical segment of the orbicularis, thus relaxing the downward pull on the eyebrow and in effect performing a denervation brow lift. This technique serves as an introduction to the idea of brow lifting and many times will delay or avoid more aggressive surgical intervention. The use of Botox (Allergan, Inc., Irvine, CA) for the lateral crow's-feet regions to reduce rhytide formation is well-described throughout the literature and will not be discussed at this time.[11,12]

Orbicularis hypertrophy, as well as skin redundancy caused by attenuation of its connections with its underlying muscle, is easily addressed by skin and muscle excision. Care must be taken to make an inferior incision 8 to 10 mm above the eyelid margin to create a natural supratarsal crease, which many times has migrated inferiorly over time. Excision of orbicularis at this level and gentle cauterization of the septum may assist the surgeon in reestablishing this crease if so desired. Care must be taken to avoid overexcision of tissue to prevent lagophthalmos (**Fig. 5.2**).

A–C

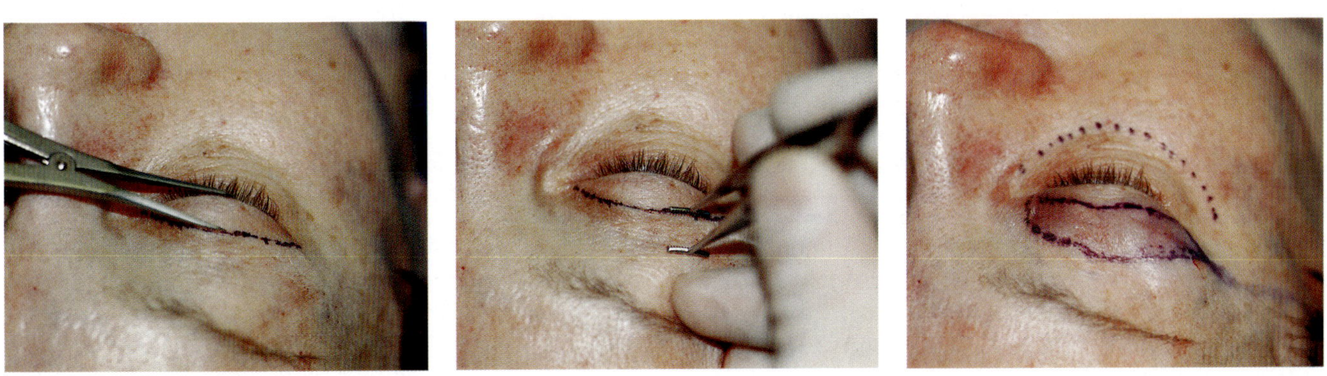

Fig. 5.2 Upper eyelid blepharoplasty, intraoperative sequence. (**A**) Measuring and marking supratarsal crease in native position; (**B**) gathering redundant skin for excision; (**C**) amount of upper lid skin resection marked and infiltrated with local anesthetic; note infraorbital rim hollow also marked for fat transfer.

(Continued on page 58)

D–F

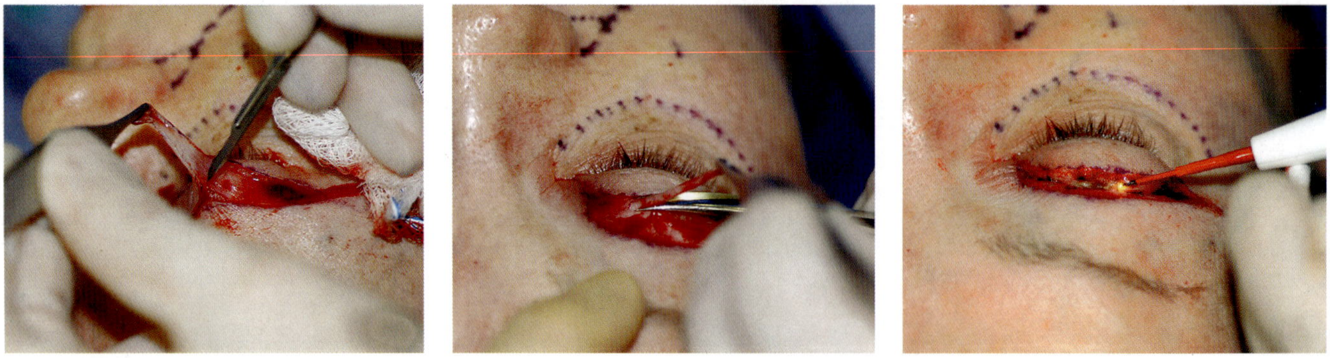

Fig. 5.2 *(Continued)* Upper eyelid blepharoplasty, intraoperative sequence. (**D**) Excision of redundant upper eyelid skin; (**E**) conservative resection of a strip of orbicularis muscle to aid in delineation of supratarsal crease; (**F**) cauterization of orbital septum to enhance tissue tightening and contracture.

Although we prefer to conserve upper eyelid fat, it is sometimes necessary to remove excess fat. This is done carefully by teasing either central or medial fat through the septum and using careful technique and cautery to avoid bleeding from retracted vessels. Lacrimal gland ptosis can also be a source of fullness in the lateral region. To correct this rare problem, suture suspension of the gland to the interior surface of the superior orbital rim may be performed.

Lower Eyelid

Lower eyelid rejuvenation is clearly more complicated in theory and practice than is upper lid restoration. Anatomic variation, as well as increased contribution of septal weakening, for which no perfect solution exists, increase the level of difficulty. Whereas the adjacent eyebrow falls into and *overlaps* with the upper eyelid, keeping it continuous but redundant, the midface descends and *separates* from the lower eyelid, creating two distinct units rather than one continuous one. Thus, techniques similar to those used to separate the eyebrow from the eyelid must be used to *restore continuity* of the lower eyelid to the middle of the face. However, midfacial suspension is arguably more difficult to perform than is brow lifting and requires more postoperative recovery time than do upper face procedures, complicating both surgical and social factors.

Again, attention to the midfacial changes provides a useful adjunctive service to lower eyelid rejuvenation. Midface lifts, performed through various approaches (deep plane facelift, transblepharoplasty, endoscopic temporal, to name a few) may be useful in restoring support to the lower lid and reestablishing confluence of these units. As well, restoring the descended SOOF to its proper anatomic location may be useful in the medial tear trough deformity.[13,14] Tarsal shortening should be used if necessary.

Perhaps the most anatomically correct technique used to reverse the "baggy eyelid" deformity is the skin and muscle flap, which continues to be the preferred modality of many surgeons for lower eyelid rejuvenation.[15] This is performed via a subciliary incision, elevation of a skin and muscle flap over the orbital septum down to the arcus marginalis, often plication of the septum, and/or the removal of excess eyelid fat through the orbital septum. Although some authors prefer to avoid the separation of the orbicularis/septum complex to avoid scarring, this technique produces predictable results when performed properly.[16] The surgeon may choose to elevate a skin-only flap inferiorly past the tarsus to facilitate earlier return of pretarsal orbicularis muscle and therefore eyelid function.[15]

The transconjunctival approach to eyelid rejuvenation has become popular over the past two decades, and as a result, surgeons began offering eyelid rejuvenation without subciliary scars (**Fig. 5.3**). Although these external scars are virtually imperceptible if placed appropriately, this approach has become quite popular and well-known to consumers. Two approaches are possible using the transconjunctival approach: one directly through the capsulopalpebral fascia into the fat compartments of the lower eyelid, and another via an incision close to the tarsus, through the coalescence of the orbital septum and capsulopalpebral fascia, and into a preseptal plane similar to a skin and muscle flap. Fat is then removed with care being taken to avoid injury to the inferior oblique muscle and intraorbital bleeding.

Theoretically, any mechanism of reducing periorbital fat can have the same effect. One such mechanism involves the injection of lipolytic substances, such as phosphatidyl choline, into the postseptal region.[17,18] The safety of such techniques must be carefully addressed and are not currently recommended by these authors given their unpredictability.

Most importantly, the general principle of fat removal is a non–anatomic correction of a sign of aging and only serves to camouflage instead of address the inciting factors. As aging is associated with continuous adipose atrophy and reabsorption, both extraorbitally and intraorbitally, it does not make "physiologic sense" to remove orbital fat in many cases. Clearly, there are indications for this technique in specific patients, but as the population ages, and as more patients live longer after fat excision procedures, surgeons are virtually guaranteed to see the results of premature orbital hollowing secondary to overexcision of orbital fat.

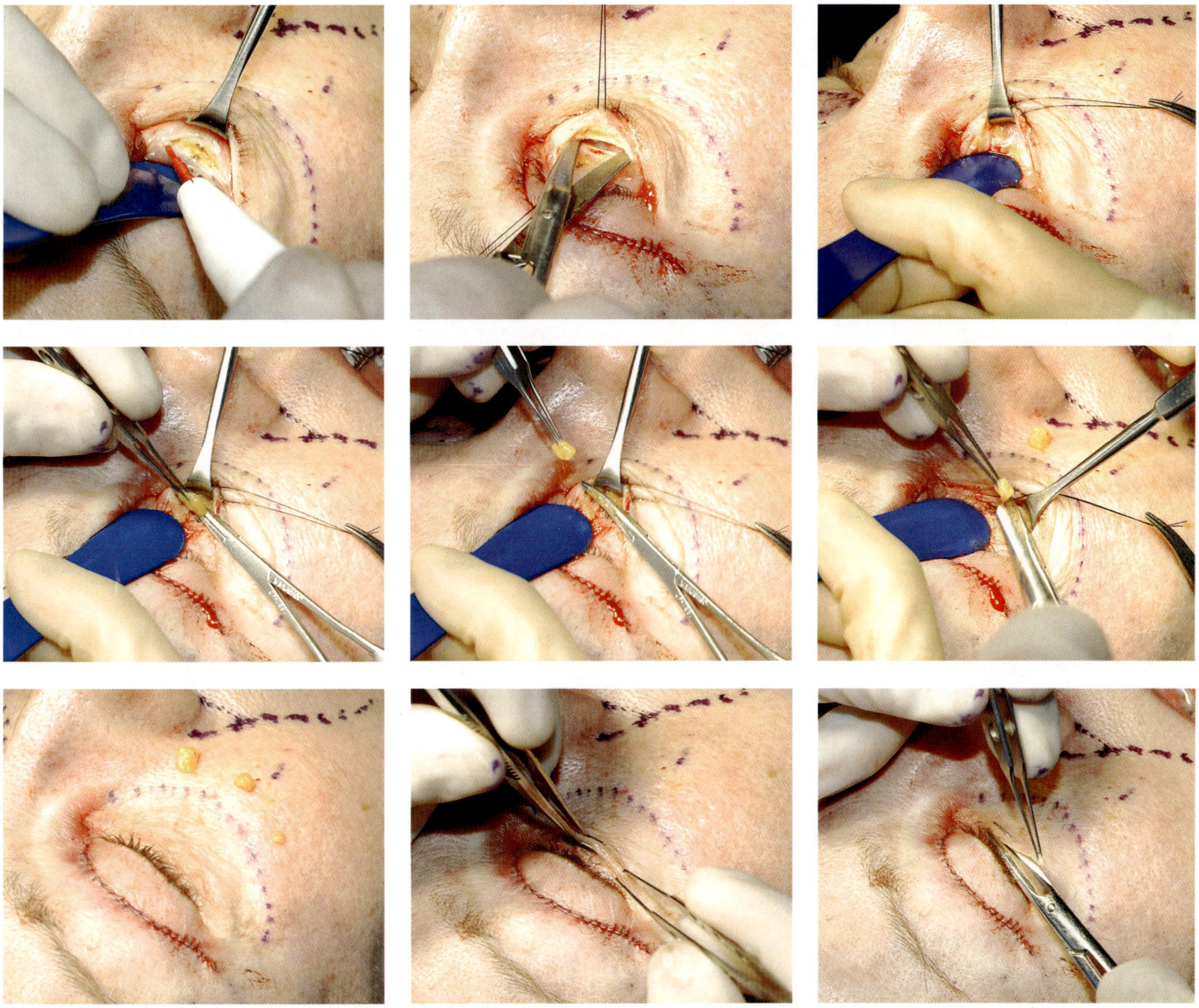

A–C

D–F

G–I

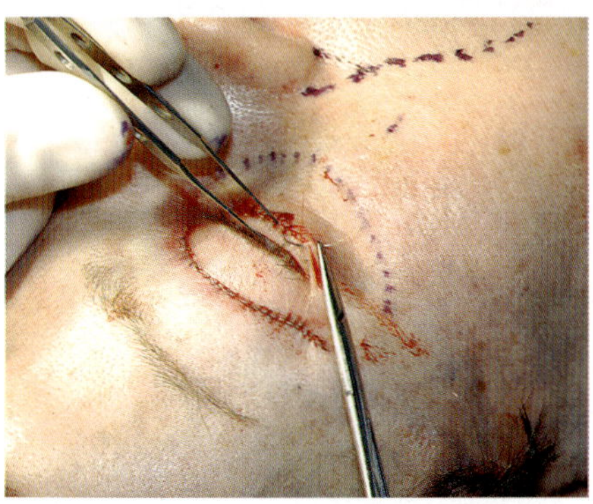

J

Fig. 5.3 Lower eyelid transconjunctival blepharoplasty with skin pinch resection, intraoperative sequence. (**A**) Transconjunctival incision with electrocautery; (**B**) retraction of conjunctiva for access to orbital fat; (**C**) exposure of inferior oblique muscle and medial fat compartment; (**D**) clamp across medial fat pocket to be resected; (**E**) fat resection; stump in clamp to be cauterized to ensure absolute hemostasis; (**F**) resection of central fat pocket lateral to inferior oblique muscle; (**G**) resected fat displayed externally; (**H**) redundant external skin gathered via conservative pinch technique; (**I**) redundant skin pinch resected; (**J**) skin closure.

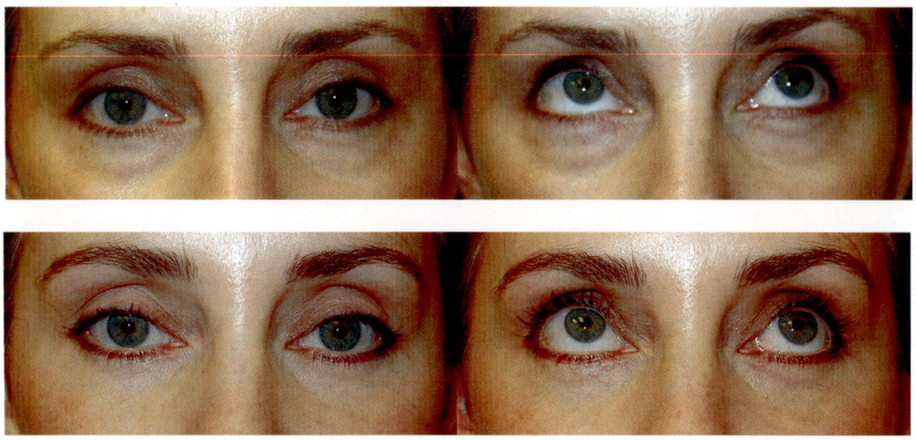

A B C D

Fig. 5.4 Eye position causing accentuation of infraorbital pseudoherniation: (**A**) forward neutral gaze and (**B**) upward gaze accentuating pseudoherniated infraorbital fat. (**C, D**) Same patient 6 months after transconjunctival blepharoplasty with infraorbital fat transfer.

Fat repositioning is yet another non–anatomic reconstruction that serves to camouflage the separation of the eyelid and either descended SOOF or malar fat rather than reapproximating the two subunits. In this technique, first described by Loeb, orbital fat is teased through the inferior septum, remains pedicled intraorbitally, and is placed either in a pocket under the tear trough deformity or over the skeletonized orbital rim.[19] This is an effective technique and may be ideal for certain patients. However, this technique again decompresses intraorbital volume, violates the septum, and may actually contribute to upper eyelid sulcus deformities, presumably by further lowering the entire globe. In one report, as many as 10% of patients had deepening of the upper sulcus.[20]

Fat preservation techniques, therefore, are enticing physiologically and have been described extensively (**Fig. 5.4**). In 1998, de la Plaza and Arroyo described the suturing of capsulopalpebral fascia to the orbital septum to replace herniated fat back into the orbit and prevent further enopthalmia.[21] Hamra also further described these techniques of fat preservation.[22] Modern-day literature includes more focus on volume restoration, such as the use of fat grafting to the lower eyelid, instead of or in addition to repositioning or fat excision (**Figs. 5.5 and 5.6**).[4,23] Fat injections (lipostructure), or the injection of fillers such as hyaluronic acid or polylactic acid, may be used to restore support and re-create orbital fullness, again placed suborbicularis (**Fig. 5.7**). This principle incited the creation of orbital implants (tear trough implant, orbital rim), which also serve to restore volume and support.[24]

Adjunctive treatments may be useful either primarily or in combination with other techniques. Laser resurfacing, both nonablative and ablative, may be useful but must be used conservatively to avoid the irreparable hypopigmentation that is a tell-tale sign of overtreatment. Many have used dermabrasion or microdermabrasion with success, and in a similar fashion chemical peels (α-hydroxyl acid or trichloroacetic acid) and radiofrequency therapy serve to increase collagen and elastin formation in the skin for a youthful look. One must not also forget the use of cosmetics to camouflage both surgical changes and those related to aging.

◆ Common Complications

When performed carefully, both upper and lower lid blepharoplasty usually produce excellent results but are not without risk. Postoperative complications are best avoided through careful preoperative planning and meticulous surgical techniques. Setting goals, establishing realistic expectations, and engaging in a thorough discussion of possible complications with patients are imperative during the preoperative consultation. In addition, identifying and managing known risk factors

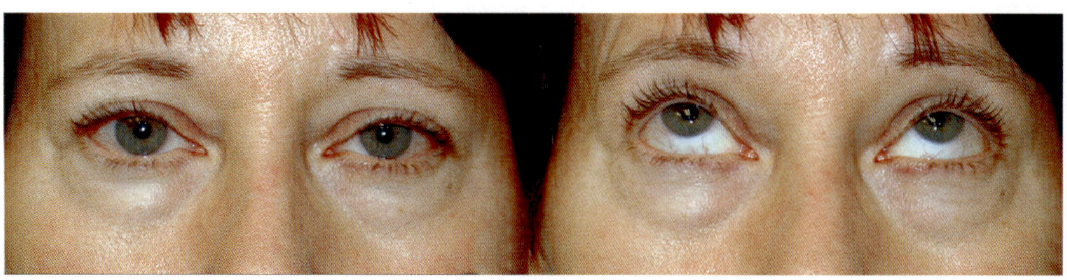

A B

Fig. 5.5 Periorbital rejuvenation. This patient underwent endoscopic brow lift and upper and transconjunctival lower blepharoplasty with infraorbital fat transfer. (**A**) Preoperative forward gaze and (**B**) preoperative upward gaze.

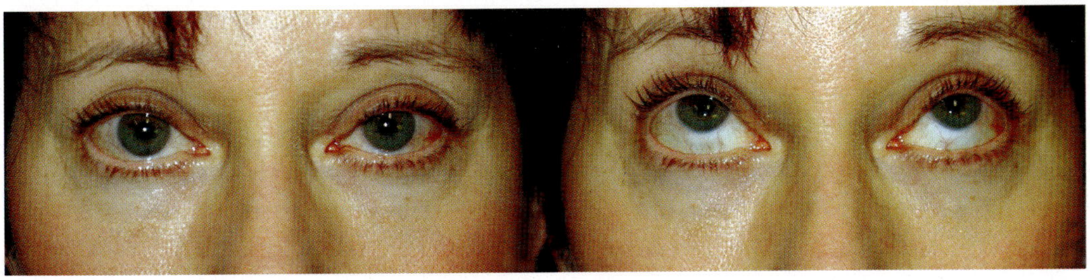

Fig. 5.6 Periorbital rejuvenation. This patient underwent endoscopic brow lift and upper and transconjunctival lower blepharoplasty with infraorbital fat transfer. **(A)** Seven months' postoperative forward gaze and **(B)** 7 months' postoperative upward gaze. Note effacement of infraorbital hollow.

(i.e., hypertension, coagulopathies, nonsteroidal anti-inflammatory drugs, antiplatelet medications) are equally important.

Common complications from blepharoplasty include edema, infection, asymmetry secondary to excessive or insufficient excision of skin, muscle, or fat, and noticeable scars. Other complications include lagophthalmos, exposure keratopathy, canthal webbing, ectropion, ptosis, chemosis, and dry eyes. Though infrequent, lower lid blepharoplasty is more commonly associated with diplopia secondary to injury of the inferior oblique muscle, as well as hematomas and blindness due to retrobulbar hemorrhage.

The newer, less-invasive volume augmentation techniques are also frequently associated with contour irregularities and asymmetries. This is often secondary to subsequent scarring and under- or overcorrection when using these fillers or grafts. In addition, the long-term results and

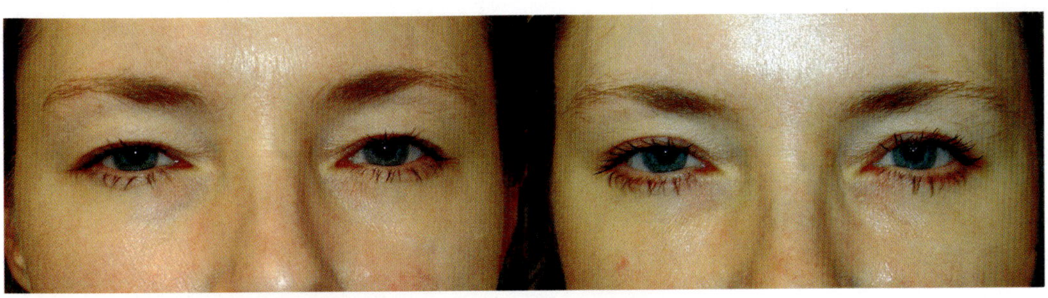

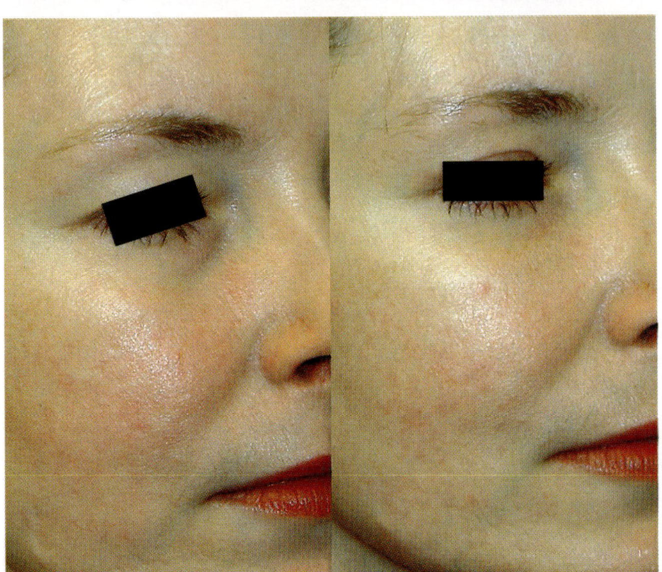

Fig. 5.7 Periorbital rejuvenation. This patient underwent upper lid skin and muscle blepharoplasty and lower lid transconjunctival blepharoplasty with fat transfer. (**A**) Preoperative forward gaze and (**B**) 1 year postoperative forward gaze. (**C**) Preoperative oblique view and (**D**) 1 year postoperative oblique view.

complications from the repetitive use of these synthetic fillers are still being studied.

◆ Conclusion

In the past, eyelid rejuvenation procedures have focused on camouflaging of the changes associated with aging rather than on true anatomic restoration. As the population of many countries ages, removal of tissue may result in long-term deficiencies and, as a result, should be avoided in many steps of eyelid surgery, most notably in the removal of intraorbital fat. Each surgeon should be comfortable with the techniques employed and continuously assess the results of intervention critically. Volume augmentation techniques may prove useful for the patient not interested in surgery, as well as for the patient undergoing surgical blepharoplasty. Attention to adjacent facial subunits and correction of their age-related changes will usually provide the best comprehensive rejuvenation. Finally, careful preoperative assessment and intraoperative technique will serve to avoid many of the common complications associated with periorbital rejuvenation.

References

1. Dupuis C, Rees TD. Historical notes on blepharoplasty. Plast Reconstr Surg 1971;47:246–251
2. Fincher EF, Moy RL. Cosmetic blepharoplasty. Dermatol Clin 2005;23: 431–442
3. Rankin BS, Arden RL, Crumley RL. Lower eyelid blepharoplasty. In: Papel ID, Frodel J, Holt GR, et al, eds. Facial Plastic and Reconstructive Surgery. 2nd ed. New York, NY: Thieme Medical Publishers; 2002: 196–207
4. Trepsat F. Periorbital rejuvenation combining fat grafting and blepharoplasties. Aesthetic Plast Surg 2003;27:243–253
5. Gallo SA, Wesley RE, Klippenstein KA, Biesman BS. Cosmetic eyelid surgery. Ophthalmol Clin North Am 2000;13:749–764
6. Fagien S. Advanced rejuvenation upper blepharoplasty: enhancing aesthetics of the upper periorbita. Plast Reconstr Surg 2002;110: 278–291
7. Mendelson BC, Muzaffar AR, Adams WP. Surgical anatomy of the midcheek and malar mounds. Plast Reconstr Surg 2002;110:885–896
8. Aiache AE. The suborbicularis oculi fat pads: an anatomic and clinical study. Plast Reconstr Surg 1995;95:37–42
9. Holt JE, Holt GR. Blepharoplasty: indications and preoperative assessment. Arch Otolaryngol Head Neck Surg 1985;111:394–397
10. Rees TD, Jelks GW. Blepharoplasty and the dry eye syndrome: guidelines for surgery? Plast Reconstr Surg 1981;68:249–252
11. Carruthers J, Fagien S, Matarasso SL. Botox consensus group: consensus recommendations of the use of botulinum toxin type A in facial aesthetics. Plast Reconstr Surg 2004;114:1S–22S
12. Carruthers J, Carruthers A. The adjunctive uses of botulinum toxin. Dermatol Surg 1998;24:1244–1247
13. Freeman MS. Transconjunctival sub-orbicularis oculi fat (SOOF) pad blepharoplasty. Arch Facial Plast Surg 2000;2:16–21
14. Farrior RT, Kassir RR. Management of malar folds in blepharoplasty. Laryngoscope 1998;108:1659–1663
15. Pastorek NJ. Blepharoplasty update. Facial Plast Surg Clin North Am 2002;10:23–27
16. Patipa M. Transblepharoplasty lower eyelid and midface rejuvenation: part I. Avoiding complications by utilizing lessons learned from the treatment of complications. Plast Reconstr Surg 2004;113:1459–1468
17. Rotunda AM, Ablon G. Treatment of lower eyelid fat pads using phosphatidylcholine: clinical trial and review. Dermatol Surg 2004;30:422–427
18. Rittes PG. The use of phosphatidylcholine for correction of lower lid bulging due to prominent fat pads. Dermatol Surg 2001;27:391–392
19. Goldberg RA, Edelstein C, Shorr N. Fat repositioning in lower blepharoplasty to maintain infraorbital rim contour. Facial Plast Surg 1999; 15:225–229
20. Schiller JD, Lin S, Neigel JM. Deepening of the superior sulcus after isolated lower transconjunctival blepharoplasty. Ophthal Plast Reconstr Surg 2004;20:433–435
21. de la Plaza R, Arroyo JM. A new technique for the treatment of palpebral bags. Plast Reconstr Surg 1988;81:677–687
22. Hamra ST. The role of orbital fat preservation in facial aesthetic surgery. A new concept. Clin Plast Surg 1996;23:17–28
23. Coleman SR. Structural fat grafts: the ideal filler. Clin Plast Surg 2001; 28:111–119
24. Flowers RS. Tear trough implants for correction of tear trough deformity. Clin Plast Surg 1993;20:403–415

6

Endoscopic Forehead Lifting

Gregory S. Keller, P. Daniel Knott, and Robert W. Hutcherson

The brow is the most important feature of the upper third of the face, representing the central facial aesthetic signature when considered in concert with the eyes and nose. The human eye is naturally drawn to this central triangle, and subtle differences in the representative sizes, shapes, and shadows of its constituent parts are immediately translated into a perception of beauty and a sense of overall chronological age.[1] Facial features distant from this core triangle carry a disproportionately lesser weight in the consideration of overall age and beauty. A thorough evaluation of ideal brow position must therefore figure prominently in any successful overall rejuvenative intervention.

The movement of the brows and the furrows created by the various brow elevators and depressors are extremely important components in facial expressivity. Whether rising with surprise, converging with uncertainty, or descending with anger, the brows translate emotion into expression. Whereas this emotional expressivity is manifest by constant change in brow position in the short term, in the long term such change becomes static. In fact, an individual's predominant expressions become steadily ingrained in the upper third of the face over time, much as a cliff face becomes chiseled over the years by the combined influences of wind and rain. Brow position and the surrounding periorbital rhytides therefore reveal the expressive muscular actions that have been etched over time. The goal of effective brow rejuvenation incorporates an understanding of these cumulative emotive influences, aiming for the establishment of a softer, more pleasing and youthful curve and shape.

◆ Brow Analysis

The position of the brows at rest necessarily represents equilibrium between the forces of agonism and antagonism.[2] The corrugator supercilii, procerus, depressor supercilii, and orbicularis oculi are the agonist muscles, which lower and corrugate the brow. The frontalis muscle is the sole antagonist that raises the brow. Gravity exerts the most important exogenous influence, inexorably leading to the stretching of the periorbital soft tissues and the loss of the resting tone of the frontalis muscle. This leads to descent of the brows in relation to the fixed point of the supraorbital rim. The effort to balance this descent leads to frontalis muscle overactivity and the creation of horizontal forehead rhytides. The process of progressive brow ptosis occurs more markedly at the lateral brow, producing lateral canthal hooding and brow overhang. Any consideration for manipulation of brow position must at its inception incorporate a cogent overall strategy encompassing eyelid function and position. The position of the brows, via attachments of the arcus marginalis to the supraorbital rim and via the septum to the tarsus and upper eyelid skin, has a defined relationship to upper lid position. Although this chapter will not focus on upper lid position, a clear understanding of these relationships must precede any operative intervention.

Aesthetic interpretation of the brow does not follow absolute standards, and surgical goals must be based on what appears correct for a given patient. Cultural, structural, gender, and age issues are factored in when preoperative goals are being planned. However, forehead aesthetic considerations can draw on quantifiable guidelines. Leonardo da Vinci outlined facial proportions with his rule of vertical thirds and horizontal fifths. In the rule of thirds, the distance from hairline to the bottom of the high point of the brow should equal the distance from the inferior brow to the nasal base, which in turn should equal the distance from the nasal base to the bottom of the chin. In the rule of fifths, the face is divided vertically into five equal columns whose width equals that of the eyelid (see Chapter 2). The eyebrow should approximate or be slightly above the superior orbital rim, and the apex of the arch should be at a point tangent to the lateral limbus, or approximately two thirds of the way from the medial brow to the brow tail. The tail of the brow should be on an oblique line from the lateral alar rim through the lateral canthus. The medial brow margin is tangent to a vertical line drawn from the lateral ala through the medial canthus. The medial and lateral brow should be in the same horizontal plane. Racial differences are often subtle, but notable. In the Asian, Latino, and African-American populations, an aesthetically pleasing origin to the medial brow is tangent to a line bisecting the nasal lobule and the medial canthus. Gender differences must also be distinguished. Female patients have a forehead height aesthetic of 4 to 6.2 cm (average 4.8 cm), whereas male forehead height typically ranges from 6 to 7 cm. Women have a smoother forehead contour from the supraorbital rim to the hairline.

Men have a more prominent lateral supraorbital rim with a tendency to frontal bossing.

Preoperative analysis and planning are critical to creating the desired surgical outcome for any procedure. In brow lift surgery, defining the goals of the surgeon and setting appropriate expectations for the patient are important parts of the operative strategy. Incorporating the visual and quantitative criteria noted above will help achieve these goals. Indications for foreheadplasty surgery are brow ptosis, glabellar ptosis, and vertical glabellar furrows. Assessment of the patient should focus on frontal hairline contour, hair density, and brow contour. Attempts have been made to objectify the analysis of brow position to optimize outcomes of endoscopic foreheadplasty. McKinney et al brought forth the concept of frame height, which is the distance from midpupil to the top of the brow.[3] Under this definition, brow ptosis exists if this distance is less than 2.0 to 2.5 cm, and a brow lift procedure is indicated. Sasaki combined the concept of frame height with the concept of brow mobility, using a "glide test" to predict the effectiveness of endoscopic brow lifting procedures.[4] The glide test is a measurement of maximal brow excursion in the medial, central, and lateral vectors under manual pressure from the examiner. Optimal results after endoscopic brow lifting were obtained when the frame height was 1.5 to 2.0 cm and the glide test values were 2 to 3 cm. These parameters are consistent with a ptotic brow with significant forehead laxity. A standard facial photographic series should be obtained.

◆ Anatomic Considerations

Brow Elevators

The principle brow elevator is the *frontalis muscle*. With its origin at the skin and superficial fascia of the orbicularis oculi muscle and its insertion into the galea aponeurosis over the crown of the skull to its connection to the occipitalis, the frontalis muscle exerts its greatest elevation centrally, with its elevation attenuating laterally. The frontalis permits movement of the scalp over the immobile pericranium, elevating the brows and, with overactivity, creates the transverse rhytides of the forehead skin. The nerve supply of the frontalis muscle is the temporal branch of the facial nerve, which travels with the temporoparietal fascia to innervate the frontalis on its undersurface. There is significant variability in frontal branch anatomy, with four branches being a common pattern. Meticulous dissection is the key to avoiding injury, and when operating in the standard planes, clinically apparent nerve injury is exceedingly rare.

Brow Depressors

The *procerus* is the only midline neuromuscular structure that acts on the brows. With its origin in the fascia of the nasal bones and upper lateral cartilages and its insertion into the skin of the medial lower forehead, the procerus depresses the medial brow, creating the horizontal glabellar rhytides. The procerus is innervated by both the frontal and zygomatic branches of the facial nerve, and therefore selective neurotomy of the frontal branch entering the procerus will have a low rate of long-term success.

The *corrugator supercilii* is an important determinant of medial brow position. It acts to medialize, corrugate, and depress the medial brow and is responsible for the vertical glabellar furrows. Its origin is the superomedial orbital rim, and its insertion is into the fascia of the lower frontalis muscle and skin of the brow. The supratrochlear and supraorbital neurovascular bundles penetrate through the corrugator muscles on their undersurface before transitioning onto the superficial surface of the frontalis muscle. The main body of the corrugator passes between these two neural structures, anterior to the supraorbital nerve and posterior to the supratrochlear nerve.

The *depressor supercilii* lies anterior to the supratrochlear nerve. Originating along the medial orbital rim and medial canthal tendon and inserting onto the medial aspect of the bony orbit, the depressor supercilii contributes to medial brow descent. The depressor is located 2 to 3 mm deep and anterior to the corrugator.

◆ Equipment

The necessary equipment for performing endoscopic forehead procedures includes the endoscope, video camera equipment, and surgical instruments. The rigid endoscope is typically between 18 and 23 cm in length, 4 to 5 mm in diameter, and with a 30-degree lens and reversed input light cable. It is equipped with a coupling device to allow visualization on a television screen. Illumination is provided by a halogen or xenon light source according to the surgeon's preference.

Most endoscopic surgical instrumentation is standardized. However, a few specialized instruments are necessary. The angled endoscopic sheath extends beyond the scope tip, permitting bimanual dissection. The sheath allows saline irrigation of the operative field, which is important to counteract cautery-related cloudiness of the lens without having to remove and wipe the lens during the procedure. While bipolar cautery is usually necessary, monopolar suction cautery is often very helpful. Periosteal elevators may be angled or straight to adjust to various forehead conformations. Sharp-tipped and blunt-tipped elevators should be available to address different degrees of periosteal adherence. A knuckle elevator is useful to dissect over the supraorbital rim. Endoscopic scissors are usually necessary to complete dissection of the dense fibrous tissue over the lateral orbital rim at the brow tail.

◆ Techniques

Brow lifting may be accomplished with a variety of techniques, yet all successful endoscopic procedures share several common features: the use of small vertical incisions, the creation of an optical cavity, the release of the brow complex, and the elevation and fixation of the brow in a more superior position.

Incisions

As endoscopic brow lifting has evolved over the past decade or two, a wide variety of incisions have been used with excellent results. As such, no single pattern may be put forward as representing the ideal. Nevertheless, each pattern of incisions must reflect a considered choice providing adequate access for tissue undermining and soft tissue fixation while keeping the absolute number of incisions to a minimum. Contemporary concepts mandate that the incisions be vertical in orientation, placed in the hair-bearing scalp, starting several millimeters posterior to the non–hair-bearing skin, in the region of nonvillous type hair (**Fig. 6.1A, B**). The length of the incisions is of lesser importance, as longer

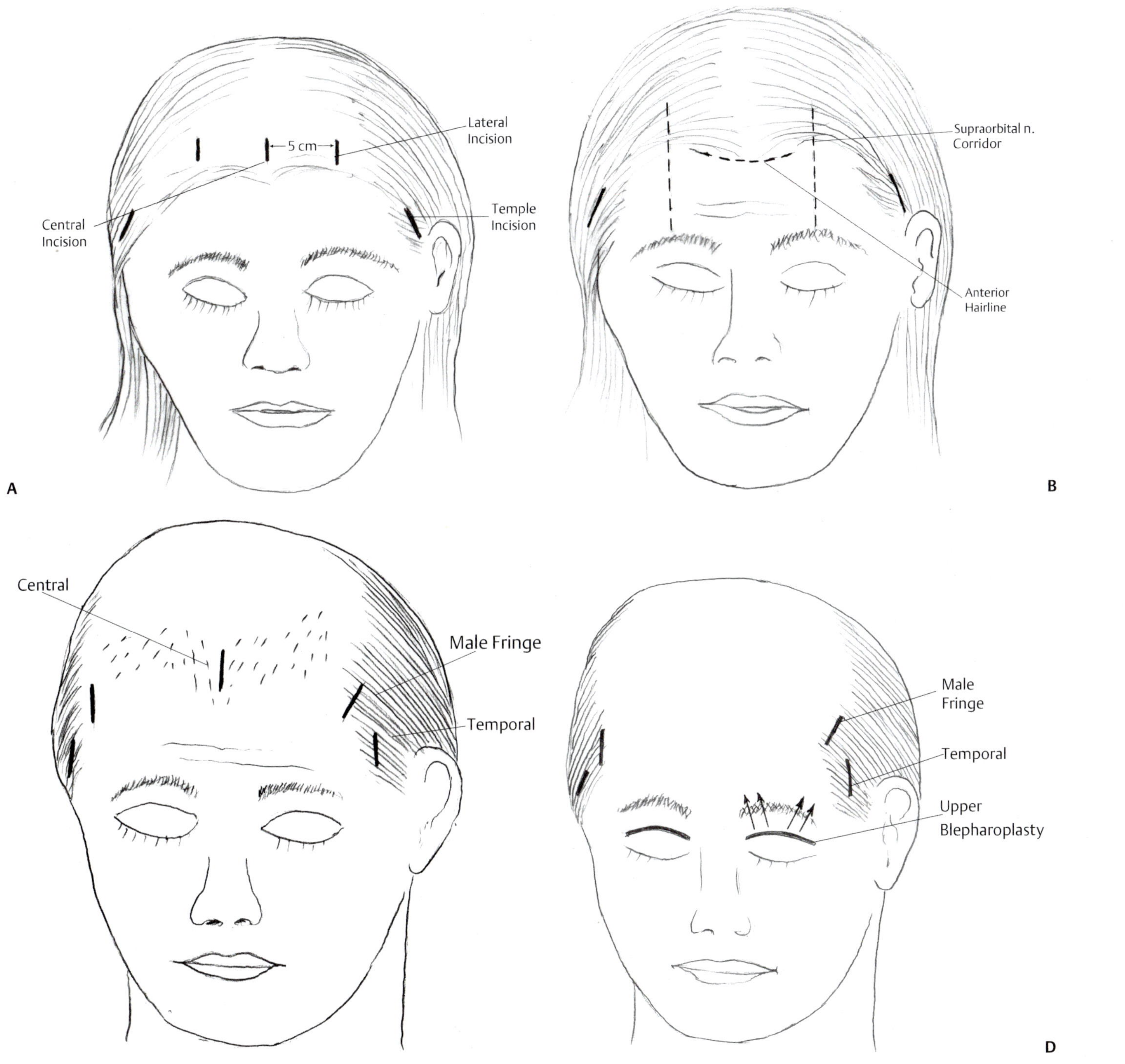

Fig. 6.1 **(A)** Standard endoscopic forehead incision. **(B)** Alternate incisions for female patients with high hairlines. **(C)** Endoscopic forehead incisions for male pattern baldness (Norwood II to V). **(D)** Endoscopic forehead incisions for male pattern baldness (Norwood VI to VII).

incisions may in fact permit less intraoperative tissue trauma and therefore improved healing and postoperative cosmesis than do smaller incisions.

Central Region

One or more incisions may be made in the central region. These anchor the dissection and are most often used for endoscope access. Although multiple incisions may be used, a single incision is usually adequate.

Lateral Region

One or more lateral incisions are usually made either a fixed distance from the central incisions (typically 4 to 5 cm) or in reference to a logical anatomic landmark of the face. The midpupillary line or the vertical tangent to the lateral limbus is often chosen for access and for endoscopic triangulation. The incision in this region is usually located medial to the superior temporal line as a bridge to the different planes of dissection. During dissection of this incision, care must be exercised to avoid injuring the lateral branch of the supraorbital nerve.

Temporal Region

A beveled diagonal incision is made 1 to 2 cm posterior to the temporal hairline through the temporal tuft over the temporalis muscle for lateral undermining and release. Oftentimes, the frontal branch of the superficial temporal artery and vein is encountered. If these structures cannot be retracted out of the way, then they should be clamped and tied to prevent postoperative hematoma.

For patients with male pattern baldness (Norwood II to V), it is often necessary to vary these incisions. If a central tuft of hair is present or may be created with hair transplantation techniques, then a 1-cm-long central incision may be made. The lateral incisions are placed along the male fringe, in addition to the diagonal temporal incisions. If the hair is very short, great care must be taken with the incisions to minimize postoperative alopecia and scar exposure, which can lead to exceedingly dissatisfied patients (**Fig. 6.1C**).

If a frontal tuft is missing and/or a patient has Norwood VI to VII baldness, the brow lift may be performed in a retrograde fashion through an upper blepharoplasty type approach.[5,6] There are a variety of fixation devices that may be placed through this approach, obviating the need for the hairline incisions (**Fig. 6.1D**). Additionally, other authors advocate horizontal incisions placed through the rhytides high on the forehead.

Optical Cavity

Effective endoscopic surgery necessitates the creation of an optical cavity. The forehead provides only potential spaces (subcutaneous plane, subgaleal plane, subperiosteal plane), and therefore the surgeon must create a cavity in one or more of these planes.[7] The subperiosteal plane is often preferred, as the dissection is often rapid, and the rigidity of the periosteum provides for the least superior mobilization of the frontal hairline.[8,9] If complete release is achieved, 1 cm of brow elevation is achieved for every 1.2 cm of superior displacement of a subperiosteal flap. The brow elevators and depressors are in the subgaleal plane, and the performance of myotomies is contingent upon accessing this plane. In the temple, the optical cavity is created between the temporoparietal fascia and the superficial layer of the deep temporal fascia. This plane preserves the temporal branch of the facial nerve and permits access to the subperiosteal plane over the zygoma, if dissection in this area is needed (**Fig. 6.2**).

Brow Release

Elevation of the brow necessarily requires release of the native fascial and periosteal attachments. Medial to the supraorbital nerve, brow position is maintained by periosteum and the procerus and corrugator and depressor supercilii. Disruption of the periosteum over the glabella and division of these muscles near their origins are widely considered as necessary for the release of the medial brow. Denervation of these muscles is also advocated by some. Selective denervation may also be employed to alter brow position to a more subtle degree.

Lateral to the supraorbital nerve, the periosteum is incised over the supraorbital rim until the conjoint tendon (fusion of the galea, periosteum, and superficial and deep temporal fascia) is reached. The retroorbital fat (ROOF) is exposed, and dissection may continue down into the upper eyelids.

In the temporal portion of the brow, the two optical cavities are joined by the division of the conjoint tendon down to the level of the superior orbital rim. A sharp, curved periosteal elevator greatly facilitates this maneuver. The periosteum must be scraped along the length of the superior temporal line to avoid injuring the frontal nerve branches, which are traveling in the temporoparietal fascia (TPF) just above. A curved endoscopic scissor is often required to completely divide the conjoint tendon at its attachment to the lateral supraorbital rim. The precanthal ligaments are divided at their origins, the lateral extension of the orbicularis is mobilized, and a horizontal release of the soft tissue over the malar eminence is performed. Elevation of the tail of the brow is made possible by this lateral release (**Fig. 6.3**).

Elevation and Fixation

Complete periosteal release is the sine qua non of effective brow elevation. Care must be taken to reassess the excursion

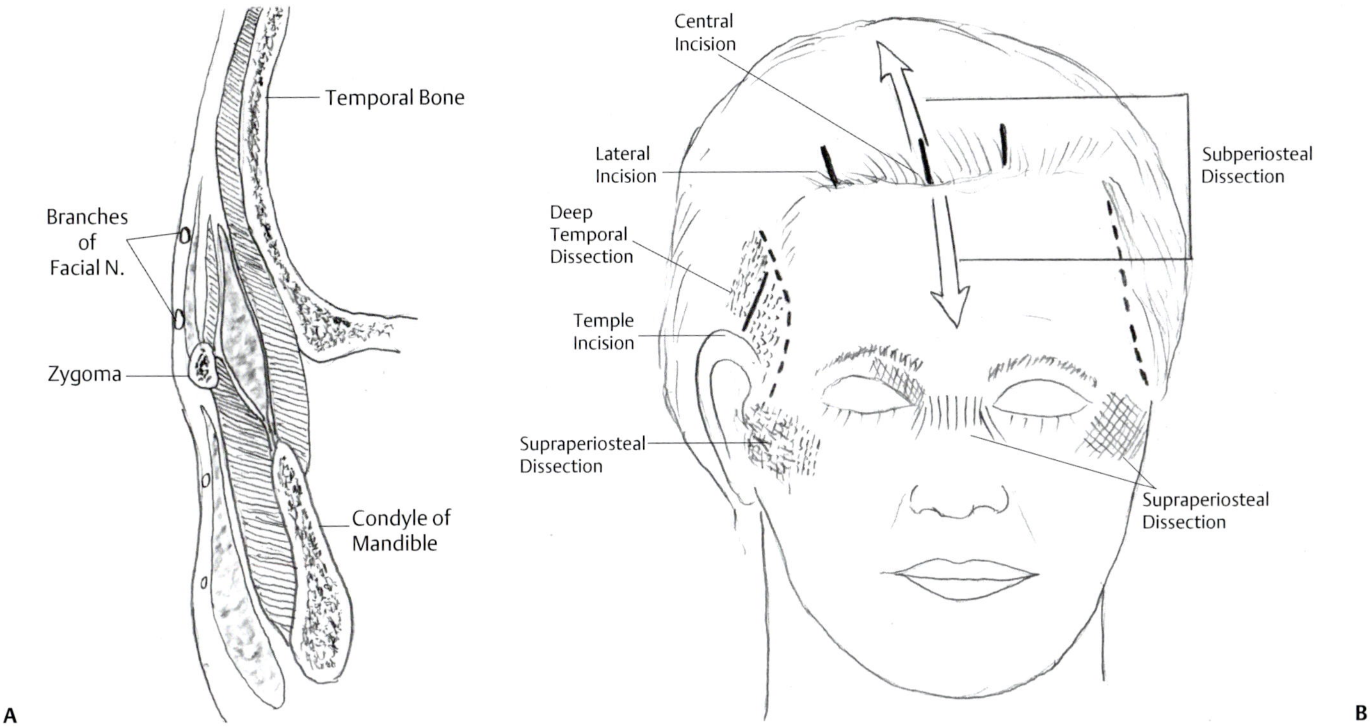

Fig. 6.2 (**A, B**) Usual composite of forehead planes used in endoscopic forehead surgery.

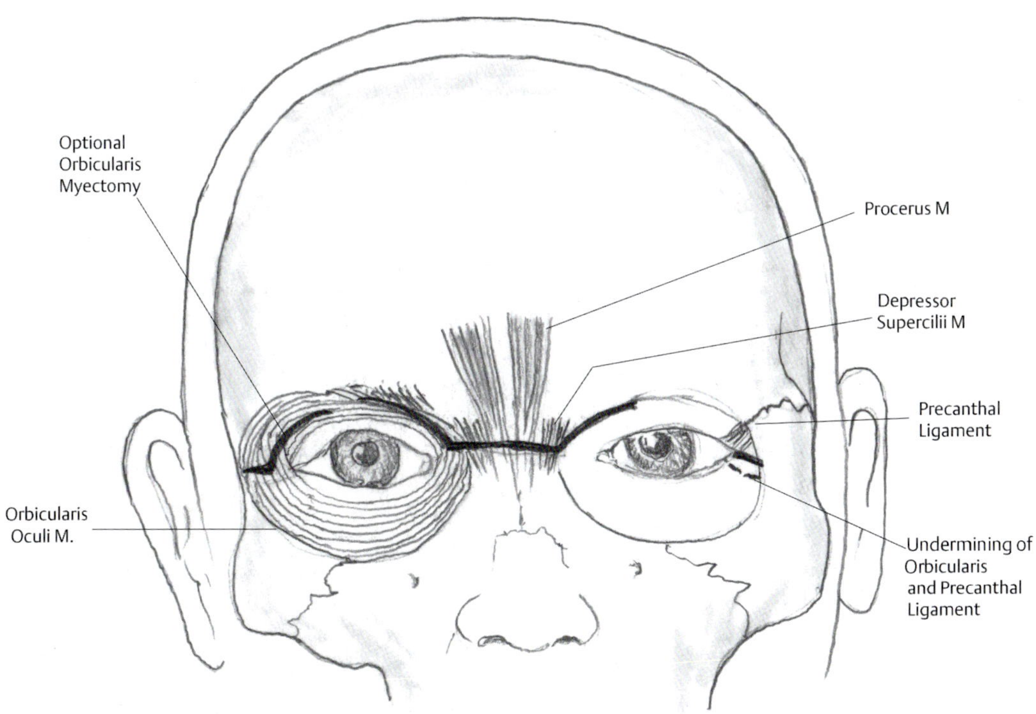

Fig. 6.3 Myotomies of the depressor muscles (corrugator, orbicularis oculi, depressor supercilii, and procerus to "release" the brow).

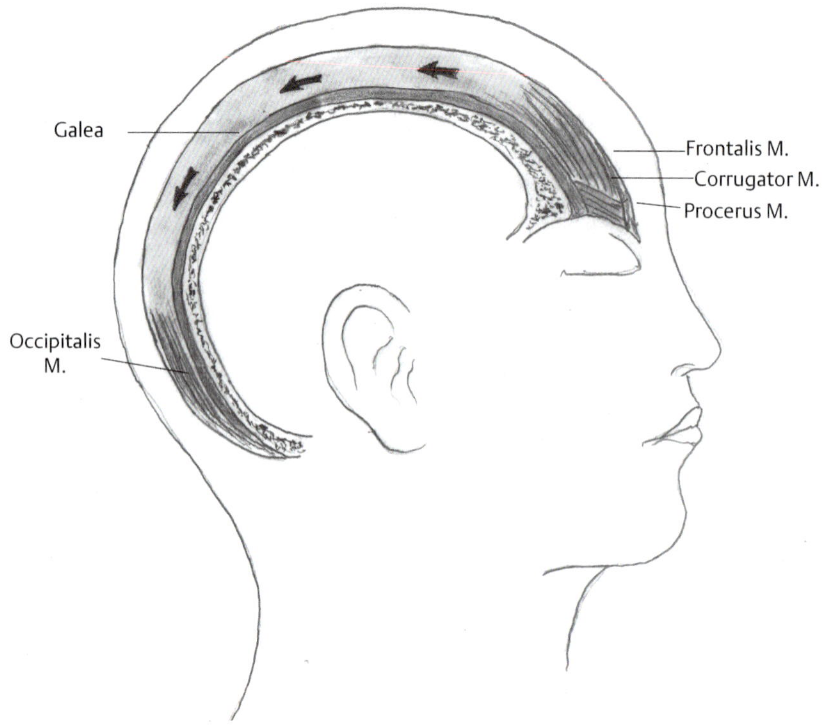

Fig. 6.4 With the release of the depressor muscles, the occipitalis-galea-frontalis sling pulls the scalp backward.

of each lateral brow complex once the release is performed to verify that it is indeed complete. Furthermore, careful comparison between the sides is essential to ensure that the release is bilaterally symmetric. Once the brows are completely released, elevation is quite simple (**Fig. 6.4**). With a complete release, care must be taken to elevate the lateral brow complex according to the aesthetic ideals of the surgeon and the patient.[10] After release, the medial brow may appear too high in relation to the lateral brow. In this instance (or in revision surgeries), the brow can be pushed downward and fixated in position with a reversed Endotine plate (Coapt Systems Inc., Palo Alto, CA) at the medial scalp. If the tail of the brow appears too low, it may be directly sutured at a higher level with a suspension suture. Alternatively, an Endotine plate may be used through an upper lid blepharoplasty incision to adjust brow position (**Fig. 6.5**).

Fixation of the scalp in a more posterior location may be achieved with a wide variety of techniques and devices.[11,12] Bone tunnels may be drilled in the bone and the scalp fixated with permanent or absorbable sutures, or permanent or resorbable screws and plates may be used (**Fig. 6.6**). Fixation is only required for a limited amount of time until the periosteum heals to the underlying frontal bone and maintains the elevation. The duration of the surgical fixation is somewhat controversial, with authors advocating from 7 days to 3 months.[13–15] In many patients, lateral soft tissue fixation is the only technique that may be required. In these circumstances, the temporoparietal fascia from the forehead flap may be sutured directly posterosuperiorly to the superficial layer of the deep temporal fascia.

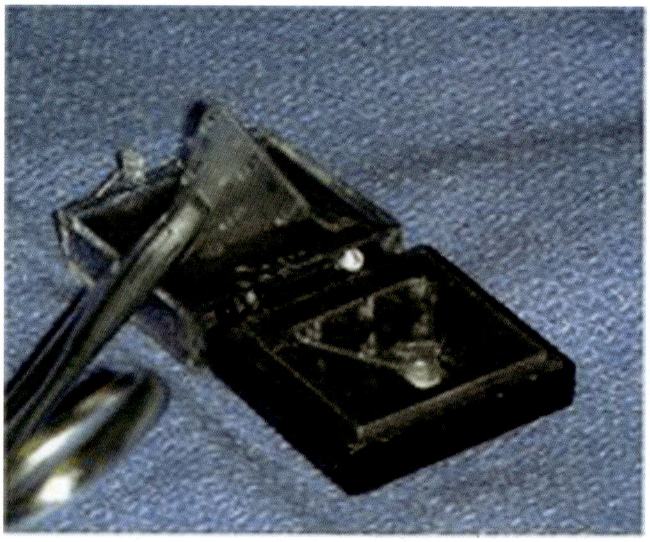

Fig. 6.5 The Endotine endobrow device permits bony placement of the resorbable anchor. (Courtesy of William H. Truswell IV, MD.)

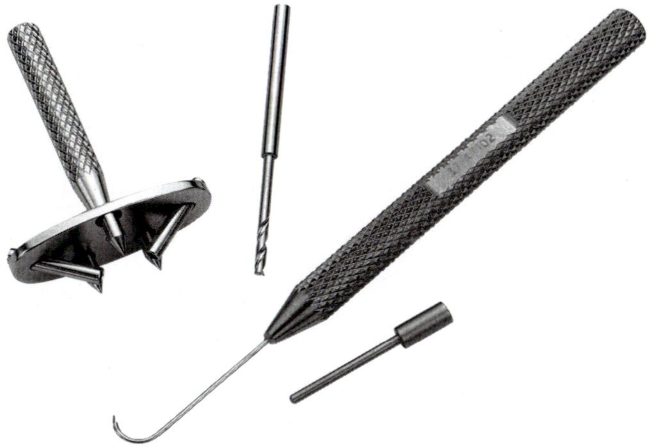

Fig. 6.6 The Medtronic ENT Browlift Bone Bridge System facilitates the creation of an angled bone tunnel through the outer table of the calvarium through which suture loops may be passed for fixation. (Courtesy of Medtronic ENT, Jacksonville, FL.)

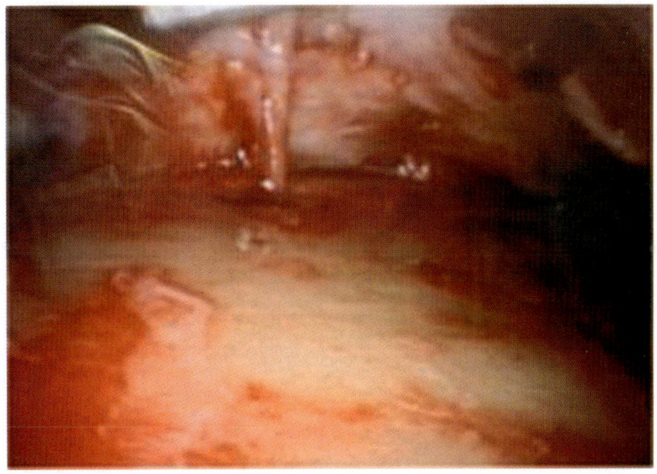

Fig. 6.7 The supraorbital neurovascular bundle emerging from a foramen. Blind undermining in this area could avulse the nerve. (Courtesy of William H. Truswell IV, MD.)

Dissection

Anesthesia techniques vary according to surgeon's preference. We prefer MAC for patients undergoing standalone forehead surgery and general anesthesia when brow lifting is performed in conjunction with facelifting or neck lifting procedures. One percent Xylocaine with epinephrine 1:100,000 mixed with equal parts 0.25% bupivacaine is used to infiltrate the incisions and to perform supratrochlear and supraorbital nerve blocks. Tumescent solution (1000 mL normal saline, 50 mL 1% plain Xylocaine, 12 mL sodium bicarbonate, and 1 mL epinephrine 1:1,000) is used to perform supraperiosteal and sub-TPF hydrodissection. Adequate time is allowed after prepping and draping for these solutions to exert a hemostatic effect.

After the hairline incisions have been made, a short-curved periosteal elevator is used to perform a circumferential subperiosteal elevation at each incision without endoscopic visualization. The elevation is limited by the dense attachments along the superior temporal line. This dissection stops 2 cm above the orbital rim to prevent inadvertent injury to neurovascular structures. If the supraorbital nerve exits the skull base in a notch, blunt elevation probably would not be harmful. However, when the nerve exits from a discrete foramen, blind elevation may lead to nerve shearing or disruption and long-term anesthesia/dysesthesia (**Fig. 6.7**).

In the midline, however, a longer elevator is used to transition through the periosteum and through the subgaleal plane to the sub–superficial musculoaponeurotic system (sub-SMAS) plane over the radix of the nose. Posteriorly, subperiosteal blind dissection is carried back to the occiput or nuchal ridge.

Under direct visualization in the temporal incisions, the innominate fascia is elevated off of the superficial layer of the deep temporal fascia, which is a white, glistening, immobile surface. The temporoparietal fascia is elevated posteriorly in a circumferential fashion, penetrating through the weaker attachments of the posterior aspect of the temporal line, thereby unifying the central and temporal optical cavities. Blunt dissection then continues to the level of the temporal hairline.

At this point, the dissection becomes more complex and must be performed under direct vision. The endoscope is placed through the temporal incision and into the loose areolar tissue between the temporoparietal fascia and the superficial layer of the deep temporal fascia, and the elevator is used to continue to sweep the innominate fascia up off of the superficial layer of the deep temporal fascia. This maneuver is critical to avoid injuring the temporal branch of the facial nerve, whose course runs through the temporoparietal fascia. The temporoparietal fat pad, lying above the innominate fascia, is often visualized and should be swept upward with the innominate fascia (**Fig. 6.8**).

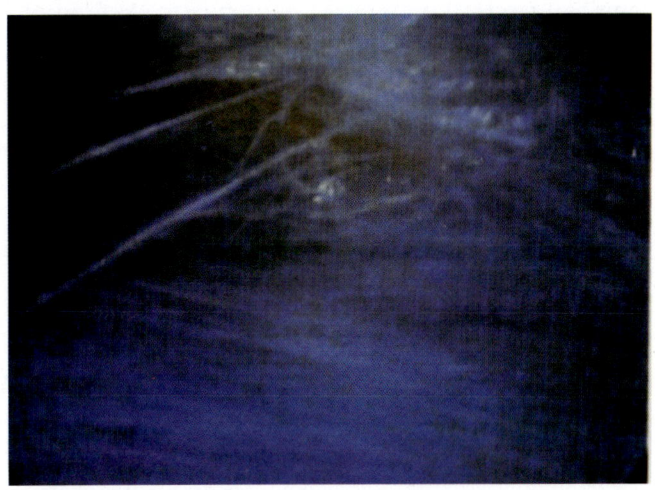

Fig. 6.8 The temporoparietal fat pad is seen above the cobweb-like stranding of the innominate fascia. (From Keller GS. Endoscopic Facial Plastic Surgery. St. Louis, MO: Mosby–Year Book Inc.; 1997:59. Reprinted with permission.)

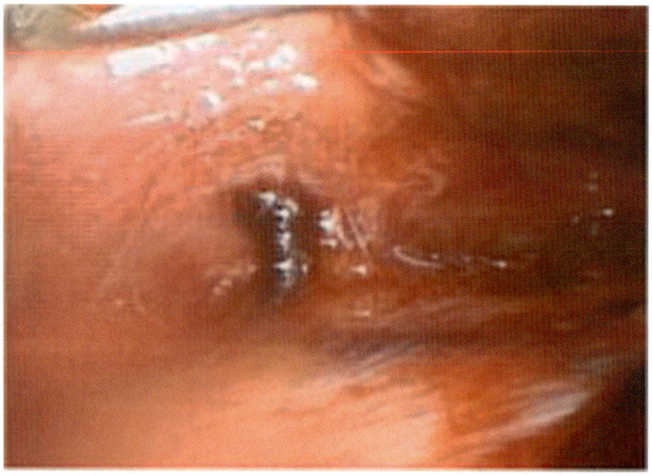

Fig. 6.9 The lateral and median zygomaticotemporal veins (sentinel veins) are visualized passing from the superficial layer of the deep temporal fascia through to the temporoparietal fascia. (Courtesy of William H. Truswell IV, MD.)

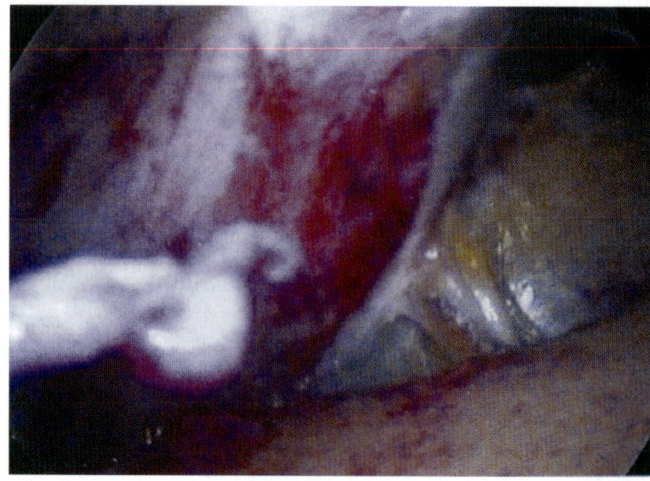

Fig. 6.10 Elevation and division of the arcus marginalis begins laterally and proceeds medially until the supraorbital neurovascular bundle is encountered. (From Keller GS. Endoscopic Facial Plastic Surgery. St. Louis, MO: Mosby–Year Book Inc.; 1997:64. Reprinted with permission.)

A second, deeper fat pad is seen as a yellow mass lying just deep to the superficial layer of the deep temporal fascia. This is the superficial temporal fat pad, which lies between the superficial and deep layers of the deep temporal fascia. The medial zygomaticotemporal vein ("sentinel vein") is most often encountered during this elevation, above the zygomaticofrontal suture. If the dissection continues laterally, the second zygomaticotemporal vein is often exposed, along with the zygomaticotemporal nerve (**Fig. 6.9**). These structures should not be disturbed. If entry into the midface is required for a concomitant midface lift, the sentinel vein should be cauterized with a bipolar cautery at its base, near the superficial layer of the deep temporal fascia. If no midface procedure is required, the sentinel vein may be preserved. The frontal branch of the facial nerve frequently runs directly above the medial zygomaticotemporal vein, and care must be taken to avoid thermal or mechanical injury.

The temporal line must then be dissected from its insertions along the frontal bone. This elevation is begun superomedially, in a safe region, at the temporal hairline. Blunt or sharp dissection may be used. Once the proper plane is established, division of these attachments may continue inferiorly. The fascial attachments of the superior temporal line coalesce into a very dense band near the lateral brow, called the conjoint tendon. For adequate brow elevation, it is imperative that this band be divided. Ideally, the periosteal attachments are stripped off of the underlying frontal bone, down to the lateral orbital rim.

The endoscope is then inserted through the central incision into the optic cavity created by the blunt periosteal elevation. Curved periosteal elevators are then placed through the lateral incisions and are used to elevate the final 2 cm of periosteum from the frontal bone above the superior orbital rims. This elevation is relatively bloodless. Starting laterally, the arcus marginalis is elevated and thereby divided above the orbital rim, exposing the ROOF. The arcus marginalis should be elevated along the whole length of the orbital rim, until the supraorbital neurovascular bundle is approached (**Fig. 6.10**). Care is taken to elevate the periosteum around the bundle, exposing the corrugator, which is usually located inferomedially. At this point, the supratrochlear neurovascular bundle must also be identified. It is 1.7 to 2.2 cm lateral to the midline. Variations in anatomy are the norm instead of the exception with these structures. Anything from a single dominant nerve that ramifies in the overlying muscle to multiple branches exiting from multiple foramina should be expected and indeed will be encountered with regularity. Veins traveling with these nerves should be carefully dissected free and cauterized with either the bipolar cautery or the suction monopolar cautery.

Once both neurovascular bundles have been identified, the dissection proceeds to the division of the brow depressors. Elevating and protecting the neurovascular bundles, first the corrugator and then the procerus is either stripped or cauterized and divided. The corrugator travels inferomedially, and when the optical cavity is tented, the muscle fibers are easily visualized. The corrugator should be incised as close to the bony rim as possible (**Fig. 6.11**). The procerus is a thin sheet of muscle located between the corrugators in the supraperiosteal nasal tunnel. It is identified by its fibers that travel vertically upward (**Fig. 6.12**). It is usually incised at the level of the nasofrontal suture. The depressor supercilii is located anterior to the supratrochlear nerve. Its fibers also travel in a vertical orientation. The depressor may also undergo myotomy with either endoscopic scissors or cautery. A similar procedure is performed on the contralateral side.

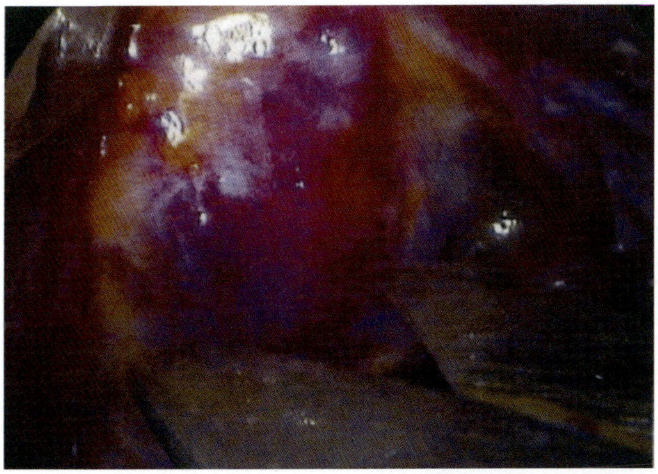

Fig. 6.11 The procerus muscle being divided with straight endoscopic scissors. (From Keller GS. Endoscopic Facial Plastic Surgery. St. Louis, MO: Mosby–Year Book Inc.; 1997:68. Reprinted with permission.)

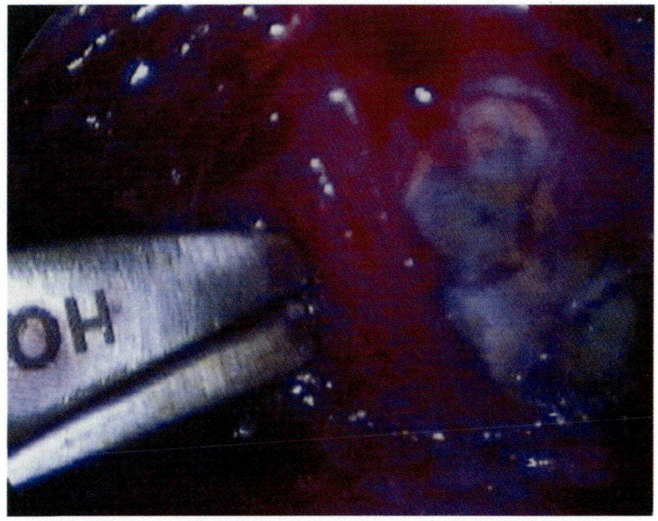

Fig. 6.12 The corrugator muscle may be identified by its oblique course between the supraorbital and supratrochlear neurovascular bundles. Here the corrugator muscle is being divided with the endoscopic scissors. (From Keller GS. Endoscopic Facial Plastic Surgery. St. Louis, MO: Mosby–Year Book Inc.; 1997:68. Reprinted with permission.)

With the brow released, suture fixation at the lateral temporal incision is often all that is necessary. If lateral fixation is not sufficient, we most commonly use scalp fixation with a screw technique (**Fig. 6.13**). Using the lateral incisions for the fixation, the optimal degree of scalp elevation is judged, measured, and marked. A hand drill is used to bore a hole in the outer table of the calvarium, and a screw is placed in the hole. The skin is pulled posteriorly, and a surgical staple is placed immediately behind the screw, fixating the scalp in position. A similar procedure is performed on the contralateral side, and the head of the bed is then raised. An assistant holds the patient's head stably in the midline, and the surgeon then inspects the brows for symmetry and harmony. Adjustments are made as necessary. The vertical incisions are then closed with additional staples after a drain is placed over the supraorbital rim. The temporal incisions are closed first with a buried, resorbable suture from the temporoparietal fascia to the superficial layer of the deep temporal fascia and then with surgical staples.

Postoperatively, the patient is treated with an appropriate oral antibiotic, cold compresses, Medrol Dosepak (unless contraindicated), and liberal lubrication of the eyes using bland ophthalmic ointment. The pressure dressing is removed in 48 hours, and the hair is washed. The screw fixation is usually removed in 14 days. The patients usually return for postoperative photographs between 2 and 3 months after the procedure (**Figs. 6.14 and 6.15**).

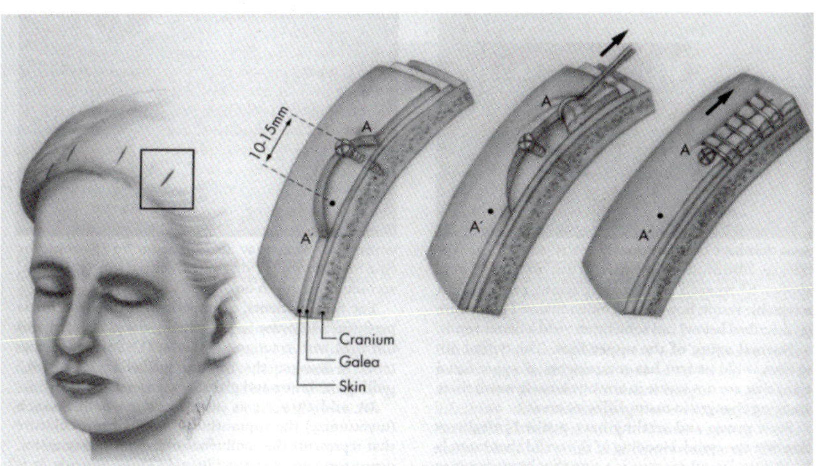

Fig. 6.13 To elevate the brow a predetermined distance (A′ to A), a screw is placed at A, the scalp is pulled so the skin initially located at A′ is relocated to A, and a staple is placed behind the screw to hold the scalp in place. (From Keller GS. Endoscopic Facial Plastic Surgery. St. Louis, MO: Mosby–Year Book Inc.; 1997:72. Reprinted with permission.)

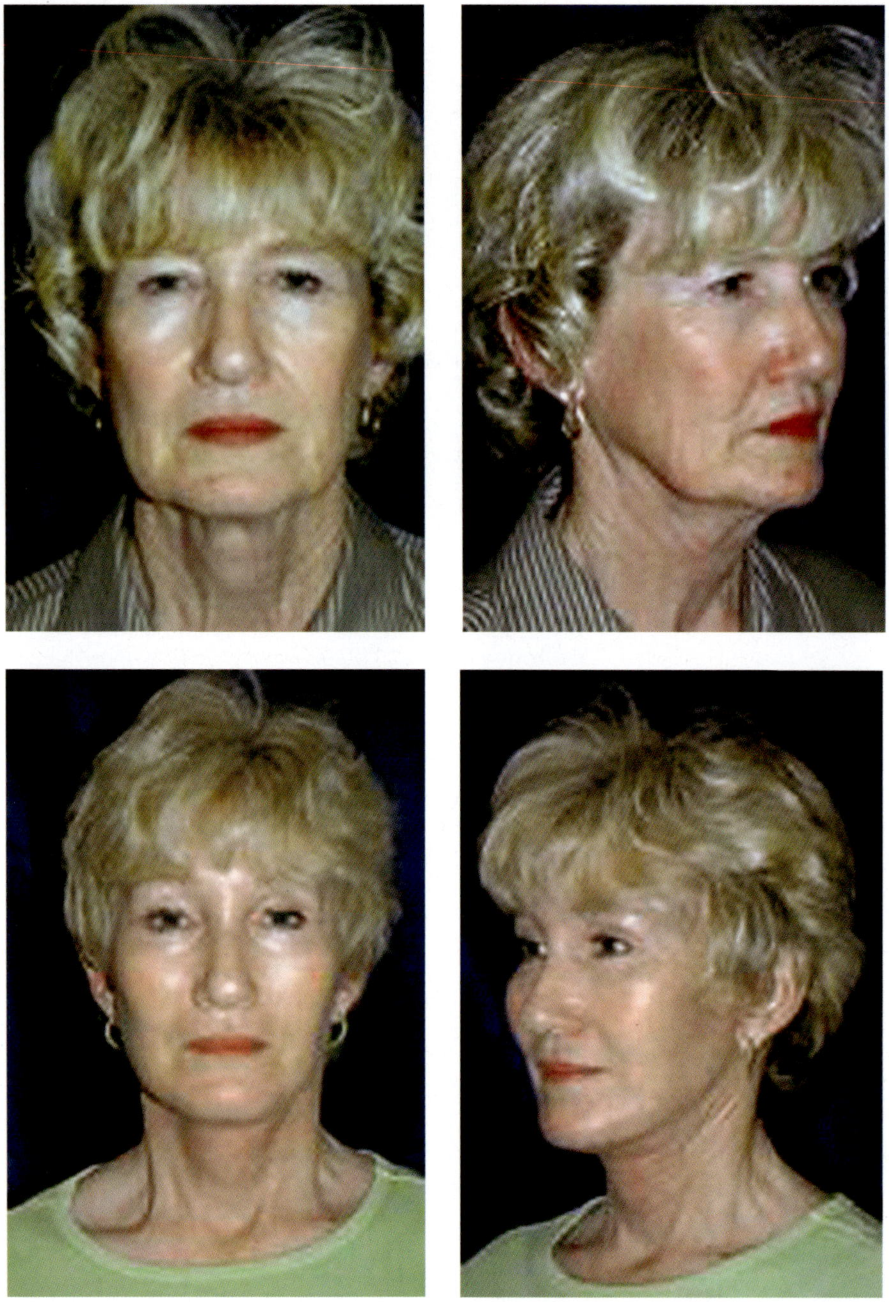

A B C D

Fig. 6.14 (**A, B**) Preoperative frontal and oblique views and (**C, D**) 3.5-month postoperative frontal and oblique views of a patient who underwent an endoscopic forehead lift in addition to a face, neck, and cheek lift. Note the subtle yet important improvement in lateral canthal hooding and the overall symmetry in brow position, yielding a more youthful, energized appearance.

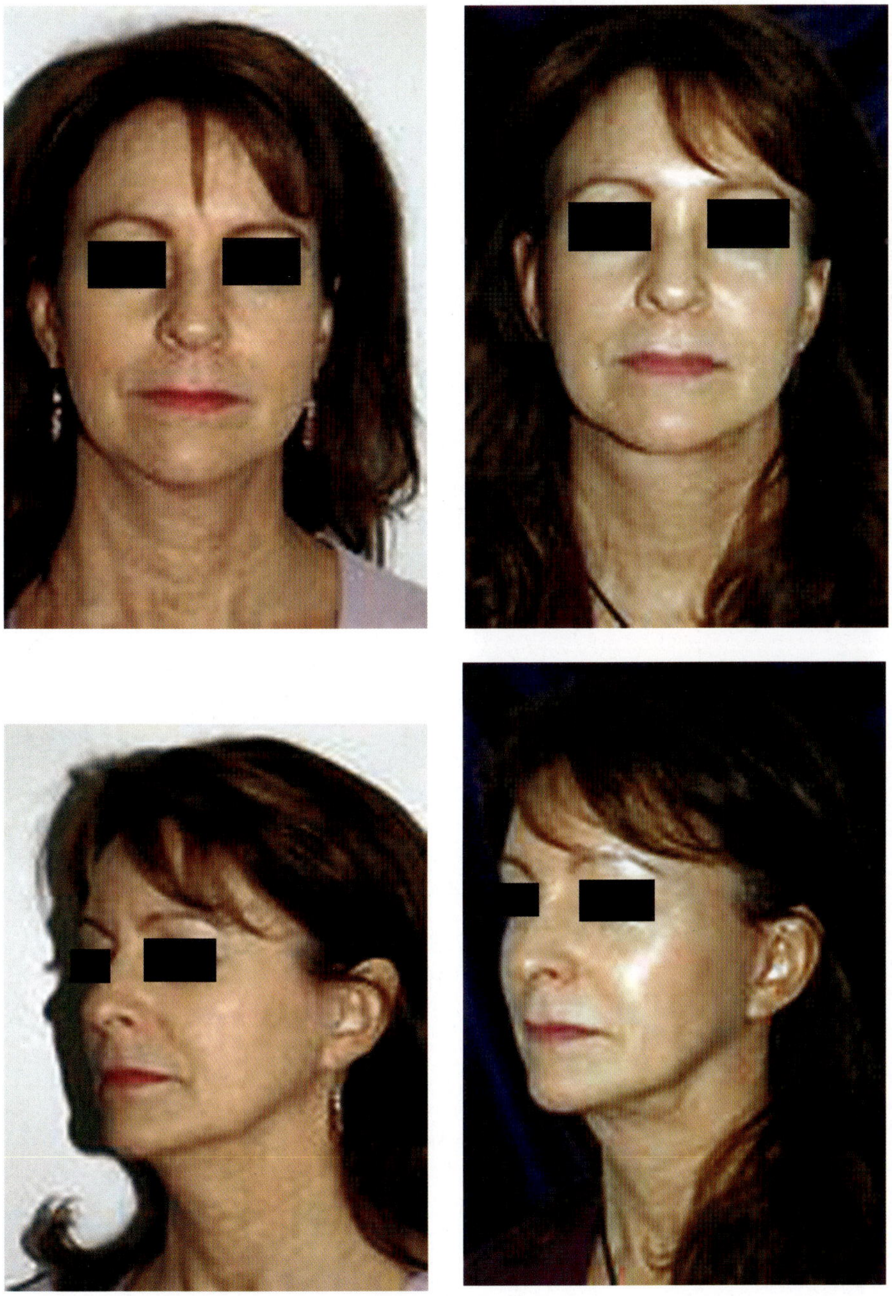

A B C D

Fig. 6.15 (**A, C**) Preoperative frontal and oblique views and (**B, D**) 3.5-month postoperative frontal and oblique views of a patient who underwent an endoscopic forehead lift in addition to a neck lift. Notice the increase in brow height without significant change in the patient's frontal hairline, as well as the excellent harmony of the brow shape.

◆ Conclusion

The effectiveness of endoscopic forehead surgery in facial rejuvenation has enabled this procedure to gain wide acceptance in the aesthetic surgical arena. Risks and complications are minimal, and a relatively brief recovery time allows the procedure to be favorably received by most patients. Ptotic eyebrows, muscle-related asymmetries, and forehead rhytides are comfortably dealt with using this approach. Its ultimate effectiveness, however, depends on a thorough understanding of forehead anatomy and familiarity with endoscopic instrumentation and the surgical principles and techniques intrinsic to this gratifying approach.

References

1. Young PA, Sinha U, Rice DH, Stucker F. Circles of prominence; a new theory on facial aesthetics. Arch Facial Plast Surg 2006;8:263–267
2. Duchene de Boulogne GB. The Mechanism of Human Facial Expression: Studies in Emotion and Social Interaction. Cutherbertson A, ed. and transl. New York, NY: Cambridge University Press; 1990
3. McKinney P, Mossie RD, Zubowsi ML. Criteria for the forehead lift. Aesthetic Plast Surg 1991;15:141–147
4. Sasaki G. Brow ptosis. In: Sasaki G, ed. Endoscopic, aesthetic, and reconstructive surgery. Philadelphia, PA: Lippincott-Raven; 1996:19–28
5. Smith J. In: Grabb WC, Smith JW, eds. Grabb and Smith's Plastic Surgery. Boston, MA: Little, Brown; 1976
6. Strahan RW, Perrott DH. Subperiosteal forehead lift: modification of the endoscopic technique using a trans-palpebral approach. In: Keller GS, ed. Endoscopic Facial Plastic Surgery. Philadelphia, PA: Mosby; 1997:97–102
7. Keller GS, Hutcherson R. Endoscopic forehead and browlift. In: Keller GS, ed. Endoscopic Facial Plastic Surgery. Philadelphia, PA: Mosby; 1997:97–102
8. Knize DM. Muscles that act on glabellar skin: a closer look. Plast Reconstr Surg 2000;105:350–361
9. Isse NG. Endoscopic facial rejuvenation: endoforehead, the functional lift. Aesthetic Plast Surg 1994;18:21–29
10. Miller PJ, Wang TD, Cook TA. Rejuvenation of the aging forehead and brow. Facial Plast Surg 1996;12:147–155
11. Hamas RS, Rohrich RJ. Preventing hairline elevation in endoscopic browlift. Plast Reconstr Surg 1997;99:1018–1022
12. Berkowitz RL, Jacobs DI, Gorman PJ. Brow fixation with the Endotine forehead device in endoscopic brow lift. Plast Reconstr Surg 2005;116:1761–1767
13. Brodner DC, Downs JC, Graham HD. Periosteal readhesion after browlift in New Zealand white rabbits. Arch Facial Plast Surg 2002;4: 248–251
14. Sclafani AP, Fozo MS, Romo T, McCormick SA. Strength and histological characteristics of periosteal fixation to bone after elevation. Arch Facial Plast Surg 2003;5:63–66
15. Kim JC, Crawford Downs J, Azuola ME, Devon Graham H III. Time scale fore periosteal readhesion after browlift. Laryngoscope 2004;114:50–55

7

Midfacial Rejuvenation

Stephen P. Smith Jr. and Edwin F. Williams III

It is well established that the process of midface aging is characterized by three components that are progressive in nature: (1) laxity of skin/soft tissues, (2) inferomedial descent of the malar fat pad, and (3) loss of facial volume. Comparison of mother/daughter photographs demonstrates the classic findings of the aging midface (**Fig. 7.1**). These are lengthening of the lower eyelid complex with pseudoherniation of orbital fat, a hollowed appearance of the lowest part of the lower eyelids and upper midcheek resulting in a skeletonized infraorbital rim, a prominent nasojugal fold, and a deepened nasolabial fold.[1–4] The aforementioned changes represent our surgical indications, and critical evaluation of the individual components of midface aging is essential for an effective approach to midfacial rejuvenation.

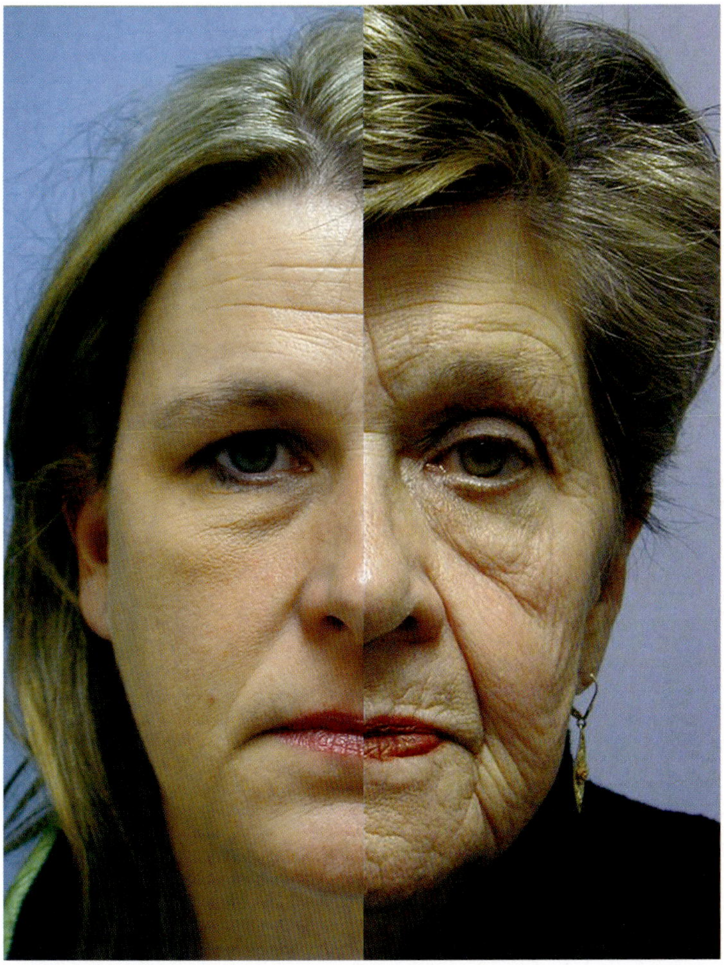

Fig. 7.1 (**A**) Daughter and (**B**) mother photograph representing nearly 30 years of facial aging.

The senior author (E.F.W.) has a vast experience with midfacial rejuvenation and has long believed that the brow and midface are intimately linked. Midfacial elevation via the temporal brow lift incision has long been the authors' preferred approach, having performed more than 850 procedures over the past 11 years.[5–7] Alternatively, other techniques are employed in the senior author's practice. Whereas other surgeons have attempted to address the midface via a rhytidectomy incision,[8–10] the authors discourage this approach, as the favored vector of lift is superolateral, which cannot be easily achieved with a laterally based incision. Additionally, we do not prefer the vertical (superior) suspension alone, but with certain indications we may suspend the midface through an extended lower blepharoplasty incision.[11,12] Percutaneous techniques have also been employed,[13–16] and in the form of barbed suture suspension by the senior author, but the technique has its limitations that will be enumerated later in this chapter. Over the past several years, our approach to midfacial rejuvenation now also routinely employs lipotransfer as an adjuvant or in isolation and represents the evolution of the senior author's approach.[17–21] This chapter will comprehensively detail the techniques currently employed in our practice for surgical rejuvenation of the midface.

◆ Anatomy

Knowledge of midface anatomy provides the facial plastic surgeon the ability to safely employ a multitude of techniques, which may require different planes of dissection. The midface is classically described as the triangular volume of tissue overlying the malar eminence. Its boundaries are the lateral canthus, oral commissure, and a line extending along the nasolabial fold to the medial canthus. The ligamentous attachments of the lower eyelid and lateral canthus have been well described, and laxity of these ligaments, particularly the subcutaneous position of the orbitmalar ligament, contributes to midface ptosis.[22]

The triangular malar fat pad is a subcutaneous structure located between the skin and the superficial musculoaponeurotic system (SMAS) with its base at the nasolabial fold and apex at the malar eminence. It is loosely adherent to the SMAS but densely adherent to the skin. In youth, the malar fat pad is seated over the malar eminence and overlies the orbital portion of the orbicularis oculi muscle (**Fig. 7.2**). With aging, the fat pad descends over the SMAS in an inferomedial direction. Hence, rejuvenation of this area involves resuspension of the malar fat pad in a superolateral direction.[23,24]

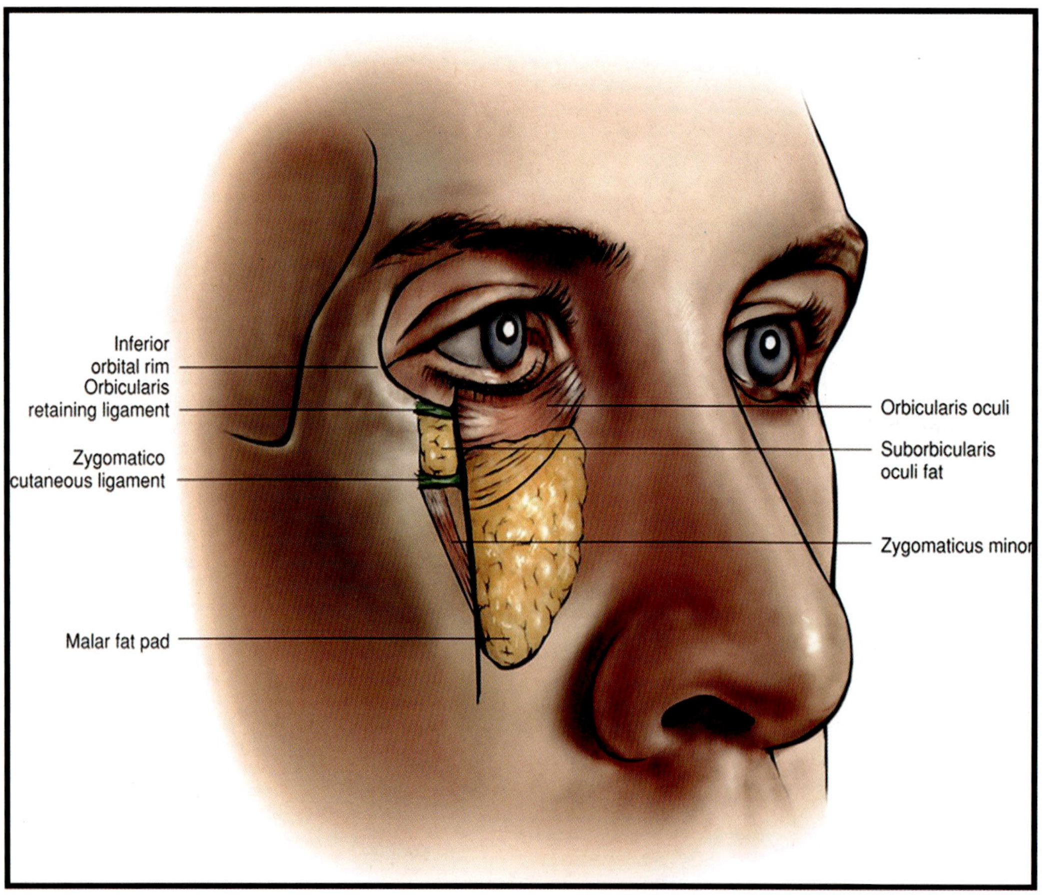

Fig. 7.2 The normal anatomy and descent of soft tissue volume is depicted. (From Krishna S, Williams EF. Lipocontouring in conjunction with the minimal incision brow and subperiosteal midface lift: the next dimension in midface rejuvenation. Facial Plast Surg Clin North Am 2006;14:221–228. Reprinted with permission.)

Midfacial suspension via the transtemporal approach also requires knowledge of the course of the frontal branch of the facial nerve. As this nerve travels in the temporoparietal fascia (TPF), maintaining a plane of dissection on the superficial (shiny white) layer of the deep temporal fascia protects this structure. Additionally, we dissect toward the midface over the zygoma, laterally to medially and in the subperiosteal plane. A well-performed dissection from the temporal region provides for precise and safe suspension in the desired superolateral vector.

◆ Techniques

At present in our practice, four main surgical techniques are considered for rejuvenation of the aging midface. The techniques may be used alone or in combination based on each individual patient's specific aging characteristics and goals, as identified in consultation. Although each of our techniques has merit, we will admit to a preferred approach. We will discuss our preference after the technical descriptions of our surgical approaches.

Brow-Midface

This surgical procedure and complications have been well described in the literature but will be comprehensively reviewed here.[5,6,25] Initially, this procedure was performed via intravenous sedation and monitored anesthesia care, but general anesthesia is now the preferred route of anesthetic delivery. Unlike in rhytidectomy, the ventilating tube does not readily interfere with surgical access.

After appropriate anesthesia is initiated, the patient's hair is secured with brown paper tape (Micropore; 3M, St. Paul, MN) to expose the planned surgical-incision sites. Patients are instructed to cleanse the hair and scalp with an antibacterial shampoo the morning of the procedure; no additional sterile preparatory solution is applied before the commencement of the procedure. Five standard endoscopic brow lift incisions are marked out with a surgical marking pen with one situated in the midline; two located lateral to the midline in the paramedian position (approximately at the lateral canthus) just posterior to the hairline; and two longer incisions located more temporally also camouflaged by the hairline and extending over a 4-cm distance above the helical crus and over the temporalis muscle and fascia. These incisions are typically placed ~1 cm posterior to the hairline.

One percent lidocaine with 1:100,000 epinephrine is then infiltrated into the above-described incision sites and along the entire orbital rim, zygomatic arch, and midface bilaterally. The forehead region, lying between the orbital rim and the incision sites, is spared local anesthesia, as hemostasis can be achieved by dissection in the appropriate avascular plane. Ten minutes are allowed to transpire prior to the first incision to ensure adequate hemostasis. As part of the surgical draping of the patient, a moistened laparotomy sponge is draped over the patient's head behind the incision sites and secured with an overlying surgical towel and clip. A moistened pad significantly absorbs any bleeding and prevents blood from trickling back into the remaining occipital hair.

If a transconjunctival lower lid blepharoplasty is planned, the procedure should be undertaken prior to midfacial suspension. After midfacial elevation, the lower lid may become excessively taut restricting ease of a transconjunctival entry to the lid. Conversely, an planned upper lid blepharoplasty should be deferred until the brow and midface are appropriately elevated so that an accurate assessment of residual cutaneous redundancy can be made.

Initially, the patient is inclined ~60 degrees in a semisitting position, which facilitates ease of bone tunneling. Proper patient positioning cannot be overemphasized as it also allows visualization of the midface using the headlight and retractor. The right paramedian incision (vertically situated in the hairline approximately above the lateral canthus) is made with a no. 15 Bard-Parker blade down through the periosteum. Monopolar electrocautery achieves hemostasis along the cut edges of the wound, being careful not to apply excessive cautery to the exposed hair follicles. The cautery device is also used to ensure that the periosteum is completely incised. A small, sharp, flat periosteal elevator is used to dissect subperiosteally for a distance of a few centimeters circumferentially around the incision site. Little additional dissection is performed posterior to the incision site beyond the initial few centimeters toward the vertex, as extensive dissection toward the occiput provides limited benefit in transposition of the brow upward. With proper wound retraction using wide-double pronged hooks, a Stryker (Stryker Leibinger, Kalamazoo, MI) hand drill outfitted with a 1.5-mm-wide × 6-mm-long drill bit is used to enter the outer calvarial table at 30 degrees (to the horizontal) and joined with an opposing entry of the drill to form a bone tunnel through which the brow-fixating suture may be passed at the end of the case. The drill should be initially aimed perpendicular with the skull to engage the drill for the first 1 to 2 mm before angling the instrument forward in the prescribed 30-degree angle. In addition, the bone tunnel should be made in the posterior aspect of the incision, as suspension of the brow upward will cover the bone tunnel if the tunnel is created too anteriorly relative to the incision. An expanded polytetrafluoroethylene (ePTFE, or Gore-Tex; W.L. Gore and Associates, Inc., Flagstaff, AZ) CV-3 needle is passed through the tunnel to ensure easy passage of the needle at the end of the case. The authors have found that a 6-mm-long recessed drill bit permits ease of bone-tunnel creation while minimizing inadvertent entry through the full thickness of the skull if the drill bit is angled ~30 degrees to the skull contour. Similarly, a 1.5-mm-wide bit will accommodate the desired caliber of needle.

A larger, sharp, flat periosteal elevator, which reduces the risk of periosteal shearing, is then introduced into the same paramedian incision where the bone tunnel was just made to elevate the remaining periosteum *toward* the arcus marginalis stopping short before actually breaking the arcus. All dissection is conducted with tactile feedback (the so-called smart-hand technique) or under direct vision with a headlight and Converse retractor. The authors have found that reliance on endoscopic equipment is both an unnecessary and time-consuming endeavor. Tactile feedback is used to elevate the central pocket (i.e., the three central incisions); whereas direct vision is needed to elevate the lateral, temporal pocket and the contiguous extension of the midface. When approaching the arcus, the smaller, sharp periosteal elevator is again used to release the arcus more definitively than can be achieved with the larger, flat periosteal elevator. When the elevator tip approaches a 1- to 2-cm distance above the supraorbital notch, the elevator is handled only in an upward, lifting motion to avoid any paresthesias or neurapraxias that may ensue from violating the supraorbital neurovascular bundle.

The midline incision is then performed to access the medial-brow complex. The principal objective is release of the periosteum at the arcus to achieve unrestricted brow elevation; and aggressive dissection of the musculature has been abandoned, as return of muscle function has been often observed despite the most meticulous removal of the procerus-corrugator complex. In addition, significant morbidity may arise from aggressive muscular resection, including contour irregularity, asymmetric brow depression, and the most dreaded outcome, frank cutaneous necrosis. Botulinum toxin type A has been the preferred method to address the medial depressor complex. The midline incision is closed with surgical clips before continuing to the left side. The left paramedian incision is then made, and the same method of bone-tunnel creation and periosteal release is performed as previously described for the contralateral, paramedian incision.

With complete dissection of the central pocket (medial to the conjoined tendons of the temporalis muscle), the longer, lateral temporoparietal incisions are performed. Dissection is carried down through the TPF so that a proper tissue plane may be achieved between the TPF and the true temporalis fascia to avoid injury to the frontal branch of the facial nerve. The incision should be situated ~1 cm behind the hairline to lie over the temporalis muscle and not more posteriorly to avoid transection of the superficial temporal artery and to minimize the long trajectory of dissection needed to reach the midface (**Fig. 7.3**). Initial dissection is performed with a large, blunt elevator over the true temporalis fascia, and then the larger, flat periosteal elevator is used to break the conjoined tendon of the temporalis muscle that divides the central and lateral pockets. Directing elevation toward the right paramedian incision and passing the instrument through that incision will ensure that complete release of the tendon has been accomplished. Three periosteal elevators are used for the entire case (the small, sharp, flat elevator; the large, sharp, flat elevator; and the large, rounded, blunt elevator). Further, we preferred elevators coated with an ebonized finish to minimize unwanted, reflective glare off the surface.

Under direct vision with a headlight and Converse retractor, dissection is taken down to the orbital rim with the small, sharp periosteal elevator, carefully looking for the presence of the sentinel vein. If the vein lies in the direct path between the upper and midface, then it may be skeletonized and cauterized with a bipolar device and transected with scissors to permit entry into the midface. Injudicious cautery of the cephalic vessel, especially if the bipolar cautery tips are aimed superficially, may jeopardize the frontal branch of the facial nerve. The arcus marginalis is then released from the superolateral orbital rim near the lateral canthus with the periosteal elevator. The assistant places a finger along the lateral margin of the orbital rim to limit the surgeon's dissection and to avoid excessive release of periosteum from the lateral canthus, which may otherwise contribute to undesirable, lateral-canthal elevation.

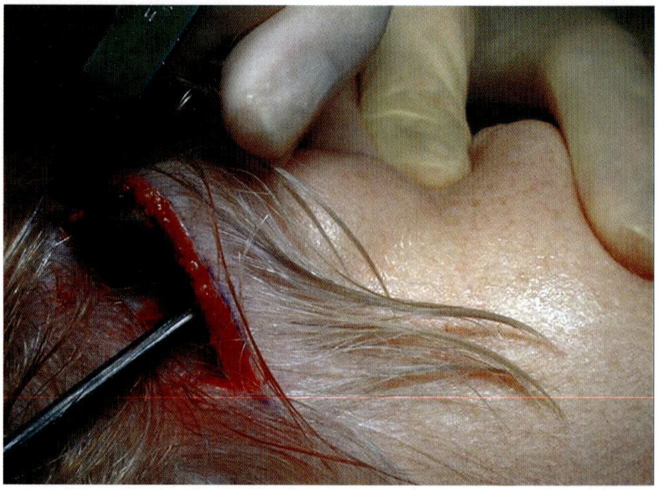

Fig. 7.3 Lateral incision approach to the midface ~1 cm behind the temporal hairline.

With direct headlight-assisted visualization, the large, sharp periosteal elevator is guided downward to enter the temporal fat pad and then to release the periosteal attachments overlying the zygomatic arch itself. This approach provides direct access to the midfacial structures. Next, the periosteal elevator is continued inferiorly over the malar eminence to release the zygomaticus major and minor muscular attachments and malar fat pad from the underlying malar bone. Although minimal, medial dissection limits both lateral-canthal distortion and potential facial-nerve injury, the dissection is continued until the midfacial structures are adequately released. Once the zygomatic muscular attachments have been severed, the surgeon should be wary of further inferior dissection and unintended masseteric elevation that may result in trismus. A CV-3 Gore-Tex suture is passed through the temporalis fascia and muscle just anteroinferior to the temporoparietal incision and then passed through the malar fat pad with a long needle driver. This maneuver is technically difficult to perform and requires a learning curve to be proficient. Pulling the suture superiorly confirms sufficient release of the midfacial tissues has been achieved. If not, then further dissection medially and inferiorly is performed until appropriate release of the midface is observed. Before the suture is fastened

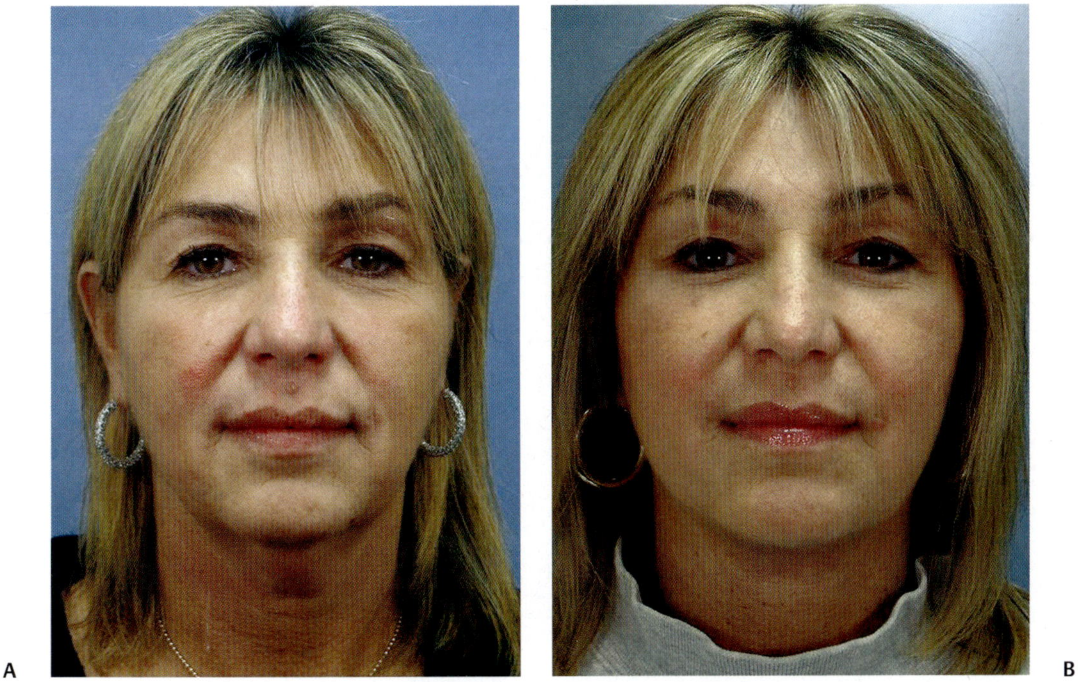

Fig. 7.4 Brow-midface technique: (**A**) preoperative frontal view; (**B**) postoperative frontal view.

superiorly to the temporalis muscle, the paramedian suture on the same side is tied down first. The paramedian suture is fixated first to relieve any tension on the suture that elevates the midface and to permit better brow positioning by suspending the most superior suture first. The CV-3 Gore-Tex suture is used to secure the overlying frontalis muscle through the bone tunnel in the paramedian incision. A technical consideration that should be observed is a generous bite of frontalis muscle needs to be grasped with the suture needle to achieve a secure and adequate suspension. The suture is secured using a square knot tied in the air, which is then fastened down. Gore-Tex permits sliding a square knot down into place. After the paramedian suspension has been completed and the incision closed, the surgeon should return to the lateral temporal incision to suspend the already distally placed suture through the malar fat pad to the proximal temporalis muscle and fascia at the incision site. The vector of suspension should be vertically oriented, and the suture through the malar fat pad should be situated more laterally over the malar prominence—both of which will minimize untoward distortion of the lateral canthus.

Next, the TPF just anterior to the temporoparietal incision is sutured to the temporalis muscle and fascia more superiorly with the CV-3 Gore-Tex suture to pull the overlying brow and soft tissue superolaterally. This suture placement is undertaken twice. All incisions are then closed with surgical clips. Suturing in the hair-bearing scalp is both unnecessarily laborious in placement and removal, and the senior author has achieved a very favorable cosmetic result with surgical-clip closure. Antibiotic ointment is applied to the external incisions, and a pressure dressing is fashioned into place. We believe this stepwise approach to the brow and midface will ensure consistent, reproducible results (**Figs. 7.4 and 7.5**).

Complications

Asymmetry Symmetry can be difficult to achieve in facial plastic surgery, especially as most patients exhibit preoperative asymmetry. The patient's underlying predisposition to the asymmetry may be difficult to overcome with our surgical maneuvers. Patients who present with an asymmetric brow during the preoperative consultation should be made aware of this finding and counseled with regard to the limitations of surgery. If gross asymmetry exists postoperatively, this may also be the result of a technical error (e.g., incomplete release of the periosteal arcus marginalis), suture dehiscence, or facial-nerve paresis.

Facial-Nerve Neurapraxia Though infrequently encountered, any facial-nerve neurapraxia is quite concerning on the part of surgeon and patient alike. Indiscriminate bipolar cautery near the cephalic vessel, improper plane of dissection in the temporoparietal region (frontal branch of the facial nerve) or possibly during midfacial dissection (zygomatico-buccal branches) should be avoided. The few cases that the authors have encountered have uniformly resolved after a period of 3 to 6 months. Frequent and amiable reassurance must be maintained throughout the postoperative course to ensure good patient rapport and support.

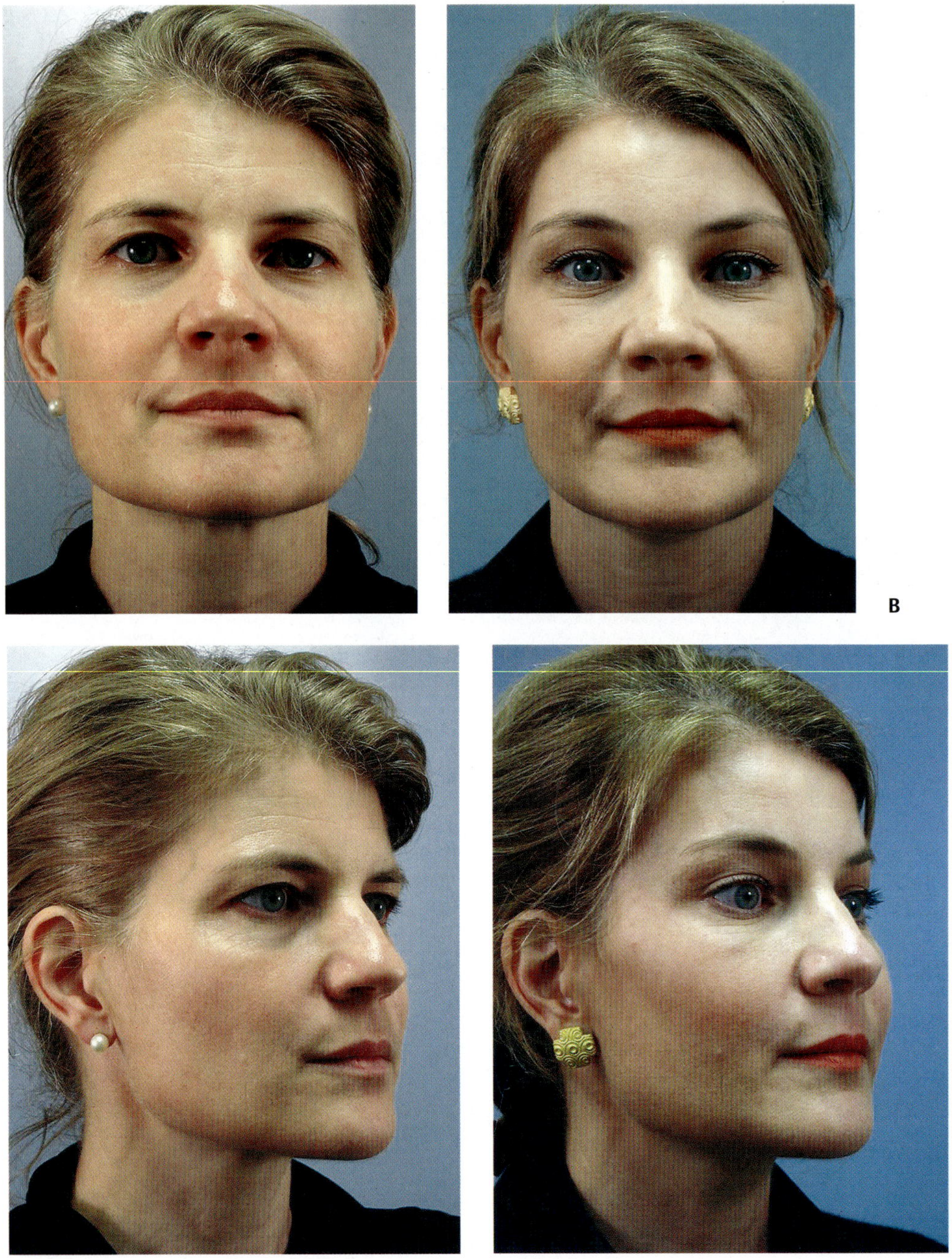

A B C D

Fig. 7.5 Brow-midface technique and upper blepharoplasty: (**A**) preoperative frontal view; (**B**) postoperative frontal view; (**C**) preoperative oblique view; (**D**) postoperative oblique view.

Alopecia and Scar Incision Alopecia We routinely adhere to three tenets to minimize this particular complication: (1) The knife blade is bevelled according to the pattern of the hair follicles: perpendicularly at the three medial incisions and posteroanteriorly for the two temporal incisions; (2) excessive monopolar cautery is limited at the wound edges; (3) tension is avoided along the incision line at the time of wound closure. The authors believe that bone-tunnel suture suspension has minimized evidence of alopecia and scarring, having previously employed a screw suspension technique. If any wound alopecia or scarring should develop, simple excision and revision of the wound should ameliorate the appearance.[25]

Lateral canthal distortion is infrequently encountered and in the senior author's experience has been uniformly transient. Having the assistant protect at this landmark with a finger during dissection has likely minimized this undesirable complication.

Dimpling is commonly encountered during the early postoperative course. Even prolonged dimpling eventually settles and should be managed expectantly.

Lipotransfer

At this point, we will describe our lipotransfer technique, as the brow-midface procedure is rarely performed in isolation. The techniques for fat retrieval, processing, and delivery have been well described and illustrated in the senior author's previous evaluations of midfacial rejuvenation,[26,27] but the technique continues to undergo subtle refinements and is included in this chapter.

Fat Harvest

The patient is placed under monitored anesthesia care (MAC) with intravenous sedation or general anesthesia. When fat transfer is performed as the sole procedure, oral sedation is an option; however, because the patients in this study are undergoing a concomitant midface lift, general anesthesia or MAC anesthesia is necessary. Prior to any surgical manipulations or infiltration of local anesthesia, the areas of planned injection are delineated with a surgical marking pen, and the estimated amount of fat needed is determined. Typically, for the four areas examined in this study, a total of 40 cc aspirated fat is sufficient. Next, the fat harvest sites are delineated with the surgical marking pen. We have found that the ideal place for fat aspiration is the inner thighs, however we commonly also access the outer thighs and the abdomen. In thin patients, we access any areas of fat accumulation, including the flanks and lateral buttocks. Once the entry sites for aspiration are determined, a single stab incision is made with a no. 11 blade. A long liposuction aspiration cannula is attached to a 20-cc syringe filled with the tumescent solution (1 mL 1% lidocaine with 1:100,000 epinephrine, 4 mL 1% plain lidocaine, and 15 mL saline). The long cannula is placed through the stab incision and directed out from the injection site in a fanlike pattern. A first pass is performed as a tunneling maneuver, and the second pass is when the tumescent solution is infiltrated. This is repeated in the other fat aspiration sites. Typically, a total of four 20-cc syringes are used to infiltrate the abdomen (two per side, from periumbilical stab incisions), and two 20-cc syringes of tumescent solution are used per inner or outer thigh. The total amount of tumescent solution used in a case is dependent on the number of aspiration sites; however, the total amount of lidocaine infiltrated is always carefully recorded. Ten minutes is allowed to elapse for maximal vasoconstrictive effect of the epinephrine. Next, the same liposuction aspiration cannula is affixed onto a 10-cc Luer-Lok syringe (Vita Needle Company, Needham, MA). The nondominant hand is used to elevate the skin and superficial fat away from the aspiration cannula, and the dominant hand is used to perform manual aspiration of the fat. A vigorous forward and backward movement of the cannula is used for optimal aspiration applying no more than "negative" 2 cc of manual pressure with the plunger. When aspirating in the abdominal area, one must be careful to stay in a relatively superficial plane to avoid any trauma to the underlying rectus muscle or untoward peritoneal entry, especially in patients with a previous history of abdominal surgery. The nondominant (or "smart") hand can be used to guide the aspiration cannula in the proper plane. After aspiration of the fat in multiple 10-cc syringes, the stab incisions are closed with a single 5-0 fast absorbing gut suture. If the abdominal area was accessed, an abdominal binder is placed. The inner and/or outer thighs are wrapped with a 6-inch Ace wrap (BD, Franklin Lakes, NJ).

Fat Processing

The plungers on the 10-cc syringes filled with aspirated fat are removed, and a metal stopper is placed on the ends of the syringes. The syringes are then passed off the table to the circulating nurse who places them into the centrifuge. The centrifuge must always be "counterbalanced" (i.e., an even number of syringes should be placed in the centrifuge directly across from each other). The fat is centrifuged for 10 minutes at 3500 rpm. At the conclusion of the centrifugation, the fat has separated into three distinct layers: the top layer consists of oil from ruptured adipocytes, the central area is the usable fat, and the bottom layer contains lidocaine, saline, and blood (serous fluid). The stoppers are then removed from the syringes to allow drainage of the serous fluid. The oil layer is then partially removed by carefully pouring it out from the top of the syringe. The remaining oil layer is removed by placing moist 4 × 4 gauze sponges (opened up lengthwise) into the tops of the syringes to wick out the remaining oil. Once the usable fat is isolated in the syringes, they are placed in a refrigerator until the conclusion of the midface procedure.

Fat Transfer Procedure

We prefer to customize our lipotransfer to each individual patient, and this can be optimized by having our patients bring in photographs from their youth. With this plan in place, the surgical technician transfers the fat from the 10-cc syringes into individual 1-cc syringes using a Luer-Lok transfer device. An 0.9-cm or 1.2-cm Tulip cannula (San Diego, CA) is placed on the 1-cc syringes, depending on the anatomic site being injected. Attention is then turned to the previously marked-out areas on the face: the lower lid complex, the tear trough, the malar eminence, the submalar region, and the nasolabial crease. An 18-gauge Nokor needle is used to create small stab incisions at the sites of entry. These entry points have been infiltrated with very small amounts of local as the fat processing is initiated. Beginning with the lower lid complex and tear trough, the stab incision is made just inferior to the infraorbital rim and lateral to the infraorbital nerve. The 0.9-cm Tulip cannula is used to inject fat along the inferior orbital rim and tear trough using multiple passes and laying down a minimal amount of fat (ideally ~0.03 cc per pass). The fat is injected at many different angles, with 1 cc superficial to orbicularis oculi and typically 2 cc deep to this muscle. At the tear trough,

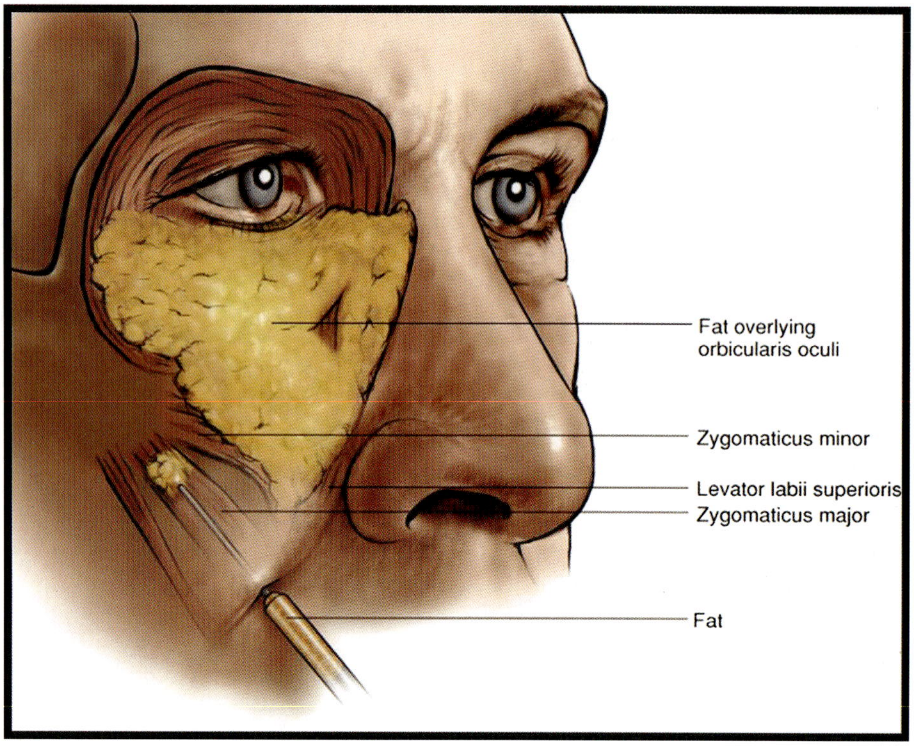

Fig. 7.6 Restoration of volume by lipotransfer is depicted. (From Krishna S, Williams EF. Lipocontouring in conjunction with the minimal incision brow and subperiosteal midface lift: the next dimension in midface rejuvenation. Facial Plast Surg Clin North Am 2006;14: 221–228. Reprinted with permission.)

however, the fat is injected only in the deep plane just superior to the periosteum. Next, attention is turned to the malar eminence. Injection at this site is focused on injecting into and along the zygomaticus major, zygomaticus minor, and levator labii superioris muscles and into the malar fat pad (**Fig. 7.3**). The entry incision is made with the Nokor needle at the inferior region of the muscles. A similar technique of inserting the blunt cannula and injecting a small amount of fat upon withdrawal is performed. Multiple passes with the cannula and injection into multiple tissue levels are performed. The submalar region may also be addressed next with injections targeting the buccinator and risorius muscles. Finally, the nasolabial creases are addressed by making the entry stab incision at the inferior-most point of the nasolabial crease. The same technique is used here except that the injection is performed solely into the subcutaneous tissue layer and not into a specific muscle. The upper white lip can also be accessed through this puncture site, if the customized lipotransfer requires augmentation in this region. After the conclusion of fat injections, the face is cleansed with saline, and a small amount of antibiotic ointment is placed on each of the stab incisions, and we then may proceed with the thread-lift portion of the procedure. The injected areas are aggressively iced for the first 48 hours to decrease edema and ecchymoses (**Fig. 7.6**). As our learning curve with lipotransfer has progressed, the result for many patients may stand alone. The concept of volume restoration in midfacial rejuvenation is reinforced by our isolated lipotransfer results (**Figs. 7.7 and 7.8**).

A

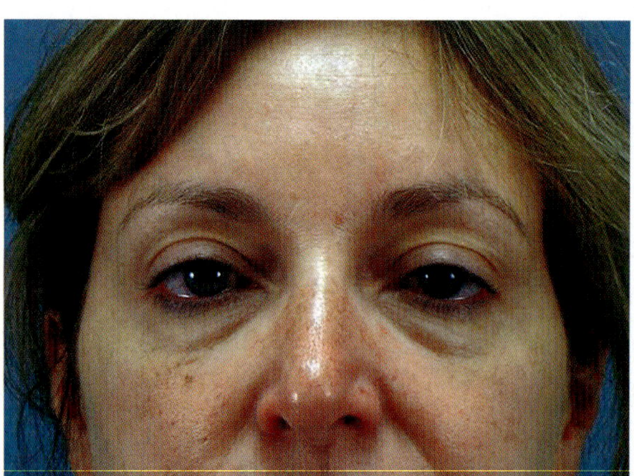

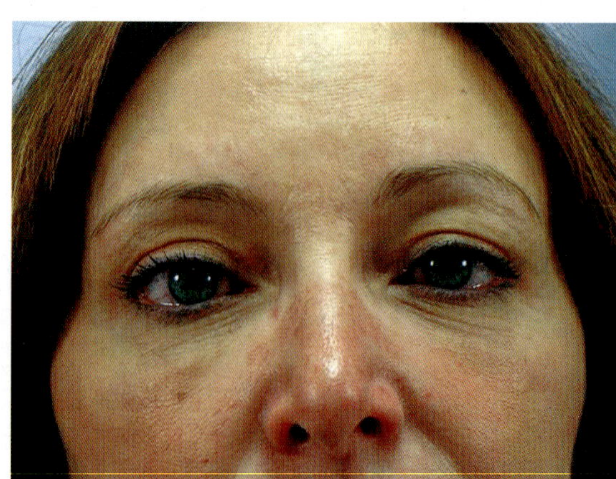

B

Fig. 7.7 Midfacial lipotransfer: (**A**) preoperative frontal view; (**B**) postoperative frontal view.

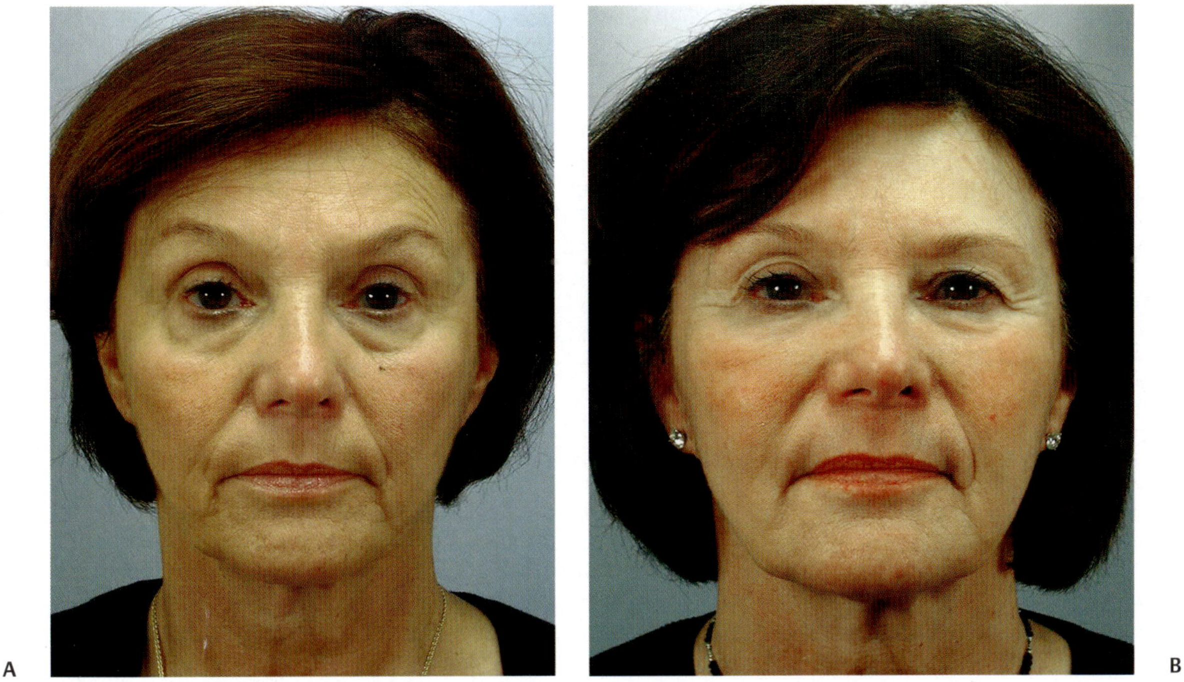

Fig. 7.8 Midfacial lipotransfer: (A) preoperative frontal view; (B) postoperative frontal view.

Complications

Postoperative Edema Postoperative edema is an expected complication from the multiple tunnels created during fat delivery to the midface. This is a self-limited process and is managed expectantly, with appropriate patient counseling.

Ecchymosis Ecchymosis is another expected sequela from the procedure, but great variation in severity has been observed. The challenge resides with the patient expecting minimal downtime and a rapid return to the social arena. We therefore recommend patients allow a week for recovery. Additionally, the senior author now offers 595-nm pulse dye laser treatment for red and purple bruising at postoperative days 6 and 7 to expedite resolution.

Asymmetry Great efforts are made to achieve precise delivery of fat. As previously suggested, it is impossible to control for perfect symmetry beyond that. Even a minimal amount of facial edema created during the procedure distorts the tissues, and baseline facial asymmetry is an expected baseline for the majority of patients.

Neurapraxia No permanent apraxias or paresthesias have been seen in the senior author's practice with either technique. He does believe, however, that the risk for transient motor apraxia is more likely with midface lipotransfer.

Hyperpigmentation Occasionally, pigmentary changes are observed after lipotransfer, particularly in the lower eyelid complex. This is presumably a postinflammation condition and is usually subtle in presentation and self-limited. For those patients with more significant hyperpigmentation changes, we will use topical hydroquinone. We have also considered the routine postoperative use of nonsteroidal anti-inflammatory drugs (NSAIDs) to minimize this complication.

Blindness A rare complication from intravascular fat injection has been reported.[28] This has not been observed in the senior author's greater than 3-year experience with this technique.

Undercorrection In reviewing the senior author's results, it seems that the results are improving even when comparing early postoperative results. The senior author believes that his evolution toward a more aggressive lipotransfer and delivery of greater volume has improved the result.

Overcorrection The goal is 20% overcorrection. Although lipotransfer is individually customized, relatively standard volume ranges are delivered throughout the midface. Otherwise, judgment may be compromised by intraoperative edema. Attempts to minimize distortion by infiltration of local anesthetic are made, as well as accurate recordings of lipotransfer volumes. Preoperative volumetric asymmetries realized preoperatively should be customized.

Extended Skin Muscle Lower Blepharoplasty with Midface Suspension

Although periorbital rejuvenation is discussed elsewhere in this text, the senior author is reluctant to address isolated lower lid aging with a skin-muscle flap technique. However, if facial analysis reveals malar descent (festooning or malar bagging) and the patient declines a brow lift/transbrow midface lift, then an extended skin-muscle flap may be recommended. If excessive lower lid laxity or frank ectropion is present, then a lower lid shortening procedure (e.g., tarsal strip) may also be required and then a skin-muscle flap is advised. For the above reasons, a skin-muscle type flap may be the approach of choice. We will describe the technical considerations[25] used to address the issue of malar descent and forego the discussion for correction of lower lid laxity.

An extended incision that follows a natural skin crease radiating from the lateral canthus should be marked out with a surgical marking pen. One percent lidocaine with 1:50,000 epinephrine is injected along the line of incision and inferiorly over the area of dissection. The appropriate 10 minutes of hemostatic time is allowed to transpire before the initial incision is made. A no. 15 Bard-Parker blade is used to make the first few millimeters of an incision ~1 to 2 mm from the inferior lid margin at the most lateral extent through both skin and muscle. A pair of iris scissors are then inserted through this incipient incision and gently spread to develop the plane of dissection below the skin-muscle flap from lateral to medial. One blade of the scissors is then inserted into the incision with the other blade remaining externally, and in this way the incision is opened laterally to medially as far as required but always lateral to the medial punctum (to minimize risk of medial-canthal web formation). The bleeding muscle edge is then cauterized with a hot-tip hand-held electrocautery.

A 6-0 silk suture is passed through the superior aspect of the incision and clamped with a hemostat to retract the lower lid upward, protecting the globe and providing countertraction. Bishop forceps or a wide, double-pronged retractor is then used to retract the skin-muscle flap inferiorly while the hand-held or monopolar cautery dissects the skin-muscle flap from the underlying orbital septum. This flap is carried downward onto the midface under the malar bag/festoon if an extended lower lid blepharoplasty is intended (**Fig. 7.9A**). If pseudoherniation of fat exists, then the orbital septum is entered and the fat clamped and removed as described previously for the transconjunctival approach. If an extended blepharoplasty is undertaken to efface a malar bag/festoon, then the malar bag/festoon is suspended to the lateral orbital rim using a 4-0 polydioxanone (PDS [Ethicon, Somerville, NJ]; Maxon [Davis & Geck, Manati, Puerto Rico]), or 4-0 Gore-Tex suture. A single pronged hook is placed into the lateral aspect of the incision to provide proper tension and alignment prior to skin-flap excision (**Fig. 7.9B**).

Any excessive skin-muscle flap is then trimmed with curved serrated iris scissors erring on the conservative side to avoid unintended lid eversion and vertical shortening, especially medially. The incision line is then reapproximated with a running, nonlocking 7-0 Prolene suture (Ethicon, Somerville, NJ). A lateral canthal suspension suture should still be considered for a standard skin-muscle blepharoplasty to lessen the probability of postoperative lid malposition. This suture is placed in a similar fashion as described for the extended technique but often with less vertical elevation (as the midface does not require suspension in this circumstance). A modest improvement of the malar bags and festoons should be noted with subtle changes appreciated with regard to midfacial descent (**Fig. 7.10**).

Complications

Postseptal Hemorrhage The most feared complication that may occur is a postseptal hemorrhage with the risk of visual loss. Albeit a rare entity, it absolutely deserves our consideration. The surgeon must attentively assess the

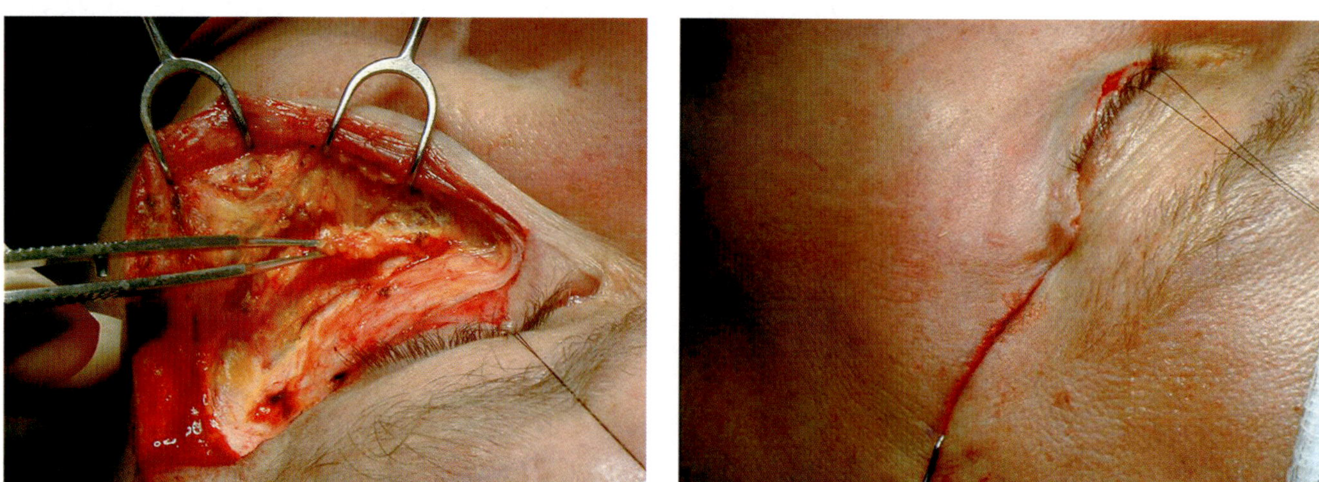

A B

Fig. 7.9 (**A**) Suborbicularis dissection for extended lower blepharoplasty with midface suspension. (**B**) Extended lower blepharoplasty with midface suspension demonstrated.

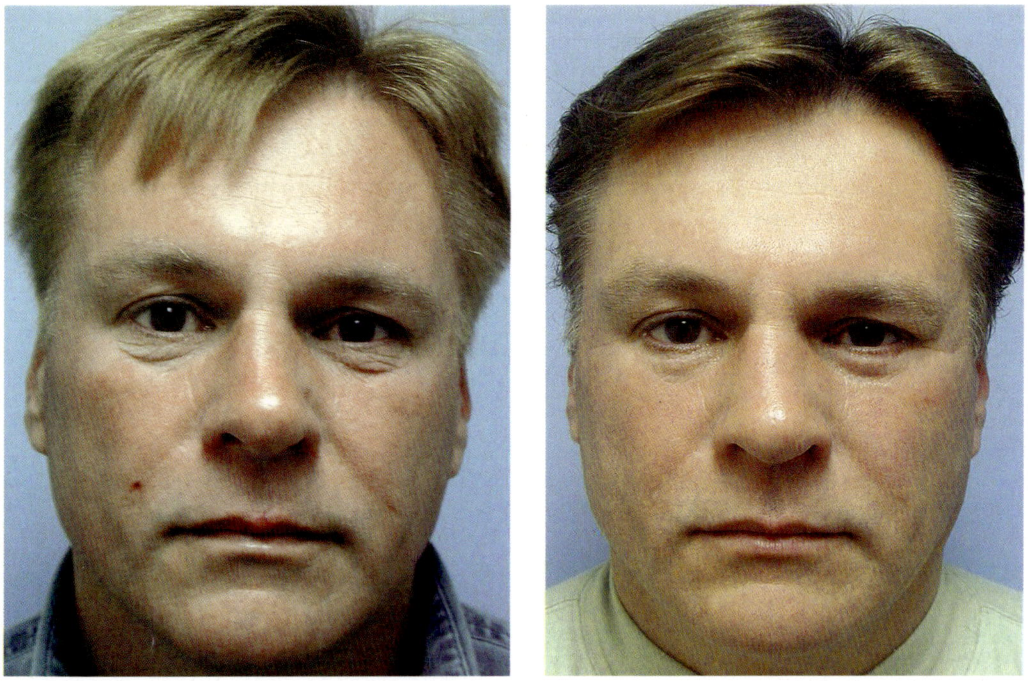

Fig. 7.10 Extended lower blepharoplasty with midface suspension: (A) preoperative frontal view; (B) postoperative frontal view.

patient's visual status, extraocular movements, pupillary response, and palpable induration of the globe relative to the other eye. If this complication is a concern, staff should make an effort to contact the most available ophthalmologist for consultation, evaluation, and further care.

Corneal Abrasion Although uncommon, corneal abrasion should be readily identified and promptly treated. The patient should also be prescribed a topical ophthalmologic ointment (e.g., tobramycin) without a steroid component to minimize an infectious complication, most commonly *Pseudomonas aeruginosa*. If no improvement is witnessed, then he or she should seek prompt ophthalmologic consultation for slit-lamp evaluation and further care.

Lower Lid Malposition Perhaps one of the most common and distressing complications that occur after blepharoplasty is lower lid malposition, whether mild lateral rounding or frank ectropion. Usually, this complication arises because of poor preoperative lid tone that worsens after transection of the lower lid retaining mechanisms, which occurs whether a transconjunctival or transcutaneous approach is implemented.

Milia Milia develop several weeks after blepharoplasty and represent epidermal inclusion cysts or pustules that form due to local irritation. They should be differentiated from suture tract marks that may manifest at the time of suture removal. A 7-0 Prolene suturing, even if retained longer than a week, rarely results in noticeable tract marks and is therefore preferred for closure.

Hypertrophic Scar/Keloid Although frank keloid formation on the face is quite rare, hypertrophic scarring may be more prevalent especially in the more pigmented ethnicities and races. Prophylactic, intraoperative triamcinolone acetonide injection (10 mg/mL) with 0.1 mL total per eyelid may be advisable in Fitzpatrick IV to VI patients, especially along the medial extent of the wound. If this complication should arise, then triamcinolone should be directly injected into the scar not more frequently than every 3 weeks to avoid dermal atrophy.[25]

Percutaneous Barbed Suture Suspension

The role for barbed suture suspension in the senior author's practice requires a patient who does not want a "surgical" lift and understands the limitations of the procedure and our lack of long-term follow-up. It should also be a patient in the midphases of aging with good tissue mobility. We believe anecdotally that the midface is the best-addressed anatomic region of the aging face by these techniques. Patients with medium-thickness skin and good elasticity are excellent candidates. Heavy faces with thick skin or patients with very thin skin and poor skin laxity are unlikely to see a desired result. At present, patient candidacy is somewhat dynamic and may continue to evolve toward more stringent selection criteria.[29]

When combining thread with lipotransfer, we sequence the thread lift after lipotransfer to avoid disruption of the threads. It is important to have marked the thread course prior to lipotransfer as facial edema is an expectation. We start by performing two stab incisions at the lower temporal region. Sharp plastic scissors are used to dissect down to the deep temporal fascia. An Adson-Brown forceps is used at the skin edge as the thread is introduced. We use, the Contour Thread system (Surgical Specialties Corp., Reading, PA). The thread is then passed through the subcutaneous tissue layers in a slightly irregular "zigzag" pathway, with great care not to capture dermis. The thread then pierces the skin at the exit site and is grasped with a small hemostat. The connected parallel thread is then passed at the adjacent premarked pathway. After the second connected thread exits, the long guide needles are aligned, the overlying tissues are adjusted in the appropriate vector, and the threads are trimmed (**Fig. 7.11**). Approximately 3 to 4 cm of thread is left at the exit site. We use four threads per side in the midface. These are left long and for sequential lifting. The threads are affixed with Steri-Strips (3M, St. Paul, MN) laterally away from the mouth at the conclusion of the case. The head is wrapped with a 3-inch Ace bandage, and the patient is taken to the recovery room.

On the 3rd postoperative day, the patient returns to the office for sequential lifting. The Ace is removed, as are the Steri-Strips. The midfacial tissue is once again gently adjusted in the appropriate direction of the thread and vector of the lift. The thread is cut at the skin so that its distal aspect may retract and minimize palpability. The patient is then discharged from the office until postoperative day 7.

On postoperative day 7, the unnatural appearing puckering is released by abrupt gentle massage in the opposite direction of the thread's lift. A similar adjustment to release puckering may again be performed, as necessary, on postoperative day 14. The surgeon and patient must be mindful that releasing the puckering restores a more natural appearance; however, the maneuver counteracts the lift. We are uncertain at this point whether a longer duration of facial distortion from the threads will provide a more durable result (**Fig. 7.12**).

Complications

Asymmetry Great efforts are made to achieve precise thread placement. It is impossible to control for perfect symmetry beyond that. Even a minimal amount of facial edema created during the procedure distorts the tissues, and baseline facial asymmetry is an expected baseline for the majority of patients.

Palpable Thread One patient has reported a palpable thread at an exit site. It eventually settled with massage and observation. With respect to extrusion, although there are reports in the literature with the Aptos (Kolster Methods, Inc., Anaheim, CA) technology,[30] the senior author has not experienced this complication in his practice.

Undercorrection In reviewing the senior author's results, it seems that the results are improving even when comparing early postoperative results. However, the most favorable results have been most frequently associated with aggressive lipotransfer. With regard to the thread component, the senior author continues to counsel patients that they will see a "noticeable" but subtle result.

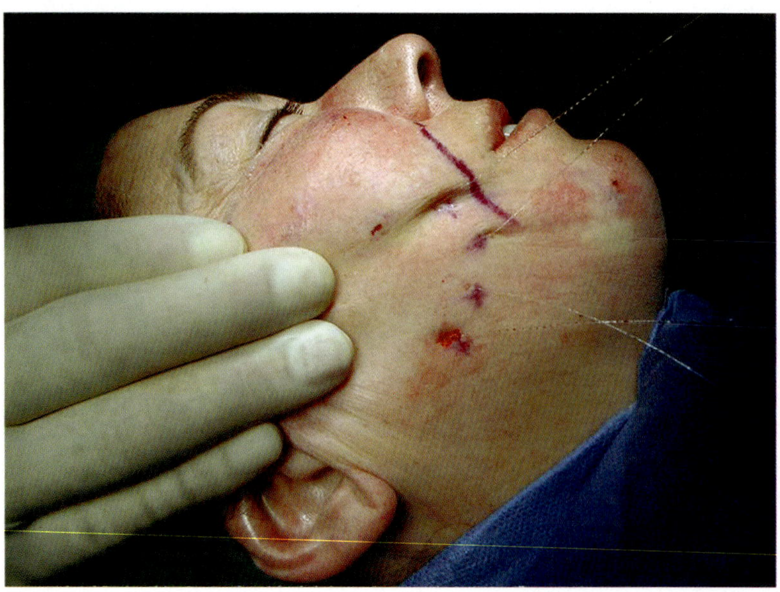

Fig. 7.11 Barbed thread suture suspension of the midface.

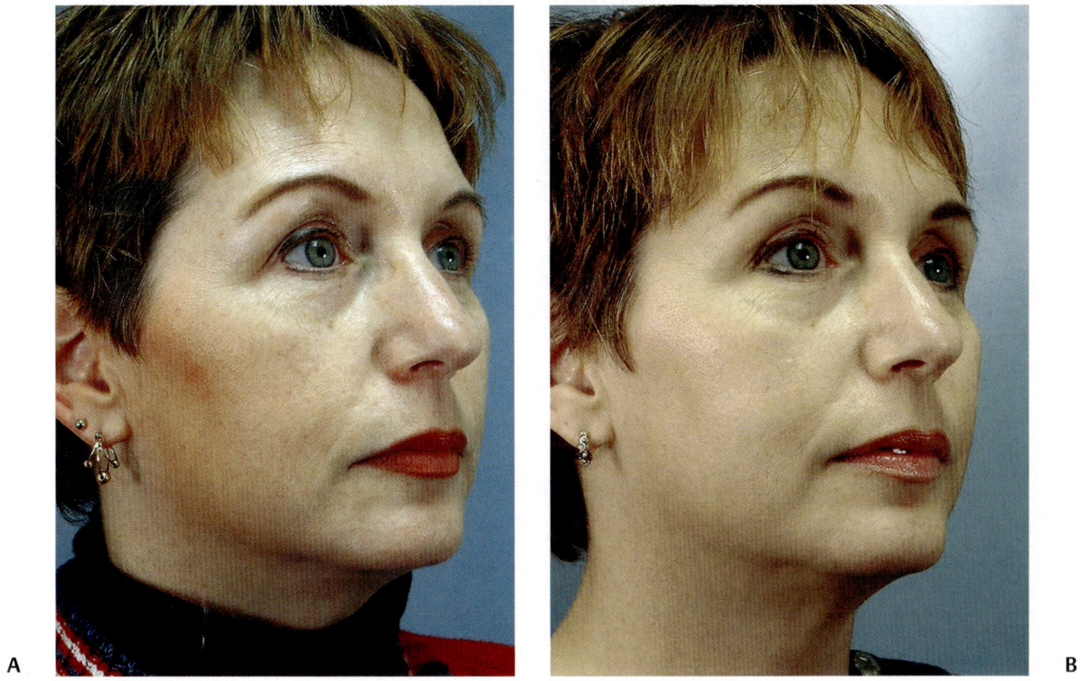

Fig. 7.12 Barbed suture suspension of midface: (**A**) preoperative oblique view; (**B**) postoperative oblique view demonstrating a limited result.

◆ Discussion

The senior author has employed a multitude of surgical techniques to address the characteristic changes seen in the aging midface. We continually and critically evaluate any technique offered for midfacial rejuvenation. In his initial review of 325 consecutive brow-midface patients published in 2003, it was observed that most patients showed the best improvements in the malar-infraorbital complex, with 70% of patients showing marked improvement.[6] Moderate improvement was noted at the jawline (with or without concurrent rhytidectomy), and little or no improvement was noted at the nasolabial fold. An additional benefit noted by the senior author is the need for lesser fat removal (if at all) with transconjunctival blepharoplasty. We also recognize the limitations of this isolated procedure for patients with poor bone structure, round faces, or festoons. Although patient and surgeon satisfaction with this isolated technique remains high, efforts have continued in pursuit of optimal results.

In our practice, the evolution of the midface lift now almost routinely includes the addition of fat transfer to the operation. We advocate the use of fat transfer to correct the tear trough deformity and the nasolabial crease at the time of the midface lift. Many patients who undergo a midface lift have a significant tear trough deformity and infraorbital skeletonization that may be enhanced with a midface lift alone. By combining fat transfer to the tear trough and infraorbital rim with the midface lift, we are able to create a youthful, convex contour between the lower lid and the cheek, which provides superior aesthetic results and long-term correction (**Figs. 7.13 and 7.14**). In addition, the nasolabial crease can be improved with fat transfer. Our early results have been published demonstrating a modest long-term improvement in our initial group of patients.[26] As our fat transfer technique has progressed, however, we are realizing even more impressive results. The technique has continued to evolve, particularly with technical considerations of fat delivery to the lower lid (upper border of the midface) complex as well as a slight increase in volume delivered. Skin textural issues aside, we believe this technique provides the most comprehensive approach to the characteristic components of midface aging. There is also discussion among clinicians that lipotransfer may potentially improve the condition of overlying skin, but this has not yet been critically evaluated. We also believe the aging temporal (brow) complex is intimately linked to the midface, and this rejuvenation method addresses that concern.

With regard to lipotransfer, the upside is tremendous with minimal morbidity. Though extremely enthusiastic with regard to its role in all of facial rejuvenation, we must temper our advocacy until our patient follow-up has matured. We truly believe the longevity of lipotransfer is significant, but we still encounter a rare patient who has not held onto a long-term lipotransfer result. Our analysis of fat will therefore continue until it is well understood in our practice.

The senior author has reserved the extended skin-muscle flap lower lid blepharoplasty with midface suspension for certain clinical scenarios, such as malar bags and

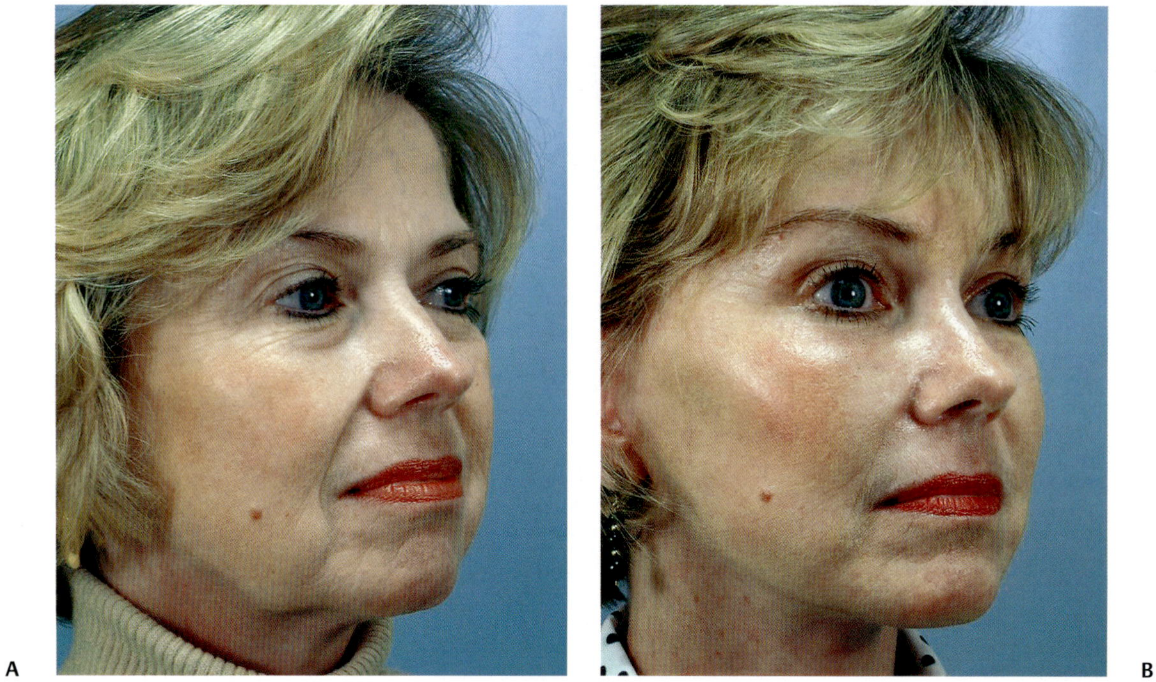

Fig. 7.13 Brow-midface technique, lipotransfer, rhytidectomy, and blepharoplasty: (A) preoperative oblique view; (B) postoperative oblique view.

festooning.[25] Even for these specific clinical scenarios, this procedure is becoming far less common in his practice, as his comfort level with lipotransfer longevity grows. The senior author has two major concerns regarding this approach to midfacial aging. One concern is the vector of midface suspension, which we believe should be superolateral. The transblepharoplasty approach is limited predominately to a vector of vertical suspension and fails to address the immediately adjacent temporal aging process. The second concern with this approach is the denervation of orbicularis oculi and resultant lower lid dysfunction. Through critical analysis of long-term patient results with

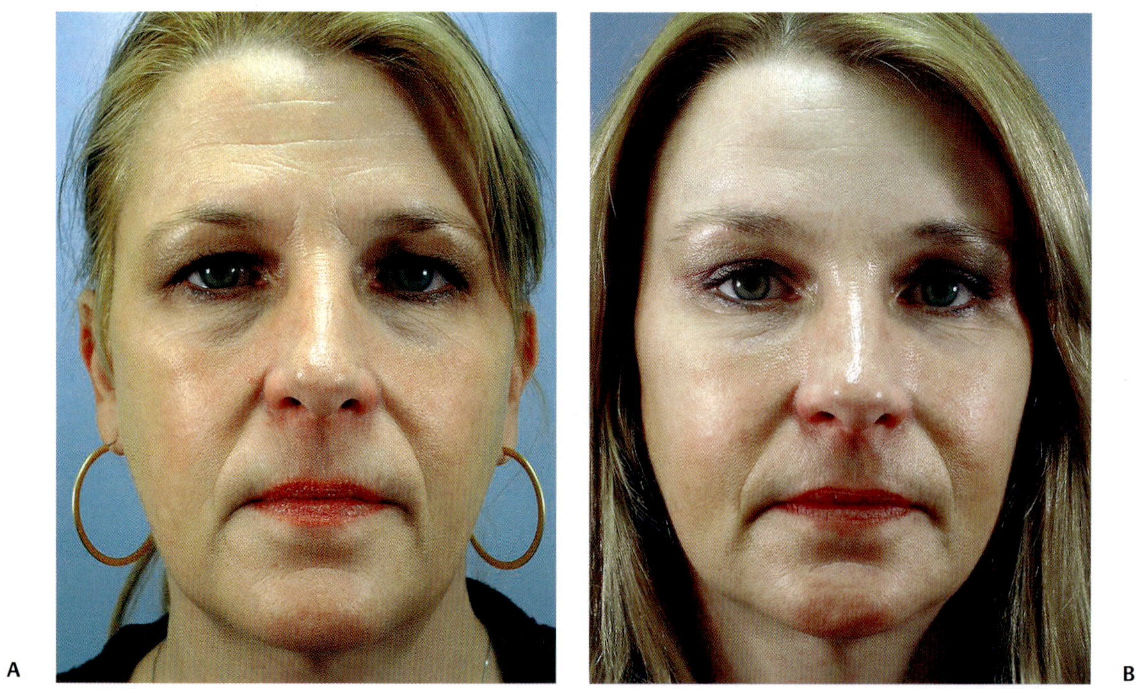

Fig. 7.14 Brow-midface technique, lipotransfer, and upper blepharoplasty: (A) preoperative frontal view; (B) postoperative frontal view.

this technique, this has become a real concern. Philosophically, trading a youthful-appearing lower lid and upper midface in the short-term for lid dysfunction in the long-term is not worthwhile when other techniques avoid this potential morbidity.

The last technique of midfacial rejuvenation used in the senior author's practice is the percutaneous midface thread-lift. The barbed suture technique has been used in our practice for approximately 1 year. The thread on its own has provided some unpredictability but seems to perform best in the midfacial region. When combined with lipotransfer, however, it has accomplished our goals of achieving a noticeable result (**Fig. 7.15**) and making patients happy; the procedure has almost uniformly been a success. We are limited by lack of extended follow-up for these patients. Despite this concern, however, there is still a patient population with the minimally invasive mindset that opts for this procedure. We are making great efforts to manage expectations and closely follow these patients long-term to better understand durability of our result. At the present

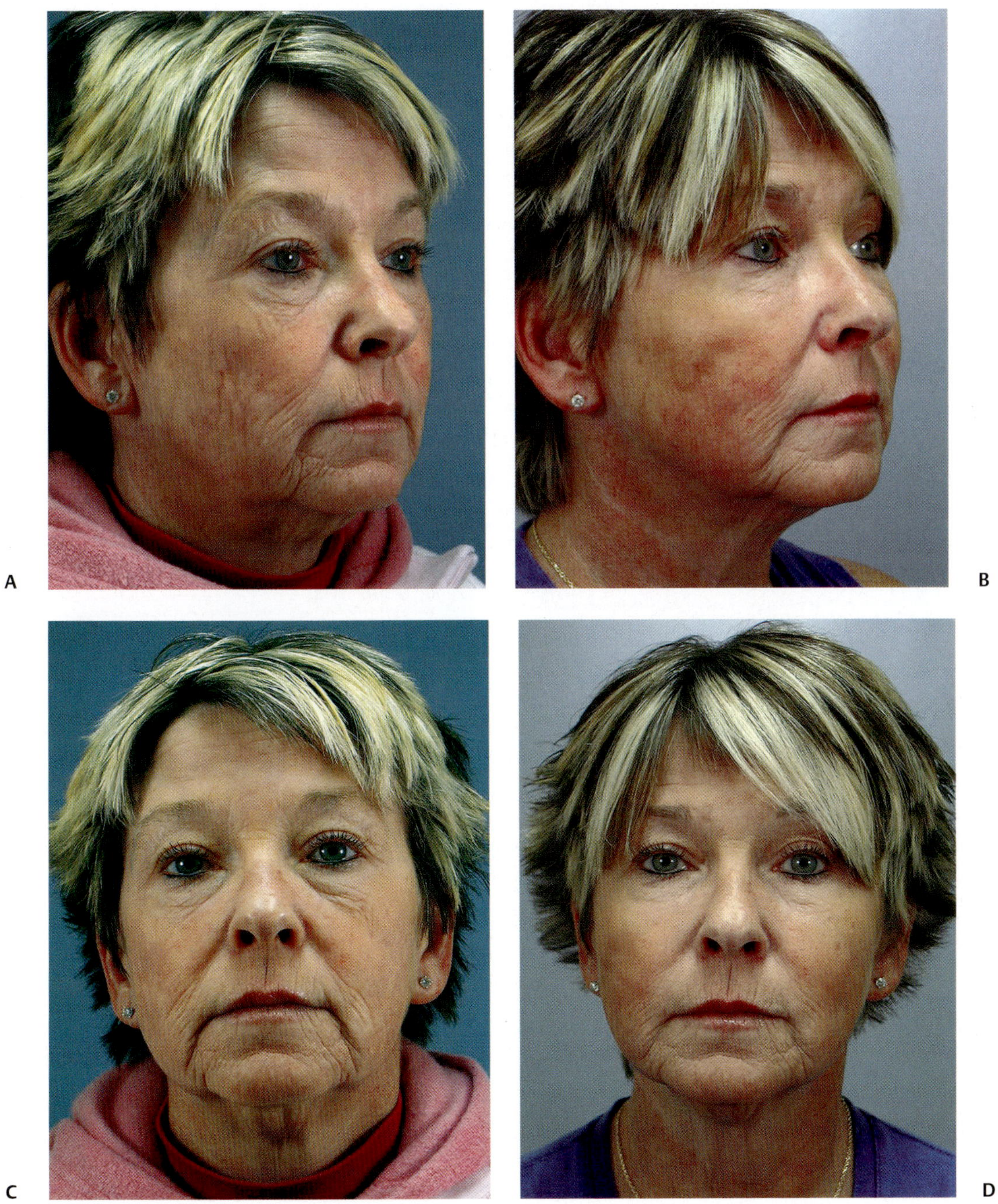

Fig. 7.15 Midfacial barbed suture suspension and lipotransfer: (**A**) preoperative oblique view; (**B**) postoperative oblique view. (**C**) preoperative frontal view; (**D**) postoperative frontal view.

time, it is difficult to ascertain whether the favorable results represent the benefit of lipotransfer independent of the thread lift. The senior author poses this question, as his results with isolated lipotransfer consistently exceed even the short-term benefits seen with thread lift alone for addressing midface aging.[29]

◆ Conclusion

Midfacial rejuvenation has long remained a challenge to the facial plastic surgeon, but only in the recent decade have effective techniques emerged. A handful of approaches and techniques have been employed by the senior author to address the characteristic changes of the aging midface, but only in the past several years does the senior author believe he has optimized his approach with the combination of brow-midface and lipotransfer. Other techniques may be evaluated in our practice, especially with the steady development of minimally invasive technologies, but until patient and surgeon satisfaction matches this surgeon's standard of care, patients must be counseled appropriately.

Acknowledgment Thank you to Samuel M. Lam, MD, Allison Pontius, MD, and Srini Krishna, MD.

References

1. Mendelson BC, Muzaffar AR, Adams WP Jr. Surgical anatomy of the midcheek and malar mounds. Plast Reconstr Surg 2002;110:885–896
2. Pessa JE, Zadoo VP, Mutimer KL. Relative maxillary retrusion as a natural consequence of aging: combining skeletal and soft-tissue changes into an integrated model of midfacial aging. Plast Reconstr Surg 1998;102:205–212
3. Ramirez OM. Full face rejuvenation in three dimensions: a "face-lifting" for the new millennium. Aesthetic Plast Surg 2001;25:152–164
4. Yousif NJ. Changes of the midface with age. Clin Plast Surg 1995;22: 213–226
5. Pontius AT, Williams EF. The extended minimal incision approach to midface rejuvenation. Facial Plast Surg Clin North Am 2005;13:411–419
6. Williams EF, Vargas H, Dahiya R, et al. Midfacial rejuvenation via a minimal-incision brow-lift approach: critical evaluation of a 5-year experience. Arch Facial Plast Surg 2003;5:470–478
7. Quatela VC, Jacono AA. The extended centrolateral endoscopic midface lift. Arch Facial Plast Surg 2003;19:199–207
8. Hamra ST. The deep-plane rhytidectomy. Plast Reconstr Surg 1990; 86:53–61
9. Hamra ST. Composite rhytidectomy. Plast Reconstr Surg 1992;90:1–13
10. Owsley JQ. Lifting the malar fat pad for correction of prominent nasolabial folds. Plast Reconstr Surg 1993;91:463–474
11. Hester TR Jr, Codner MA, McCord CD, et al. Evolution of technique of the direct transblepharoplasty approach for the correction of lower lid and midfacial aging: maximizing results and minimizing complications in a 5-year experience. Plast Reconstr Surg 2000;105:393–406
12. Gunter JP, Hackney FL. A simplified transblepharoplasty subperiosteal cheek lift. Plast Reconstr Surg 1999;103:2029–2041
13. Keller GS, Namazie A, Blackwell K, et al. Elevation of the malar fat pad with a percutaneous technique. Arch Facial Plast Surg 2002;4:20–25
14. Sulamanidze MA, Fournier PF, Paikidze TG, Sulamanidze GM. Removal of facial soft tissue ptosis with special threads. Dermatol Surg 2002; 28:367–371
15. Lycka B, Bazan C, Poletti E, Treen B. The emerging technique of the antiptosis subdermal suspension thread. Dermatol Surg 2004;30:41–44
16. Lee S, Isse N. Barbed polypropylene sutures for midface elevation: early results. Arch Facial Plast Surg 2005;7:55–61
17. Ellenbogen R. Free autogenous pearl fat grafts in the face: a preliminary report of a rediscovered technique. Ann Plast Surg 1986;16: 179–194
18. Illouz YG. Present results of fat injection. Aesthetic Plast Surg 1988; 12:175–181
19. Illouz YG. Adipoaspiration and "filling" in the face. Facial Plast Surg 1992;8:59–71
20. Coleman SR. Facial recontouring with lipostructure. Clin Plast Surg 1997;24:95–110
21. Amar RE. Microinfiltration adipocytaire (MIA) au niveau de la face, ou reconstruction tissulaire par greffe de tissue adipeux. Ann Chir Plast Esthet 1999;44:593–608
22. Muzaffar AR, Mendelson BC, Adams WP Jr. Surgical anatomy of the ligamentous attachments of the lower lid and lateral canthus. Plast Reconstr Surg 2002;110:873–884
23. Donofrio LM. Fat distribution: a morphologic study of the aging face. Dermatol Surg 2000;26:1107–1112
24. Lucarelli MJ, Khwarg SI, Lemke BN, et al. The anatomy of midfacial ptosis. Ophthal Plast Reconstr Surg 2000;16:7–22
25. Williams EF III, Lam SM. Upper and midfacial rejuvenation. In: Williams EF III, Lam SM, eds. Comprehensive Facial Rejuvenation: A Practical and Systematic Guide to Surgical Management of the Aging Face. Philadelphia, PA: Lippincott Williams & Wilkins; 2004: 54–84
26. Pontius AT, Williams EF. The evolution of midface rejuvenation: combining the midface-lift and fat transfer. Arch Facial Plast Surg 2006;8:300–305
27. Krishna S, Williams EF. Lipocontouring in conjunction with the minimal incision brow and subperiosteal midface lift: the next dimension in midface rejuvenation. Facial Plast Surg Clin North Am 2006;14: 221–228
28. Teimourian B. Blindness following fat injections. Plast Reconstr Surg 1988;82:361
29. Williams EF, Smith SP. Minimally invasive midfacial rejuvenation: combining thread-lift and lipotransfer. Facial Plast Surg Clin North Am 2007;15:209–219
30. Silva-Siwady JG, Díaz-Garza C, Ocampo-Candiani J. A case of Aptos thread migration and partial expulsion. Dermatol Surg 2005;31: 356–358

8

The Thread-Lift Technique of Cervico-Facial Lifting

David A. F. Ellis, Lorne Segall, and Kristina Zakhary

The first rhytidectomy procedures, reported as early as 1901, consisted of only elevation and redraping of the facial skin.[1] Since then, the concept of the cervico-facial rhytidectomy has evolved and improved. With the definition of the superficial musculoaponeurotic system (SMAS) in 1976 by Mitz and Peyronie and the increased understanding of facial anatomy and the pathophysiology of aging came an increased sophistication and complication of facelift surgery technique.[2] Cervico-facial rhytidectomy procedures began to involve larger incisions and more extensive soft tissue dissection.[3]

Recently, the pendulum has swung back, and patients have begun to seek minimally invasive approaches for cervico-facial rejuvenation, with more rapid healing and less risk of morbidity.[4–7] In fact, in the United States, the number of traditional plastic surgeries declined by 5% over the past 5 years, whereas minimally invasive cosmetic procedures increased by 53%, according to a report from the American Society of Plastic Surgeons.[4] Some patients would even readily accept a more subtle result in exchange for a rapid recovery and return to normal activities. This demand has prompted surgeons to develop techniques that can be performed in an outpatient setting and can achieve equally successful results with less aggressive procedures, smaller skin incisions, and shorter recovery times.[5–7] The ideal cervico-facial lifting procedure combines safety, minimal morbidity, and high patient satisfaction.[8]

Soft tissue suspension with barbed cables or sutures is a novel, minimally invasive technique for correction of face and neck involutional aging changes.[9] These sutures were popularized by Sulamanidze in the late 1990s and termed *Aptos* ("antiptosis") sutures or threads, but the patent is held by Ruff who concurrently developed these barbed threads in the early 1990s and named them Contour threads.[10–12]

The barbed polypropylene sutures must be inserted in the subdermal SMAS plane to elevate the brow, midface jowls, and neck and be fixed to the deeper fixed structures.[9] This provides an effective, relatively atraumatic method of correcting the facial soft tissue ptosis associated with aging. The suspension cables simplify the facial lifting procedures by shortening surgical incisions and eliminating the need for extensive undermining and surgical manipulation of the SMAS. This simplistic barbed suture suspension procedure can be performed under local anesthesia, through needle insertion into the subcutaneous tissue, and lifting with vectors of superoposterior suspension.[13] This reduces operative time, the need for intravenous anesthesia, postoperative recovery time, as well as the various risks of rhytidectomy complications including hematoma, flap necrosis, infection, nerve damage, and scarring.[14] The major benefits to the patient over the more traditional face- and neck lifting procedures include the lack of extensive tissue undermining and trauma and a lack of significant patient morbidity. The procedure is conservative and time-sparing, requiring less than an hour to perform, and allowing most patients to return to work immediately or within a few days.[15]

◆ The Aptos Thread

The Aptos thread (Kolster Methods, Anaheim, CA) was popularized by Sulamanidze in the late 1990s. The term *Aptos* is derived from the Greek words *anti* and *ptosis*.[10] The Aptos thread suspension is based on the concept that the skin can be lifted and held in a suspended position with barbs alone without affecting the underlying muscle or bone. It is essentially a 2-0 polypropylene, nylon suture with barbed projections in opposite directions that adheres to the dermis (**Fig. 8.1**).[11] The proximal side of an Aptos thread has barbs that extend forward in the direction of its movement through the tissue, and the distal side has barbs extending in the opposite direction, against the direction of the suture's movement through the tissue.

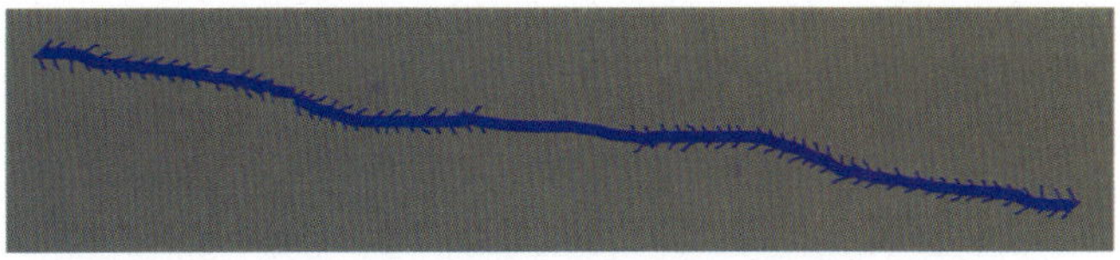

Fig. 8.1 Aptos suture with bidirectional barbs.

The bidirectional design of the suture barbs enables the suture to travel one way within the soft tissue and prevents the suture from moving in the opposite direction. This provides a uniform and symmetric gathering of the soft tissues, with the suture remaining fixed in a specific position, uplifting the soft tissue and creating a new facial contour.[10,11]

◆ The Contour Thread

Another device, the barbed Contour thread (Surgical Specialties Corp, Reading, PA), developed by Dr. Gregory Ruff who holds the patent, evolved in concept over the early 1990s. In 1995, the Contour thread received U.S. Food and Drug Administration approval in the United States for lifting of cheek, jowl, and brow.[12] Using the model of the porcupine quill, Ruff designed a multibarbed, unidirectional monofilament suture that maintains a grasp on soft tissue through an even, spiral distribution of barbs on each quill. The Contour thread is essentially a 25-cm 2-0 polypropylene barbed suture that is wedged onto a 7-inch straight needle with a tapered cutting tip on one end to facilitate suture passage through tissues. On the opposite end of the Contour thread is a 26-mm, 0.5 circle tapered needle, used for suture fixation (**Fig. 8.2**).[14] The Contour suture differs from the Aptos thread in that it has unidirectional barbs and is necessarily anchored superiorly to a fixed structure. More recently, double-armed Contour threads are available, which no longer need to be sutured to soft tissue or fascia for proximal support.

◆ A Physiologic Basis for Thread Lifting

In an attempt to clarify the mechanism of tissue ptosis correction by the barbed sutures, Sulamanidze and co-workers performed an experimental study of the tissue morphologic changes in response to implantation of barbed polypropylene sutures.[16] Histopathologic studies were performed in which barbed polypropylene sutures were inserted subdermally in rats and compared with nonbarbed polypropylene suture in control rats. The tissues were examined with special stains for collagen, fibroblasts, and vascular response, with serial skin biopsies taken regularly for up to 6 months. A difference was noted between the barbed suture and its control, in that the smooth nonbarbed polypropylene suture elicited minimal or no vascular, inflammatory, fibroblastic, or collagen response. The barbed suture, in contrast, demonstrated an early inflammatory response followed by a vascular proliferation and fibroblastic reaction, which created a collagen cuff with laterally extending bands around the barbs. It was concluded that this collagen cuff accounted for the maintenance of the grip of the barbs to the subdermal tissues and the correction of soft tissue ptosis. It was also postulated that cervico-facial immobilization after suspension cable placement was necessary in order to allow initiation and early maturation of the collagen response.[16] Further studies were performed to evaluate the tensile strength of the barbed sutures, which demonstrated that they can maintain greater tensile strength measured in pounds per square inch (4 to 5 lb/in^2).[17] These results form the basis for the scientific principle behind the clinical results seen with the barbed suspension cables.

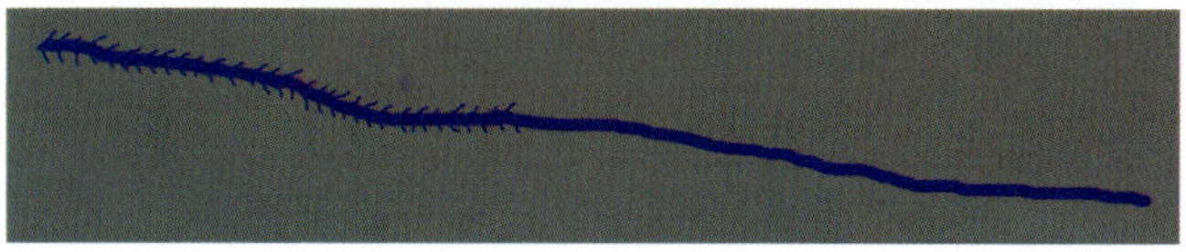

Fig. 8.2 Contour suture with unidirectional barbs.

◆ Indication for the Thread-Lift Procedure

1. The correction of cervico-facial ptosis with *only* cable suspension sutures is indicated in select patients who were reluctant to undergo traditional face and neck lift procedures.
2. The thread-lift procedure can be used as an adjunct to SMAS imbrication in patients undergoing cervico-facial rhytidectomy.

◆ Head and Neck Sites Amenable to Thread Lifting

1. Nasolabial (lip-cheek) groove
2. Melomental groove
3. Lateral eyebrow
4. Platysmal bands in the neck

◆ Patient Selection

The ideal patient is either a younger person who does not have a full face with heavy soft tissues, many rhytides, and much redundant skin, or a facelift patient whose surgical result may be enhanced or further supported by the placement of these subdermal suspension cables. Patients with excessive skin redundancy and heavy, ptotic facial and/or neck soft tissue are not suitable candidates for the cable suspension technique as the sole procedure due to poor longevity of results and a higher risk for complications. These patients would most likely be best treated by other cervico-facial rejuvenation modalities, such as more traditional facelifting procedure and/or laser skin resurfacing techniques.

◆ Surgical Procedure

Preoperative Marking and Anesthesia

A map of vectors is marked on the patient's face and neck while the patient is in a seated position to determine the pathways of the suspension cables and the number of

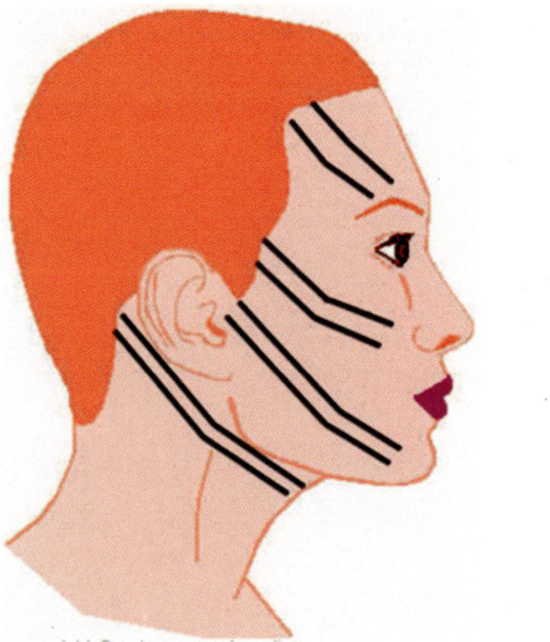

Fig. 8.3 Examples of marking the vector of pull of the suspension cables.

cables needed to obtain the necessary elevation (**Fig. 8.3**). The surgical site is prepped with chlorhexidine, and the procedure is performed in a sterile fashion. Appropriate surgical drapes are placed.

Local anesthesia is used; 1.0% lidocaine with 1:100,000 epinephrine solution is administered subdermally at the area of the entry of the suspension cable, along the area of the cable passage, and at the exit site. An average of 0.5 to 1 mol of local anesthesia is used for each suspension cable. This is sufficient anesthesia for painless placement of the suspension suture. When the suspension cables are placed in conjunction with cervico-facial rhytidectomy, the procedure is performed under either intravenous sedation or total intravenous anesthesia.

Thread-Lifting Using the Aptos Threads

After administration of anesthesia, a small, 1-cm transverse skin incision is made at the proximal aspect of the cable entry site, and the 8.5-cm-long Aptos suture is introduced into the subcutaneous tissue, 1 to 2 mm deep to the skin, through an 18-gauge or 20-gauge spinal needle, from the superior point of suspension and advanced along the mapped pathway with a serpentine pattern (**Fig. 8.4**). This changing of direction is meant to increase the tissue area of barbed contact and create a stronger barbed attachment. The Aptos suture within the subdermally placed spinal needle is advanced to the lower limits of ptotic tissue, exiting the skin beyond the area of desired lift. As the spinal needle is removed, the inferior portion of protruding thread is clamped with a hemostat for security. After this, superoposterior traction is placed on the suture proximally, and the ptotic tissue is compressed upward against the direction of the suture barbs, allowing the barbs to open up and adhere to the lifted subcutaneous tissue (**Fig. 8.5**). This holds the tissue in the new elevated position. The proximal portion of the Aptos suture is threaded through a 26-mm, 0.5 circle tapered Keith needle, and is anchored to the temporoparietal fascia, mastoid fascia, or parietal periosteum to support the following areas: bucco-zygomatic, melomental, jowls, neck, or lateral eyebrow, respectively (**Fig. 8.6**).

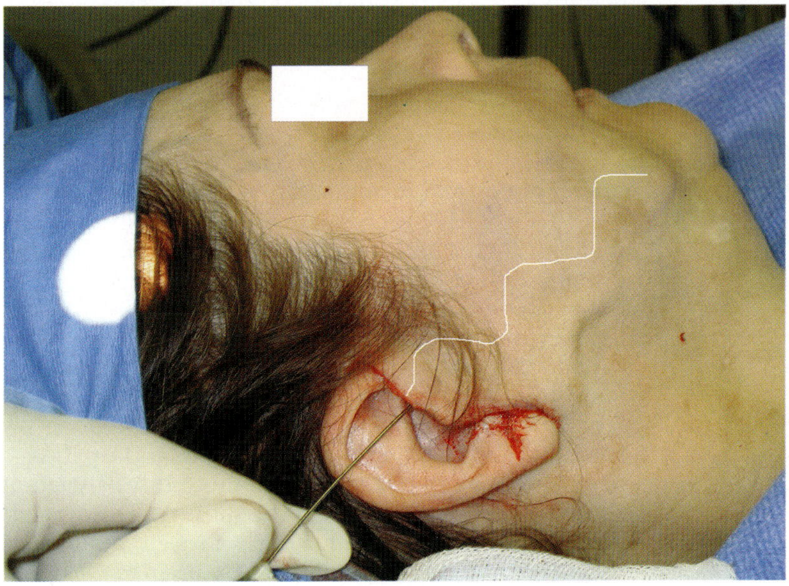

Fig. 8.4 Serpentine insertion of suspension cable through a small incision.

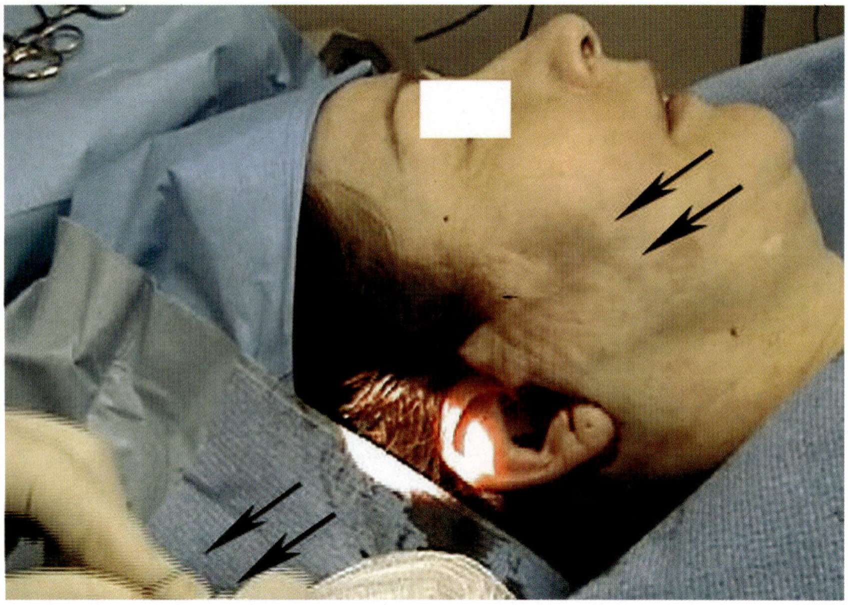

Fig. 8.5 Superoposterior traction placed on the suture proximally and the ptotic tissue compressed upward.

Thread-Lifting Using the Contour Threads

The contour threads are inserted through an initial skin incision made superiorly, and the straight needles are threaded through the subcutaneous tissue in a serpentine pattern and exit the skin immediately distal to the area to be lifted (**Fig. 8.4**). The sutures are used in pairs with the pathways descending anteroinferiorly in an inverted "U" pattern. Each pair of threads is sutured to each other proximally. At this superior point, the curved fixation needle is used to anchor the sutures in the temporal fascia, mastoid fascia, or parietal periosteum, depending on the areas to be lifted. As the threads are pulled downward, the tissues to be lifted are massaged upward (i.e., "contoured") into the proper position.

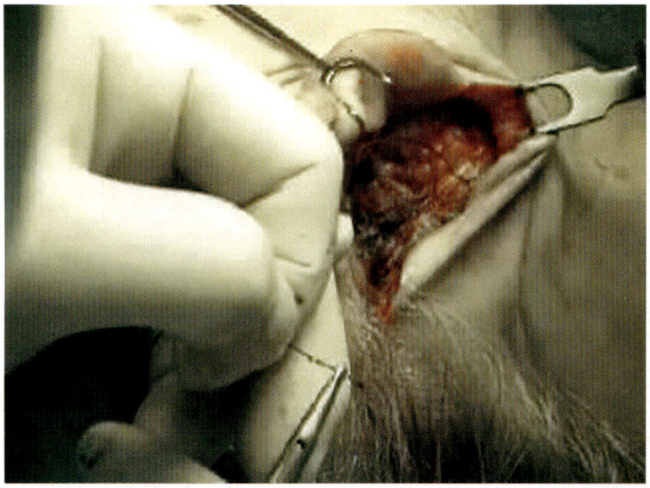

Fig. 8.6 Suture the proximal cable to a fixed structure such as mastoid fascia.

Final Adjustments

The suspension cables are then adjusted for symmetry and natural appearance, with the patient awake, in a seated position, while checking for patient approval and satisfaction. Once satisfactory results are achieved, the distal protruding portion of the suspension cables are cut at the skin surface and tucked into the subcutaneous tissues. In more recent cases when the thread-lift is performed in conjunction with surgery, we have a small segment of the distal suture (~3 cm) protruding from the skin, so that final adjustments, contour tightening, and trimming of the suture can be performed on the 3rd to 5th postoperative day once some of the tissue edema has resolved. In these cases, the distal ends of the barbed suture are covered with Steri-Strips (3M, St. Paul, MN). The proximal incision is then closed with skin sutures. Finally, a protective gauze or Ace bandage (BD, Franklin Lakes, NJ) is applied to immobilize the tissues.

◆ Postoperative Care

Postoperatively, the patients are advised to avoid excessive facial animation and manipulation for 2 weeks in order to prevent dislodging of the barbs and negatively affecting the correction. This is especially important in women during the application of makeup. Mild postoperative analgesics (acetaminophen with codeine) are given. No postoperative antibiotics are routinely administered.

For patients in whom the barbed sutures were left protruding from the skin distally, follow-up visits occur on the 3rd to 5th postoperative days. In these patients, the involved soft tissue is lifted and adjusted under the patient's supervision. Then the distal ends of the sutures are cut at the skin surface and tucked into the subcutaneous tissues.

All patients are then seen postoperatively at 1 week, 2 weeks, 1 month, and then every 6 months up to 1 year.

◆ Our Thread-Lift Results

From July 2004 until July 2005, 87 patients underwent this procedure, with a total of 299 cable-lifting suture placements. The patients ranged from 37 to 75 years of age, with the mean age of the patients being 58 years. The majority of these patients were women (88.1%). Of our patients, 61 underwent placement of the suspension cables as the sole method of cervico-facial lifting (208 cables). The other 26 patients had the suspension cables placed as an adjunct to other cervico-facial rhytidectomy procedures, such as facelift or neck lift (91 cables). Suspension cables as the sole method of cervico-facial lifting were performed in less than an hour.

This method was mostly used to correct ptosis of the bucco-zygomatic areas (27%) (**Fig. 8.7A, B**), anterior neck platysma bands (25.4%) (**Fig. 8.7C, D**), melomental soft

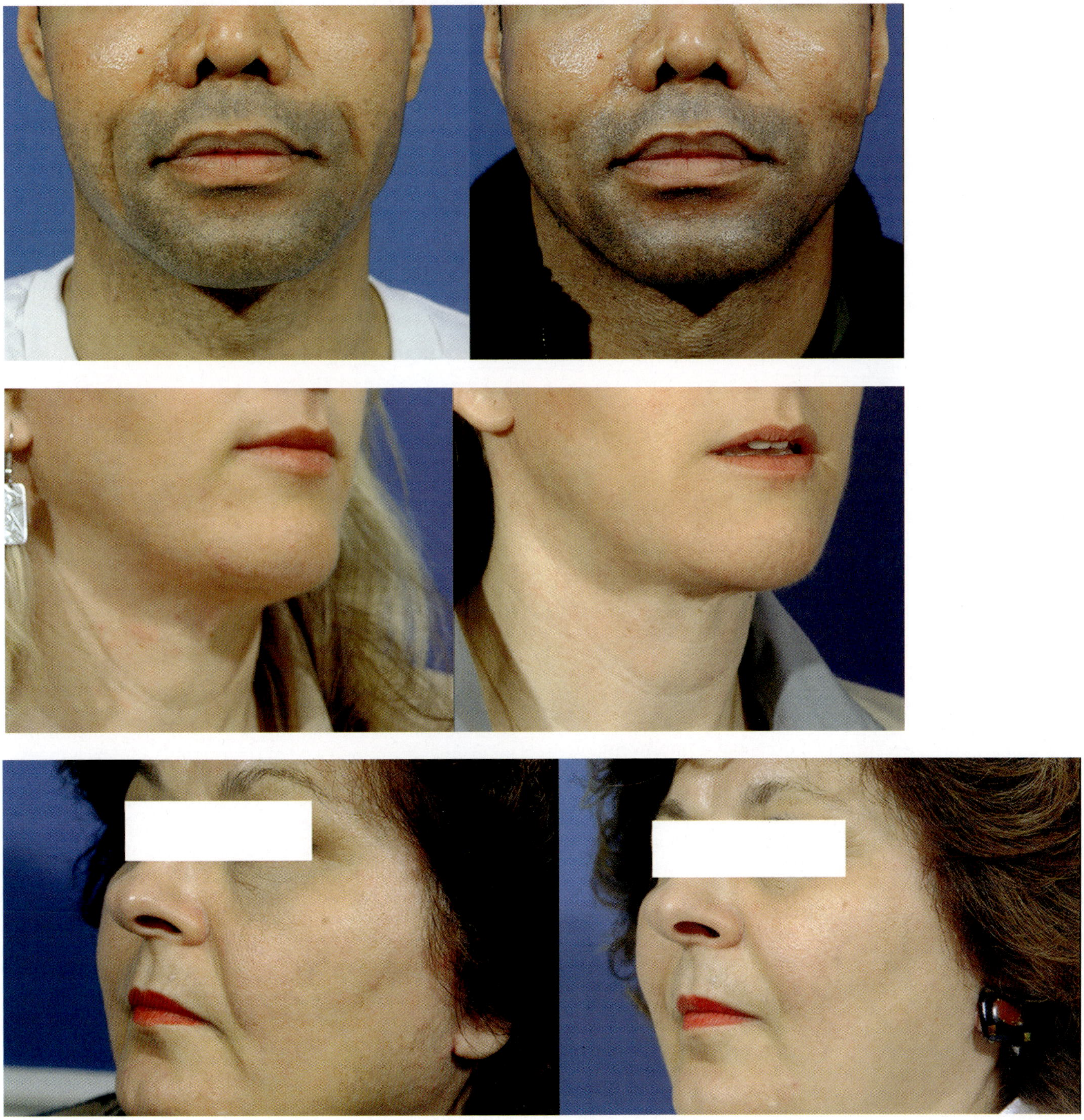

A–B

C–D

E–F

Fig. 8.7 Bucco-zygomatic tissue ptosis correction with suspension cables (**A**) before and (**B**) after. Neck platysma band correction with suspension cables (**C**) before and (**D**) after. Melomental fold correction with suspension cables (**E**) before and (**F**) after.

(Continued on page 96)

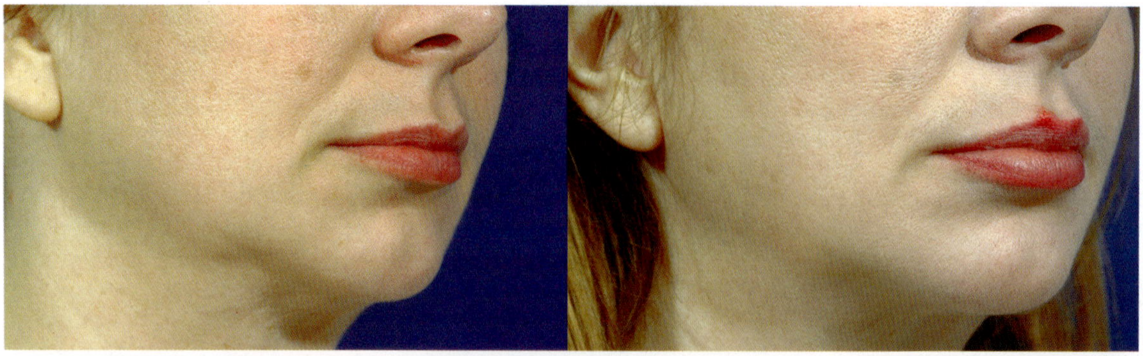

G–H

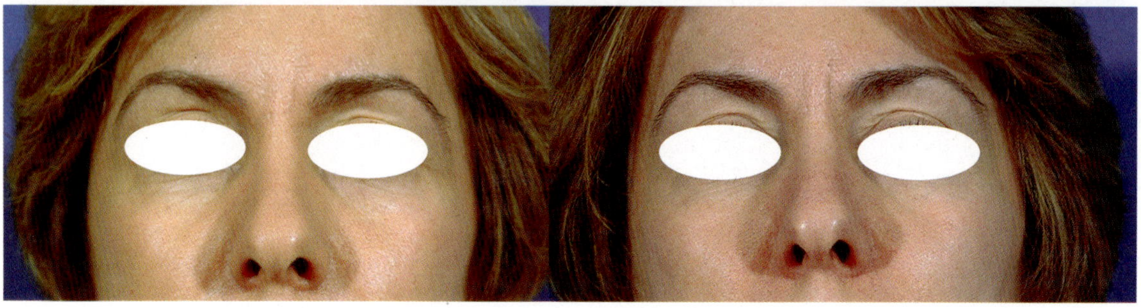

I–J

Fig. 8.7 *(Continued)* Jowl correction with suspension cables (**G**) before and (**H**) after. Asymmetric left eyebrow correction with suspension cables (**I**) before and (**J**) after.

tissues (21.4%) (**Fig. 8.7E, F**), jowls (19%) (**Fig. 8.7G, H**), and lateral eyebrow (7.1%) (**Fig. 8.7I, J**).

In all cases, the visible facial rejuvenation was seen immediately with an initial 100% patient satisfaction rate, and the patients who underwent suspension cable lifting alone were able to return to work within 1 to 2 days.

◆ Patient Satisfaction

In general, our patients were satisfied with the procedure. In total, 49.4% of our patients described a very favorable improvement, 26.7% described an acceptable improvement, and 23% were not satisfied with their improvement. In the group who underwent the thread lift as the sole cosmetic procedure, the majority of the patients were very satisfied with the cosmetic outcome (**Fig. 8.8**). The authors' experience with this technique suggests that it can work as a solitary procedure or can be combined with other procedures, including traditional cervico-facial lifting techniques, to support the lift and obtain optimal results. It is, however, technique sensitive and does require proper training and experience.

The true test of the procedure, however, is patient satisfaction. Because the facial plastic surgeon's success depends on patient satisfaction, treatment plans to correct the effects of the aging face should be developed while considering the patient's concerns and expectations.[18] Perhaps the high satisfaction rate with the cable suspension techniques stems from the desire, in an increasingly prominent segment of the population, for positive results combined with the efficacy, relatively low morbidity, and minimal downtime offered by this procedure.

◆ Longevity

To determine the longevity of the cable suspension procedure, we followed our patients for a period up to 21 months. Most patients have maintained 85 to 100% of the correction achieved at the time of surgery. Most cases of treatment failure occurred in patients who were older than 50 years of age. We did notice that forehead suspension had a poor longevity with a high rate of treatment failure by 6 months after the procedure, unlike other head and neck sites.

Both Sulamanidze and Lycka reported in two independent series that the cosmetic correction can been maintained for 2 to 3 years if early immobilization is achieved.[11,13] These results are promising, but further studies are still needed to determine the best areas for treatment and the optimal technique to maximize the longevity of the results.

◆ Complications Involving the Thread-Lift Procedure

Numerous complications are possible, including:

1. Bleeding related (hematoma, bruising)
2. Infection (cellulites, abscess)

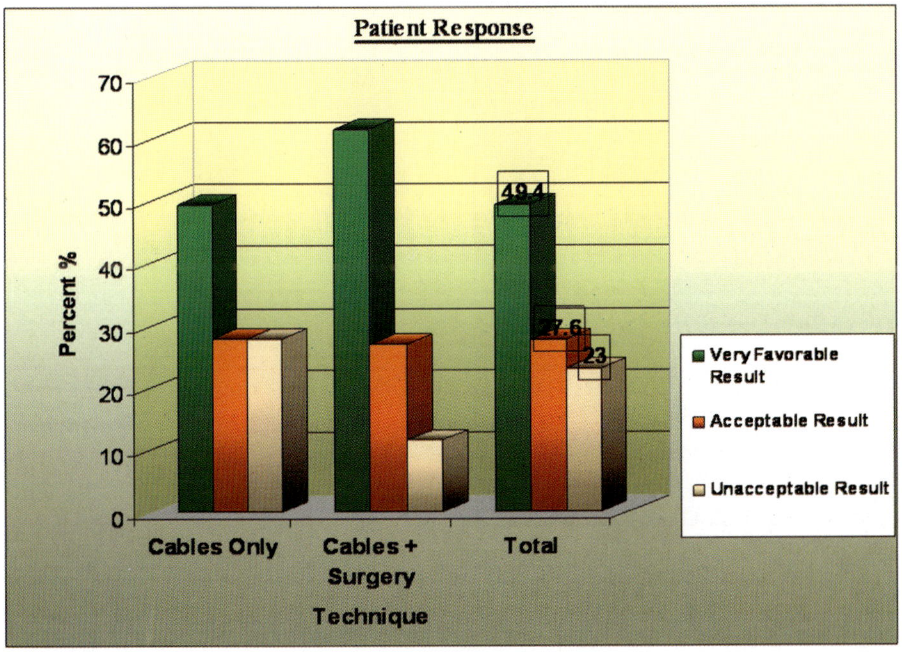

Fig. 8.8 Patient response bar graph.

3. Seroma
4. Contour irregularities (dimpling, visible cables, asymmetry, palpable suture knot)
5. Nerve injury
6. Scarring (hypertrophy, hyperpigmentation)
7. Fracturing of suture with extrusion

The risks associated with the procedure, however, are low compared with those of other existing procedures. There are a few minor complications, which can occur in the immediate postoperative period, but these usually resolve spontaneously within the first 2 weeks. These minor complications may include asymmetry, visible threads, palpable knots, dimpling, suture breakage, and prolonged ecchymosis.

Symmetry problems must be addressed at the conclusion of surgery and during early postoperative visits by using gentle tissue manipulation to correct an overly corrected side. It is important to assess the patient during the first week to evaluate the results. Suspension cables may be visible early on, especially in a patient with thin skin and little subcutaneous tissue and when using the blue-colored Aptos threads. This usually improves spontaneously within the first 2 weeks. If it persists to the patient's dissatisfaction after 2 weeks, the barbed suture can be removed. Suture migration or splitting at the skin surface has been seen. This can be corrected by easily removing the extruded portion and then replacing it with another barbed suture.

In our experience, in the immediate postoperative period, there were a total of 36 complications (16.1%). These included 5 cases of seroma or hematoma (5.7%) and other minor complications including 1 cable suture that produced prolonged bruising (0.3%); 12 cables that were visible (4.0%), meaning that the pathway of the suspension cable was discernible subcutaneously; 8 cables that caused dimpling (2.7%); 4 cables that fractured and broke intraoperatively (1.3%); and finally, 2 cases of asymmetry (0.7%) occurred, which necessitated revision of the procedure and placement of additional suspension cables. Most of these complications resolved spontaneously within 2 weeks, and in the cases of persistent dimpling, temporary injectable fillers were used to correct the dimples. There were no observed complications of infection or significant postoperative pain. In the month after the procedure, 54 cables (18.1%) fractured and migrated to the skin surface, requiring removal and performance of a second procedure to replace the extruded cable. All of the cases of cable extrusion occurred in patients with fuller, heavier cervico-facial soft tissue and/or significant skin redundancy. Most of the cases of suspension cable extrusion (25.6%) occurred with placement of the larger Aptos cables in the first 9 months of the study. The extrusion rate decreased steadily over the following 12 months, dropping to 9.1% in the final 6 months of the study with the use of the Coherent suspension sutures (**Fig. 8.9**).

Complications with Cable Suspension Alone

When the suspension cables were used as the sole method of cervico-facial lifting, there were no major complications. In the immediate 14-day postoperative period, minor complications included 1 cable suture that caused prolonged ecchymosis (0.5%); 6 cables that were visible (2.9%); 8 cables that caused dimpling (3.8%) necessitating deep dermal fillers to temporarily correct the dimples; 4 cables that broke intraoperatively (1.9%) and were replaced immediately; and finally, 2 cases of asymmetry (3.3%), which required revision of the procedure and placement of additional cables. These minor

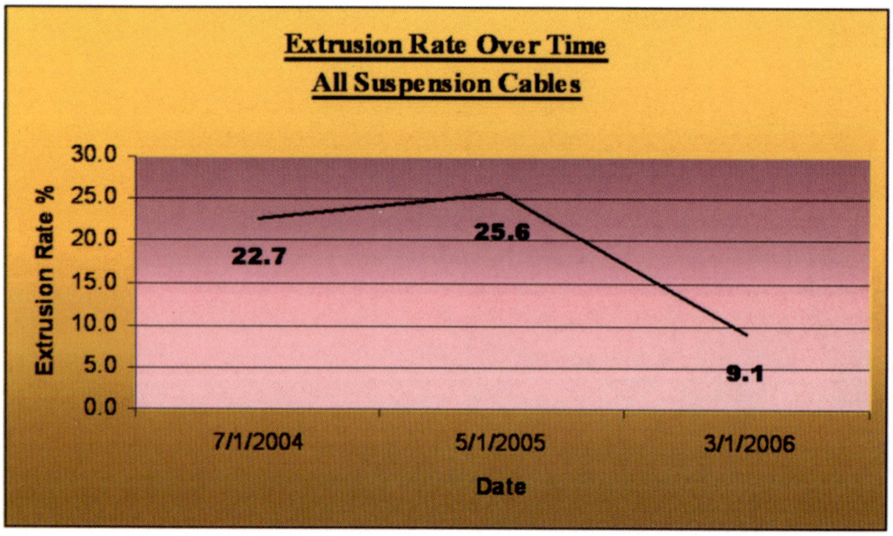

Fig. 8.9 Extrusion rate over time: all suspension cables.

complications resolved spontaneously after 2 weeks. In the month after the procedure, 48 cables (23.1%) disrupted and extruded through the skin, requiring a second procedure to replace the extruded cable. Most of the cases of suspension cable extrusion (33.3%) occurred during the first month after the procedure and decreased steadily over the next 12 months, dropping to a 12.9% extrusion rate in the final 6 months of the study (**Fig. 8.10**).

Complications with Cable Suspension in Conjunction with Surgery

When the suspension cables were used in conjunction with other cervico-facial surgical rejuvenation techniques such as a facelift or neck lift, major complications included two seromas (7.7%) and three hematomas (11.5%). In the immediate 14-day postoperative period, the only minor complication involved six visible cables (6.6%), which resolved spontaneously within 2 weeks. There were no observed cases of dimpling, broken cables, asymmetry, or infection. In the month after the procedure, six cables (6.6%) disrupted and migrated to the skin surface. Again, most of the cable extrusions occurred in the first 9 months with the use of the Aptos cables (34.9%), dropping to a 5.4% extrusion rate in the final 6 months of the study with the use of Coherent cables.

◆ Conclusion

The latest trend in facial plastic surgery has been to use minimally invasive treatments to correct the aging face and neck. A recent innovation in minimally invasive facial rejuvenation has focused on the use of modified polypropylene barbed sutures to treat soft tissue ptosis in

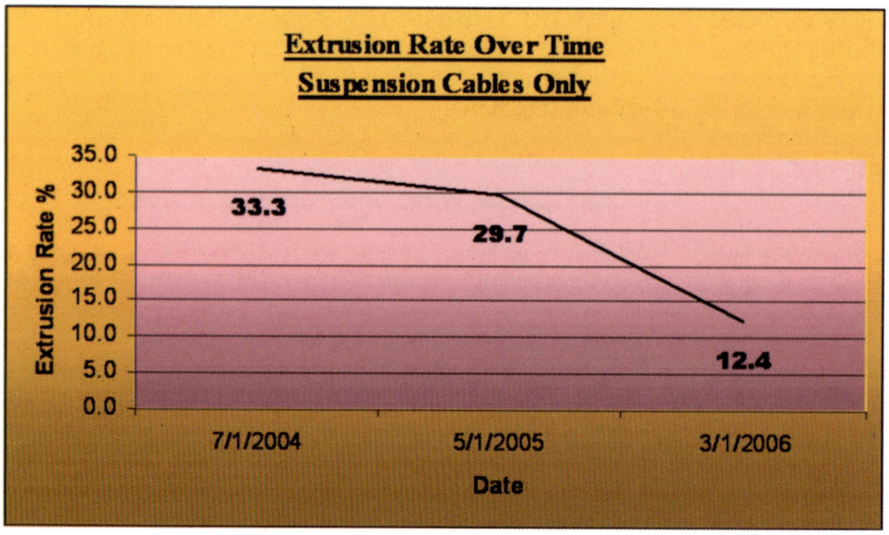

Fig. 8.10 Extrusion rate over time: suspension cables only.

the cervico-facial region. It is a simple and conservative procedure that is becoming increasingly popular among patients who are searching for results with minimal morbidity and downtime. These procedures can be performed alone under local anesthesia or as an adjunct to traditional face and neck lifting procedures to achieve optimal results. Further scientific study and clinical experience will determine optimal technique for placement of the suspension cables and their role in the myriad of other facial rejuvenation techniques.

Patient selection plays a pivotal role in achieving both successful results and patient satisfaction with this treatment, like any other cosmetic surgical procedure. The thread-lifting technique has a role in facial rejuvenation when used for the proper indications in properly selected patients. The use of these polypropylene barbed sutures as a single procedure does not replace the traditional cervico-facial lifting procedures and should not be performed in patients who would best be treated with a facelift procedure.

References

1. Passot R. La chirugie esthetique des rides du visage. Presse Med 1919;27:258–262
2. Mitz V, Peyronie M. The superficial musculoaponeurotic system (SMAS) in the parotid and cheek area. Plast Reconstr Surg 1976;58:80–88
3. Ivy EJ, Lorenc ZP, Aston SJ. Is there a difference? A prospective study comparing lateral and standard SMAS face lifts with extended SMAS and composite rhytidectomies. Plast Reconstr Surg 1996;98:1135–1143
4. Peck P. Nearly four million Botox treatments performed in a year. MedPageToday 2006;March 16
5. Ansari P. Elimination of the retroauricular incision in face-lifts. Aesthetic Surg J 2003;23:14–19
6. Baker DC. Minimal incision rhytidectomy (short scar face-lift) with lateral SMASectomy. Aesthetic Surg J 2001;21:68–79
7. Saylan Z. The S-lift: less is more. Aesthetic Surg J 1999;19:406–409
8. Hamra ST. Discussion: is there a difference? A prospective study comparing lateral and standard SMAS face lifts and extended SMAS and composite rhytidectomies. Plast Reconstr Surg 1996;98:1144–1147
9. Lee S, Isse N. Barbed polypropylene sutures for midface elevation: early results. Arch Facial Plast Surg 2005;7:55–61
10. Sulamanidze MA, Fournier PF, Paikidze TG, et al. Removal of facial soft tissue ptosis with special threads. Dermatol Surg 2002;28:367–371
11. Sulamanidze MA, Paikidze TG, Sulamanidze GM, et al. Facial lifting with "APTOS" threads: featherlift. Otolaryngol Clin North Am 2005;38:1109–1117
12. Leung JC, Ruff GL, Megaro MA. Barbed, bi-directional medical sutures: biomechanical properties and wound closure efficacy study. Presented at: Society for Biomaterials 28th Annual Meeting; April 25, 2002; Tampa, FL
13. Lycka B, Bazan C, Poletti E, et al. The emerging technique of the antiptosis subdermal suspension thread. Dermatol Surg 2004;30:41–44
14. Monheit GD. Suspension for the aging face. Dermatol Clin 2005;23:561–573
15. McCarty ML, Brackup AB. Minimal incision facelift surgery. Ophthalmol Clin North Am 2005;18:305–310
16. Sulamanidze M, Sulamanidze G. Experimental morphological and functional feasibility study of the Aptos method. Dermatol Surg 2004;30:48–56
17. Silva SJG, Ocampo CJ. Correccion de flacidez facial con hilos APTOS. Dermalogica CMQ 2003;1:224–229
18. Zide BM. What you can do is not what they want. Plast Reconstr Surg 2003;111:1753–1755

9

Facial Skeletal Implants

Michael S. Godin and Jason S. Hamilton

The ability to augment cosmetically deficient areas of the face is a powerful tool for the facial plastic surgeon to employ. The surgeon may spend hours improving the nose, for example, only to later find that the greatest cosmetic benefit he gave the patient at surgery was the chin implant, which took less than 30 minutes to place. Aging face surgery often *turns back time*, generally by resuspending fallen tissues in a more youthful position and removing the sagging excess. Facial skeletal implants can actually *stop time* by providing a permanent augmentation that will not change as the patient ages.

What follows is a description of the more common ways implants are used to augment the facial skeleton. For the purposes of this discussion, synthetic implants will be emphasized. The surgeon must always realize that biologic alternatives such as autologous (derived from the patient), homologous (derived from other humans or cadavers), and xenographic (derived from animals) implants are usually available and must be considered.[1] Such materials include bone, cartilage, dermis, dermal fat, free autologous fat, and acellular dermis.

Prior to considering the variety of materials available for implantation into the human face, it is valuable to consider what the qualities of the ideal implant material would be (**Table 9.1**). When selecting a material for implantation, the surgeon is wise to consider how it measures up against such a list of characteristics, bearing in mind the context in which it is to be used.

The material should first and foremost be highly compatible with any type of tissue into which it is likely to be placed. These tissues are bone, muscle, fat, dermis, and occasionally the submucosa of the oral or nasal cavity epithelium. The material should be readily available and not prohibitively expensive. It should not be capable of transmitting disease, which is to say that if it is derived from an animal or human source, steps must have been taken to ensure that the material cannot harbor bacteria, viruses, or prion proteins. The implant material should be inherently resistant to infection. It must feel natural in the area it is placed. It is ideal if the implant will fix in place strongly enough to prevent migration but not so much that it cannot be removed if infection necessitating its removal occurs.[2] The ideal material would be easy to shape and secure. Finally, the ideal implant material would have a long history of safety and longevity after implantation into human tissue.

Table 9.1 Ideal Implant Characteristics

Biocompatible
Natural feel
Resistant to infection
Not capable of transmitting disease
Resistant to migration
Readily retrievable
Easy to shape and secure
Long record of safety and reliability

◆ Choice of Materials

A great variety of synthetic materials have been used to augment the face with varying degrees of success, including paraffin wax, metals, ceramics, and plastic polymers.[3] Though the focus of this chapter is on indications for and techniques of implant insertion, a description of the more commonly used synthetic implants follows.

Silastic (Polymethyl Silicone)

Silastic (Dow Corning, Midland, MI), or solid silicone, is a high-viscosity, vulcanized form of dimethylsiloxane, which is the repeating unit in injectable medical grade silicone.[4] Silastic is well tolerated by the body, which forms a fibrous capsule around the implant shortly after it is placed. While the Silastic is encased in the capsule, it is not bound to it in any way, and therefore displacement of the implant is possible. Persistent seromas have also been reported,[4] and these in combination with the lack of firm fixation may lead to extrusion, especially after implantation into the nose or auricle.[5] Despite these concerns, Silastic remains a popular choice for nasal augmentation, especially in Asian countries. It certainly may be easily shaped, and fenestrated implants that allow ingrowth of fibrous tissue for stabilization have been manufactured. Silastic is manufactured in varying degrees of firmness, known as *durometers*. A 10-durometer implant is often chosen for mandibular augmentation.[3]

Gore-Tex (Expanded Polytetrafluoroethylene)

At the time of this writing, W.L. Gore (Flagstaff, AZ), the manufacturers of Gore-Tex, have announced the decision to discontinue the manufacture of Gore-Tex implants for facial cosmetic and reconstructive applications. According to company officials, this decision reflected no problems with clinical use of the material or, for that matter, with its popularity. The company will continue to manufacture expanded polytetrafluoroethylene (e-PTFE) for medical use and has shifted its entire focus to cardiac and vascular surgery applications. This comes as a bit of bad news for surgeons, the authors of this chapter included, who have come to rely on e-PTFE as a facial skeletal implant because of its excellent durability, natural feel, supreme ease of contouring, and biocompatibility. Gore-Tex is microporous, with an average internodal space of 30 μm, which allows sufficient ingrowth of tissue to prevent migration while preventing more robust tissue incorporation, as would occur with a porous implant or mesh material. Therefore, if there is a problem necessitating removal, it can be removed without undue trauma to surrounding tissues. Gore-Tex does well on bone and when contacting fat or muscle. It should not be placed in contact with dermis as an inflammatory reaction frequently occurs. Gore-Tex has been used successfully in nasal augmentation with follow-up of more than 10 years reported.[6] It also has an enviable record of reliability in chin augmentation. A 2003 report of pooled data by six facial plastic surgeons revealed a complication rate of less than 1% in 324 patients.[7] Gore-Tex has been an excellent implant material that is close to the ideal in many ways. It is hoped that a similar type of implant will become widely available to take its place.

Medpor (Porous High-Density Polyethylene)

Medpor (porous high-density polyethylene [HDPE]; Porex Surgical, Newnan, GA) is a firm skeletal implant material with pore size in the 100-μm range and a pore volume in the range of 50%, as measured by mercury intrusion porosimetry.[8] Medpor can be carved with a standard surgical blade, and thin sheets of it may be sutured together to add thickness where desired. It is available in blocks and sheets. The material's shape can be molded by submersing it in hot sterile saline (above 180°F per the manufacturer) for several minutes then bending it to the desired shape and allowing it to cool. The use of a cold sterile saline bath can accelerate the cooling process.[8] Romo et al reported good results using HDPE in 187 rhinoplasty patients. Both primary and revision cases were included, and follow-up ranged up to 3.5 years. Five (2.6%) of the implants required removal due to infection or breakdown of overlying skin.[9]

Of the implants described, HDPE is the only one that can truly become a *skeletal* implant. Osseous ingrowth occurs with mature bone existing in the surface pores at approximately 1 year after implantation.[2] At this point, the hard implant is essentially a fixed extension of the bone and is not subject to displacement, which occurs more frequently with the Silastic material.

◆ Chin Augmentation

If a facial plastic surgeon were allowed to incorporate only one area of facial skeletal augmentation into his or her practice, that surgeon would be wise to choose the chin. Placement of such an implant in a patient with chin retrusion works wonders in improving appearance. Bringing the chin forward can balance the facial profile, changing what is a convex shape in the lower face to a straighter, more aesthetic one. **Figure 9.1** illustrates this point. Augmentation of the chin can balance the appearance of a strong nasal profile. The large nose is made to look less imposing because it is balanced by more projection in the lower face. Chin augmentation is also a powerful tool in aging face surgery. When a retrusive chin is augmented, there is a lengthening of the entire jawline. The geometry of the cervicomental angle is altered, and a more aesthetic neck and jawline appearance emerges. **Figure 9.2** illustrates this effect in a patient who underwent revision rhinoplasty. The only other procedure performed was the chin implant. The effect on the cervicomental angle is readily apparent.

A chin implant can also greatly improve the effect of a facelift in the properly selected patient. By lengthening the short jawline, the surgeon has a better framework on which to position the facial soft tissues. **Figure 9.3** demonstrates the use of mental augmentation in a facelift patient with a retrusive chin. The lengthening of the jawline and forward pull on the submental skin clearly contributes to the positive quality of the result. **Figure 9.4** illustrates how the chin implant may be used in a patient with a more normally projecting chin who has a very difficult neck and desires as much improvement as the surgeon can possibly give. In this instance, bringing the anterior projection of the chin forward creates the platform on which through submental liposuction and firm posterior and superior repositioning of the platysma muscle a significant change in the cervicomental angle can be established.

Operative Technique

A pertinent history and physical examination should be performed. In the course of this preoperative analysis, the physician may perceive that the chin is underprojected and that augmentation may be called for, even thought the patient may not realize this. In this case, the surgeon should examine the patient's dental occlusion and ask about problems pertaining to temporomandibular joint (TMJ) function. Pain on chewing, popping or cracking noises emanating from the TMJ area with mouth opening or closing, or even chronic headache can all be signs that there is a problem

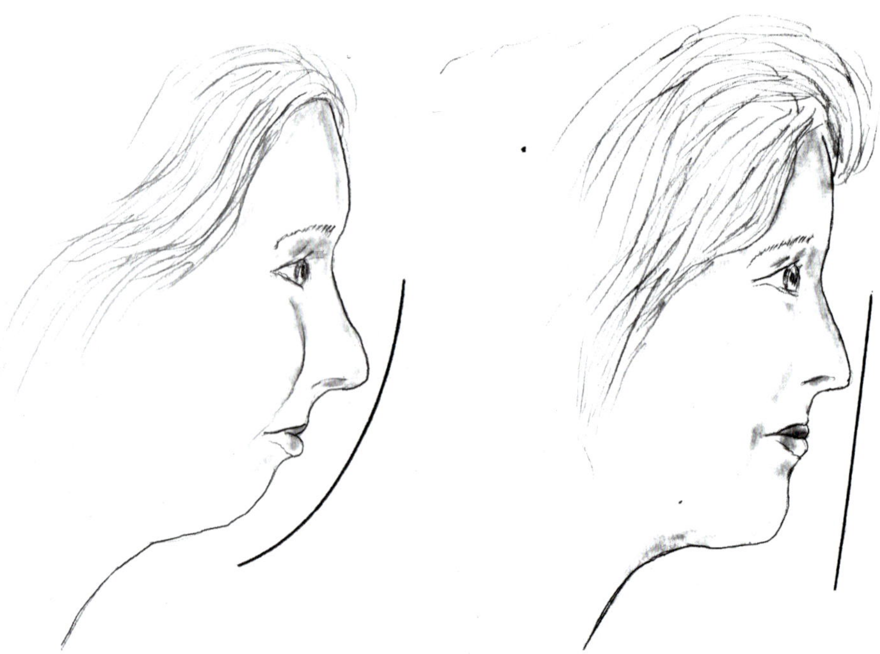

A

B

Fig. 9.1 (**A**) Convexity of the facial profile is aesthetically undesirable. (**B**) A chin implant can help straighten the profile and improve appearance.

with the patient's bite. If this is the case, the patient requires referral to an oral/maxillofacial surgeon for evaluation of the relationship between the maxilla and mandible and perhaps orthognathic surgery.

A complete set of photographs (front, oblique, and lateral views) should be taken and reviewed with the patient as part of the consultation. It is vital that these be shot with the patient's head in level position to avoid misjudging the projection of the mentum relative to the rest of the face. The patient should be lined up in the Frankfort plane, whereby the top of the external auditory canal is at the same height as the inferior orbital rim. When looking at the soft tissues, this equates to the top of the tragus being at the same height as where the bony orbital rim is seen or palpated to be. The lateral view is the most powerful tool to demonstrate to the patient, when appropriate, that the chin is retrusive and that an implant may be helpful. Before-and-after views of patients for whom the surgeon has performed such an implant will serve well to demonstrate the profound effect the procedure can have. Front and lateral

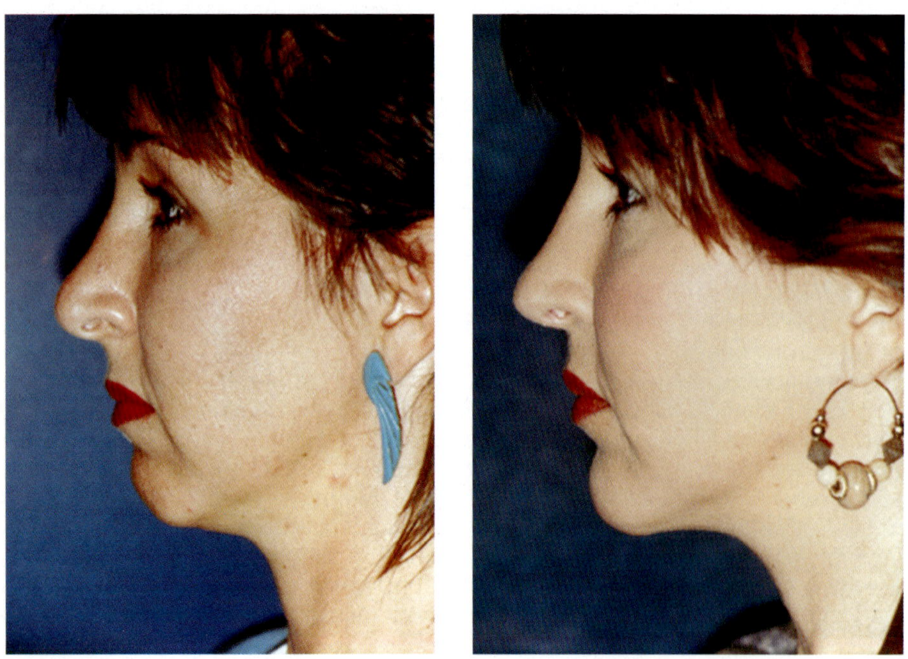

A

B

Fig. 9.2 (**A**) Before and (**B**) after revision rhinoplasty with a Gore-Tex chin implant.

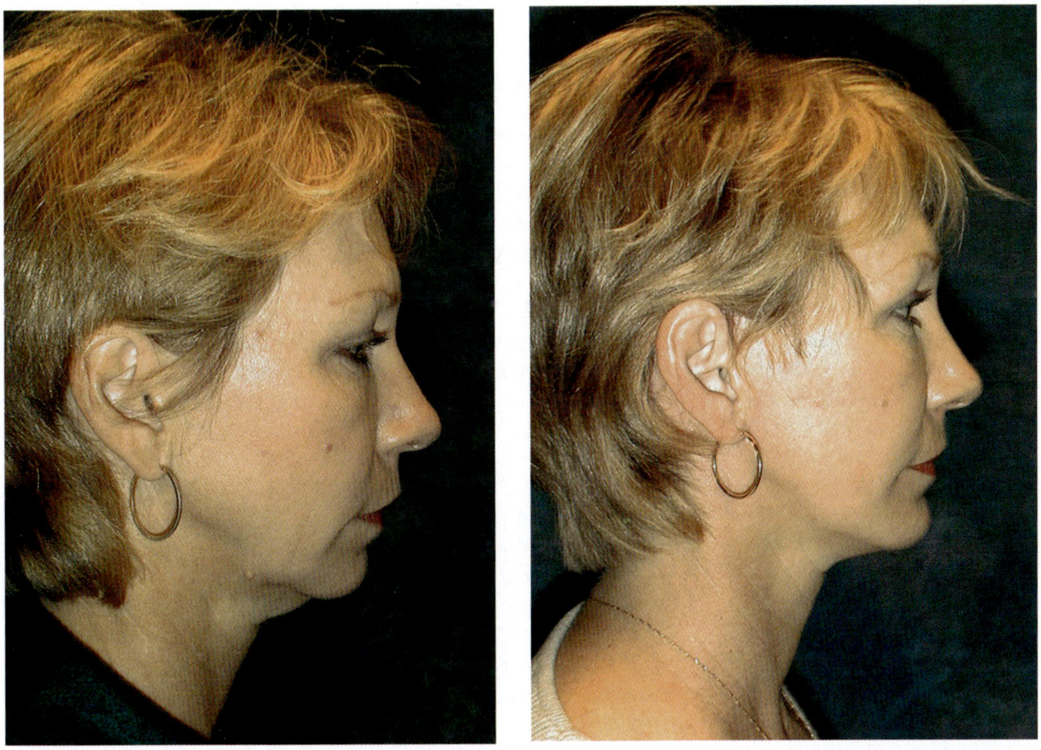

A B

Fig. 9.3 (**A**) Before and (**B**) after facelift, Gore-Tex chin implant, and brow lift. Chin augmentation enhances the facelift result.

views are helpful in assessing the width of the chin and also looking at the groove or depression that occurs along the jawline anterior to the jowl and is termed the *prejowl sulcus*. A chin implant can be fashioned to not only project the chin but also to help fill in this sulcus. It is important to talk with the patient about this effect as well as the estimated change in the width of the chin that will result from the procedure.

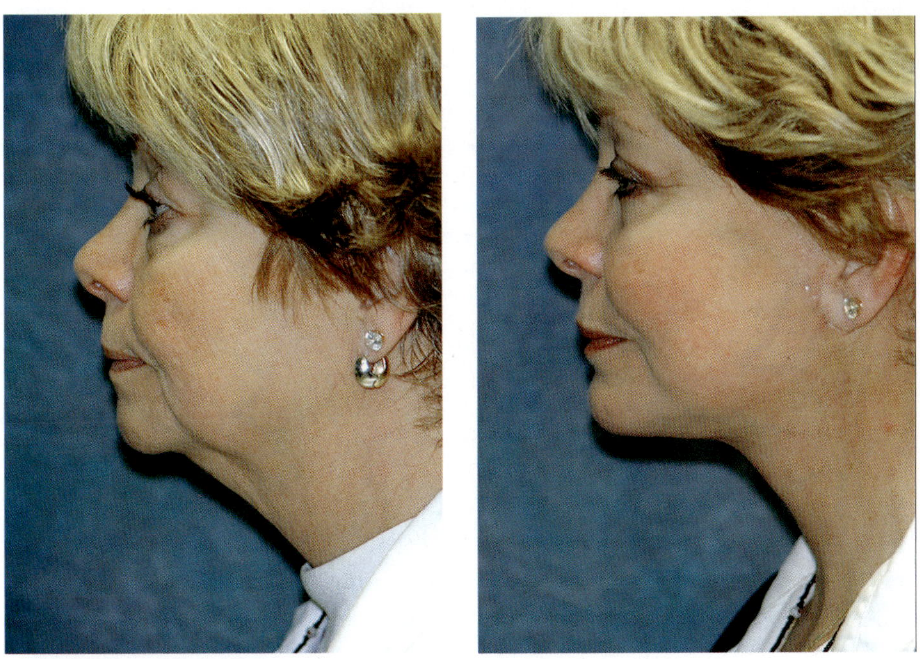

A B

Fig. 9.4 (**A**) Before and (**B**) after facelift, Gore-Tex chin implant, and upper and lower eyelid blepharoplasty.

Selection of Size

Choosing the best implant size is a crucial factor in delivering a result that the patient will enjoy. It is easy for the inexperienced surgeon to use chin projection on the lateral view to determine how large an implant to use, only to realize later that a different size should have been used. In general, the patient's overall size and especially head size help determine how large an implant to use. For example, a large implant, unless extensively modified (carved down), rarely looks good on a small woman, regardless of how retrusive the mandible is. Whereas such a patient could end up with a beautiful improvement on the lateral view, she could also have an excessively widened chin on the frontal view, which happens to be the only view she looks at in the mirror each day. In such a case, the patient would be justifiably unhappy and the surgeon headed back to the operating room to exchange the implant for a more suitable size.

Another error that can be made is to place an implant in a patient whose chin is retrusive but possesses a strong forward curve. These patients usually have occlusal abnormalities and require orthognathic surgery rather than simple chin augmentation (**Fig. 9.5**). Placement of an implant in this setting might result in overprojection of the chin resulting in a shelf-like effect that is unaesthetic. In both of the above scenarios, the point is that the surgeon must consider the chin, jawline, and neck from all views and in three dimensions to anticipate the effect of the implant and make the correct decision.

Exposure

The patient is marked, prepped, and draped in a sterile fashion. Chin implants may be placed through intraoral or submental incisions. Each approach has its advantages and drawbacks. An intraoral approach avoids an external scar. A submental approach allows for a truly sterile procedure, by preventing oral contaminants from coming into contact with the implant and surgical site. A submental approach also avoids disruption of the labiomental crease and the possibility of labial insufficiency should healing in the area be less ideal than expected. For the latter two reasons, the authors prefer the submental approach, which is described below.

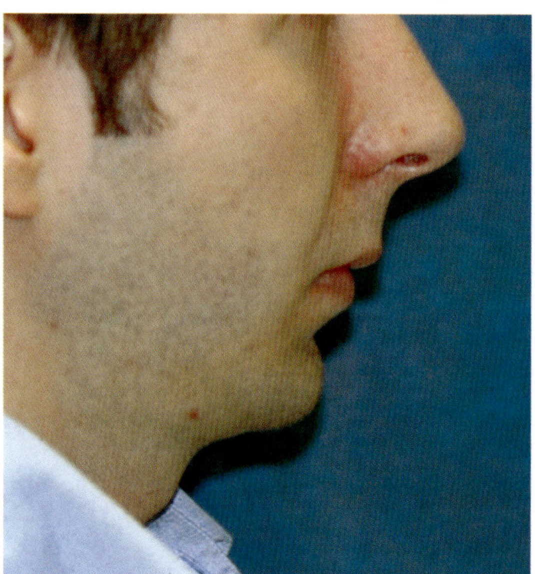

Fig. 9.5 Patient with mandibular retrusion who exhibits a normal forward chin curve. Orthognathic surgery may be required to balance the profile. A chin implant may actually worsen his appearance.

An existing submental crease is selected for the incision site, if one is available. In younger patients without a defined crease, the surgeon need simply have the patient bend his or her head downward toward the chest, and the future crease site will emerge. It is important to realize that the implant will pull the submental skin forward, and for this reason, the incision is marked slightly posterior to the desired eventual location. When several creases exist, which is usually the case, one of the more posterior ones may yield a less conspicuous scar. The eventual location of the incision site after the implant has been placed should be well posterior to the anterior point of the chin.

The submental tissues to be incised, anterior surface of the midline mandible, and parasymphyseal areas are injected with local anesthetic. The authors' preference of 1% lidocaine with 1:100,000 epinephrine mixed in equal quantities with 0.25% Marcaine (Hospira, Inc., Lake Forest, IL) (bupivacaine) with 1:200,000 epinephrine (as bitartrate) yields a long-lasting anesthesia with excellent vasoconstrictive effect.

Dissection is carried through the skin and subcutaneous fat. It is worth taking the time to carefully cauterize any bleeding vessels at this point to ensure good visualization of the surgical site during the rest of the procedure. Dissection is continued through the thin muscular layer as the incision is retracted upward over the symphysis using a rake retractor. Dissection is carried down to the periosteum layer by layer, cauterizing bleeding vessels as necessary.

The midline periosteum is preserved to give a strong structure to which the implant may be sutured and also to help prevent erosion of the mandible, which may occur if a solid implant, such as Silastic, is used. A vertical incision is made in the periosteum, 1 cm lateral to the midline on both sides, and subperiosteal tunnels running along the inferior portion of the anterior surface of the mandible are developed. A lighted Aufricht retractor provides ideal exposure and illumination for this purpose (**Fig. 9.6**). It is important for these to lie low on the mandible and for them to be no larger than the implant ends that they will contain. Excessive degloving of the mandible serves no purpose other than to allow migration of the implant. The surgeon should strive for precise pockets that would keep the implant immobile, even in the absence of fixation sutures.

Implant Modification and Insertion

The implant should arrive in sterile condition from the manufacturer and is opened shortly before needed in the procedure. It may be soaked in an antibiotic solution (such

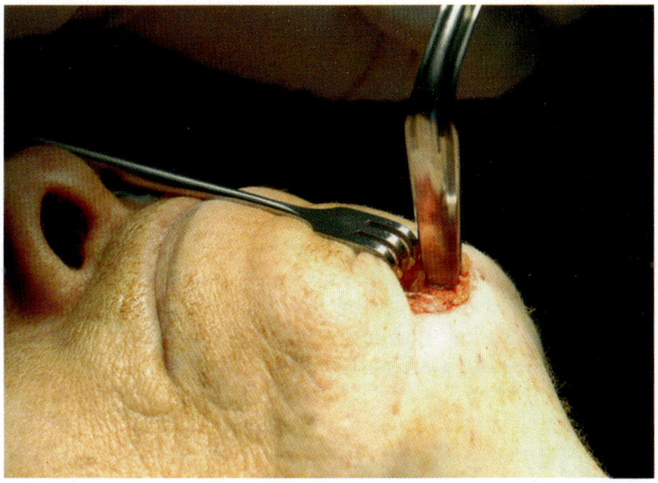

Fig. 9.6 A lighted Aufricht retractor provides ideal exposure to place a chin implant.

as bacitracin 50,000 units in 1 L sterile saline) prior to insertion. The same solution may be used throughout the procedure to irrigate the insertion site. If the implant requires modification prior to placement, this may be achieved using a sterile cutting block and a no. 10 blade in a precise shaving motion. The goal is to carve an implant that is the appropriate size for the patient's face in all dimensions. It is also important to carve the ends of the implant if they are bulky or the patient's tissue thin, so that an abrupt transition between the implant and the mandibular surfaces cannot be seen or even palpated. To ensure that this is so, the skin overlying the implant is made wet with sterile saline after the implant has been inserted and the surgeon carefully feels this area by gliding his fingertips over the area where the end of the implant lies. When no transition is felt, the implant ends have been carved correctly.

It is often necessary to place and remove the implant several times with modifications made to it gradually. This approach, while time consuming, is far better than placing the implant on the first try through creating too large a pocket or excessively thinning the implant. Once the implant appears to be the proper size and shape, it is inserted, one end at a time, into each of the subperiosteal pockets (**Fig. 9.7**). A surgical marking pen may be used to create a midline indicator stripe on the implant to assist with accurate placement. The lighted Aufricht retractor and Senn retractor are used for exposure, and a Freer elevator is used to help place the implant and move the soft tissues out of the way. Great care is taken during dissection of the pockets as well as the implant placement to avoid damage to the mental nerve, which exits the bone from its own foramen in the vicinity of the first premolar. It is for fear of damaging this nerve that the dissection must be kept low on the mandible and always done under direct vision. After the implant has been placed and the ends examined and palpated one last time to ensure correct position and a smooth transition, the implant may be secured and the incision closed. The implant is secured with one or two permanent sutures (the authors' choice is 4-0 monofilament polypropylene) to the midline periosteum.

Closure, Dressing, and Postoperative Care

The wound is closed in layers using absorbable suture (4-0 chromic gut) in the muscular and subcutaneous layers and permanent, everting sutures (5-0 monofilament polypropylene) in the skin. Failure to achieve a layered closure and good eversion of the skin can lead to an indented, unsightly scar. The wound is dressed with antibiotic ointment, nonadherent Telfa (Tyco Healthcare Group, Mansfield, MA) gauze, and adhesive strips. The dressing is removed by the patient 1 day after surgery and local wound care instituted. The patient receives intravenous antibiotic during surgery (cefazolin 1 g intravenous drip) and takes oral antibiotics (cephalexin 250 mg every 6 hours) for 3 to 5 days.

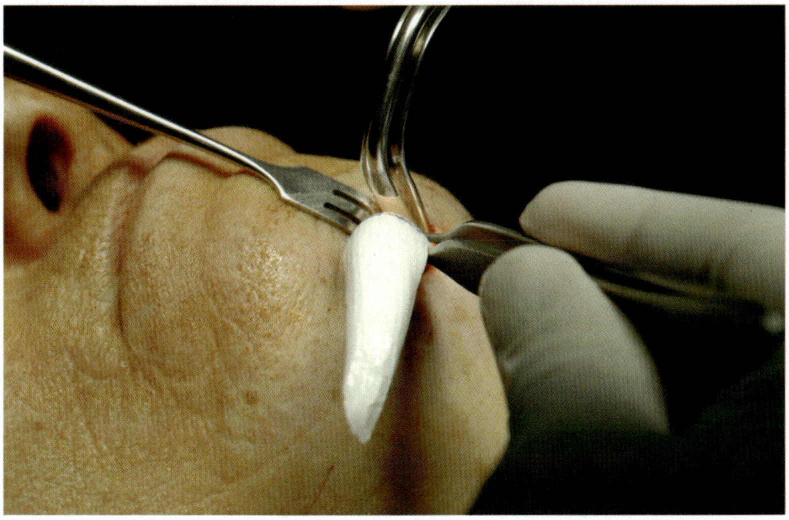

Fig. 9.7 Placement of the implant into the subperiosteal pocket under direct vision using a smooth forceps.

Complications

Complications are rare when a chin implant is properly performed. *Dislocation of the implant* out of the proper position is unlikely with a porous material such as Medpor or Mersilene (Ethicon, Inc., Somerville, NJ) mesh, where ingrowth of the surrounding tissues fixes it in place. Microporous implants such as those made of e-PTFE also fix into place due to limited ingrowth of cells and the attachments they form. A nonporous implant, such as one made of Silastic, will be the most likely to displace, as the thin capsule that forms around it and the fixation sutures that were placed at surgery are not as strongly resistant to movement as tissue ingrowth or fixation. As mentioned above, it is crucial during surgery to develop precise pockets that hold the implant in the desired position.

Improper placement of the implant is another adverse situation that may become apparent postoperatively. If, for example, the subperiosteal pockets were not evenly dissected or the ends of the implant were bent on themselves at the time of surgery, the chin may still look and feel right while swelling is present. But as edema resolves, these problems will become evident. The surgeon and patient must make a determination as to whether the problem is bothersome enough to require surgical revision; it often is in this situation. In the course of the revision, the pockets must be made even and the implant ends smoothed. New fixation sutures can be placed to maintain the improved position.

Mental nerve injury with anesthesia of the ipsilateral lower lip can be very disturbing to the patient. Such an injury can affect speech as well as the ability to eat, drink, and even manage saliva. This complication is prevented by good visualization of the bone as the subperiosteal pockets are being developed. If the surgeon is fairly certain that the nerve was not directly injured during surgery, then another possibility that should be considered is pressure of the implant on the nerve at the mental foramen. This situation may be able to be confirmed radiographically, and if it is strongly suspected, the implant could be moved or removed.

Infection occurs infrequently but can result in loss of the chin implant. The risk of infection necessitating removal ranges from less than 1% to 2.6%.[7,9] Sterile technique must be maintained during surgery. Bleeding must be controlled prior to implant to prevent hematomas that can become secondarily infected. If the implant is to be placed transorally, copious irrigation of the surgical site must be performed before and after it is secured. The patient must be careful to avoid hard foods that can damage the suture line and to rinse the mouth after eating or drinking. If a submental approach is used, the wound should be kept clean and antibiotic ointment applied frequently. The skin sutures should be removed when the wound is strong enough to remain closed. The authors will usually remove every other suture on the 5th to 7th days and take out the remaining sutures on the 9th or 10th day. After sutures are removed, a skin glue such as Collodion (Paddock Laboratories, Inc., Minneapolis, MN) as well as paper tape are placed on the incision. The glue and tape are changed every 3 to 5 days and are maintained for approximately 2 weeks. During this time, the patient must keep the area dry.

Persistent pain or erythema at the incision site is a sign that infection may be brewing. Pain is not unusual immediately after the chin implant, but it should abate significantly in the first week. If pain or erythema persists, the patient should be placed on an appropriate antibiotic and seen back frequently. If there is any pus draining or pointing, cultures should be performed immediately and antibiotic coverage adjusted based on their result. If the collection appears to be limited to the incision site, which does not directly overlie the implant, then it should be drained in a way that does not disturb the implant or provide a pathway from the infected site to it. This does occasionally occur, and in this setting the implant can be saved. If the infection occurs in the area surrounding the implant, then drainage, local wound care, and appropriate antibiotics may save the day. If, however, the situation does not improve, the patient will need to be brought to surgery and the implant removed. The wound bed is irrigated and, if necessary, débrided carefully. The wound is closed in layers. Removal of the implant and appropriate postoperative care almost always result in resolution of the infection. It is worth remembering that the capsule and scar tissue that remain after such an event can actually provide a degree of permanent augmentation.

Late infections of chin implants can also occur but are rare. Given the proximity of the implant to the mouth and the possibility of bacteremia after dental procedures (even regular cleanings), it is the authors' preference that the patient receive prophylactic antibiotics when undergoing such procedures.

◆ Nasal Dorsal Augmentation

Whereas the use of synthetic materials for augmentation of the chin is well accepted, the same cannot be said for the area of the nasal dorsum. Augmentation of the nose with man-made materials remains an intensely controversial subject. Many excellent rhinoplasty surgeons argue strongly against it.[10] Autogenous cartilage is the gold standard for grafting in rhinoplasty. Adamson[11] wrote, "cartilage contributes the dual functions of volume filling and structural support where needed. Alloplasts should be used only for volume filling because extrusion rates are unacceptably high when they are used for structural support." The authors heartily agree with this. Alloplastic grafts can be used when indicated for alignment of the profile (i.e., raising the dorsum, either partially or in its entirety) and for filling in and camouflaging defects or asymmetries in the nasal contours, but they should not be used for tip support. Autogenous or homograft tissues, most notably cartilage from the nasal septum, auricle, or rib, are more appropriate choices for providing support of the nasal tip or vault when indicated. When tip support is not required from the implant and the vault is structurally sound, however, a synthetic implant can be considered.

Choice of Materials

The array of synthetic materials available to the surgeon is similar to those for the chin. The nasal dorsum is a far more demanding location, however, and careful thought must go into making the correct decision for the patient. Whereas there is normally an abundant thickness of soft tissue to lie over a chin implant, this is often not the case in rhinoplasty. The thicker the nasal skin, the more forgiving it will most likely be when an implant is placed beneath it. Great care must be taken to choose the best material and to shape it to an inconspicuous implant that blends well with the rest of the nasal bone and cartilage in thin patients with thinner skin. This is also true in revision cases where scar tissue obscures planes of dissection and where the implant may lie in close proximity to or even contact the dermis. Autogenous materials are almost always preferable in this situation. On the other hand, in primary rhinoplasty patients with normal or thick skin who require significant dorsal augmentation, a synthetic implant can be very helpful. One study of e-PTFE implants revealed a 5.4% incidence of graft removal necessitating infection for revision patients that was more than 4 times greater than the incidence of infection (1.2%) in patients undergoing primary rhinoplasty.[6] The same authors reported a high rate of complications in patients with preexisting septal perforations and regarded them as an absolute contraindication to placement of synthetic dorsal grafts.

Aesthetic Analysis

A thorough aesthetic analysis includes a detailed history, examination of the nasal interior and exterior, and review of front, oblique, lateral, base, and reverse nasal views with the patient to understand his or her preferences and expectations. If dorsal augmentation is selected, a determination should be made concerning whether the entire dorsum or only a portion of it requires augmentation. The most common partial augmentation that the authors perform is a radix graft, which is used to fill in a gap from the nasion to the upper slope of the bony hump (**Fig. 9.8**). Because of the relatively small area involved, autologous septal or conchal cartilage is almost always used. It is important to consider the appearance not only from the lateral aspect but also from the front and lateral views when carving this graft, because it is easy to leave it too wide and create a visible edge. When augmentation of all or most of the dorsum is required and the skin is thick enough to cover well, a synthetic graft can be a good choice.

Technique

Dorsal implants can be introduced though a closed or open approach. It is the authors' preference to place most of these through an open approach, but if a closed one is chosen, certain safeguards must be taken. It is important to place the intranasal incisions in such a way that they do not lie directly beneath a synthetic graft. Thus, an intracartilaginous incision is not appropriate if the entire dorsum is being grafted. If transnasal placement is desired, an infracartilaginous incision can be made and dissection performed over the lower and upper lateral cartilages and bony dorsum to create a pocket for the implant. Antibiotics are used in the same way as described above in the section on chin augmentation. The implant is carved to the appropriate shape and placed on the dorsum so that it extends from the nasion to the anterior septal angle (**Fig. 9.9**).

A

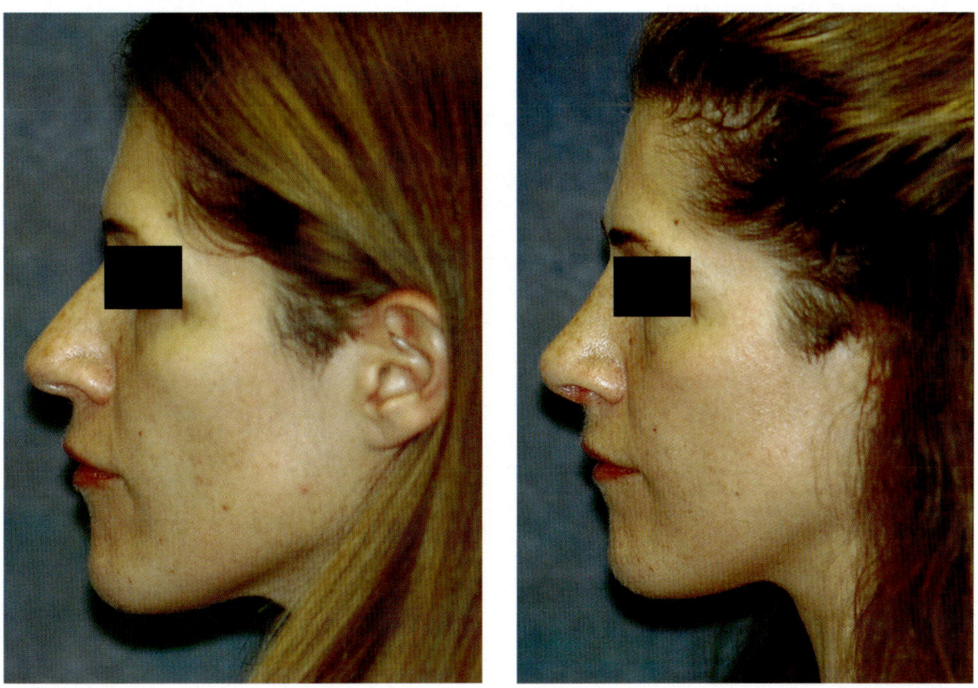

B

Fig. 9.8 **(A, B)** Patient who required augmentation of the upper portion of the dorsum with a radix graft.

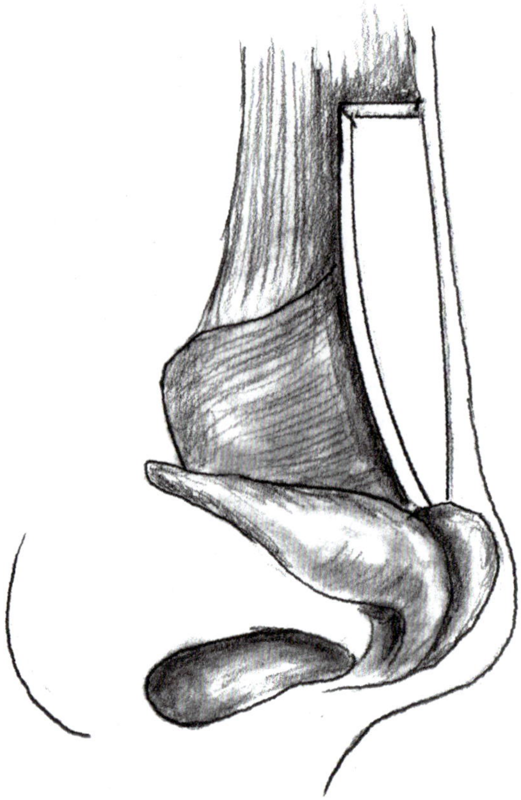

Fig. 9.9 Location of placement of a carved Gore-Tex implant onto the nasal dorsum.

Prior to placement of the implant, any dorsal irregularities, including small humps, can be reduced. It is important to remember that the dorsal skeleton must have a somewhat convex shape to appear straight when the skin, which is thin at the rhinion, but thicker in the supratip and at the nasion, lays upon it. A 4-0 monofilament polypropylene suture is used to secure the caudal end of the implant to the cartilage of the anterior septal angle. This end should not project above the lateral crurae and domes. It is also important to make the implant inconspicuous by creating a bevel along the edges of whatever type of material is chosen using a blade and sterile carving block (**Fig. 9.9**).

Complications

The most feared complications of dorsal augmentation are extrusion and infection resulting in loss of the implant. The occurrence of this has been reported to be as low as 2.6% with Medpor, 3.2% with Gore-Tex, and 9.7% with Silastic. The patient is aggressively treated with antibiotics and drainage if infection occurs. If extreme thinning of the skin develops and extrusion seems imminent, or if the infection cannot be controlled, removal of the implant with as little trauma to the nasal skin as possible should be considered. If the implant can be removed through the nose, additional trauma to the skin may be avoided. Healing usually occurs quickly once the implant is removed, and the patient will require reassurance during this period. As with autologous and homograft materials, displacement of the implant or gradual thinning of the skin with increased prominence of the graft and visible telangiectatic vessels in the overlying skin may also occur.

◆ Midface and Mandibular Augmentation

Contemporary facial rejuvenation is multimodal and focuses on restoring all layers involved with the aging face. Skin, subcutaneous tissues, and skeletal elements are treated simultaneously to produce the best aesthetic result. Alloplastic implantation allows for permanent volumetric change and can be used for bony and subcutaneous insufficiency. This is in contrast with facial fillers, which currently allow only temporary change. Deficiencies in the midface and mandibular regions are excellent platforms for the use of preformed synthetic implants. A well-defined jaw line and prominent, full malar region project youth and beauty. A flat hypoplastic cheek and weak jawline convey an aged, gaunt, and tired look. Deficiencies in the malar region are most commonly due to aging, bony hypoplasia, congenital asymmetries, trauma, and surgical defects. The midface has historically been a difficult area in which to achieve consistently excellent results in facial augmentation. Surgical correction of inherent deficiencies or asymmetry and rejuvenation of the aging ptotic midface requires a full understanding of all anatomic components involved in this region. Periorbital changes, midface descent, volume loss, and inherited hypoplastic bony components all contribute to a poor aesthetic appearance in the malar/cheek regions. Newer techniques in midface lifting, synthetic and autogenous volume replacement, and customized preformed alloplastic implants have significantly improved our ability to enhance the appearance of this complex region.

Patient Selection

The patient evaluation begins with a thorough history and physical examination; a detailed discussion of the patient's primary areas of concern and a methodical and comprehensive preoperative facial analysis will assist in selecting the ideal candidates for alloplastic rejuvenation. As with all cosmetic surgery, vigilant preoperative planning increases the probability of a good outcome. Open communication is critical to ascertain expectations and to identify and amend unrealistic hopes. Criteria for accurate selection of alloplastic implants based on skeletal and topographic midface features have been well described in the literature.[12,13] In addition to implant selection, consideration should also focus on the sum total correction of midface volume loss and descent, periorbital aging pathology, inherent asymmetries, and hypoplastic skeletal elements. Combined procedures that reposition soft tissues, augment volumetric loss, along with alloplastic augmentation should maximize the aesthetic result in the properly selected patient. This comprehensive approach will prevent dissatisfaction among patients who may not have considered how these elements contributed to an overall poor appearance. Blepharoplasty, midface lift, and skin resurfacing may be necessary to achieve the desired result. Younger patients who have inherited skeletal or soft tissue insufficiency, trauma or surgically created defects, or congenital asymmetries may only require alloplastic correction.[14] Various preformed alloplastic implants are readily available for correction of the malar, submalar, and tear trough regions.

Midface Analysis

Implant selection is based on preoperative facial analysis. Photographic documentation is a mandatory adjunct to making an accurate evaluation. Patients can be classified by five distinct midfacial topographic contour deficits based on the prominence or insufficiencies of the malar skeletal and soft tissue components. Type I patients demonstrate adequate soft tissue development with bony malar hypoplasia. Type II patients have adequate malar development but have ptotic or atrophic soft tissues in the submalar region. Type III patients have a pronounced malar bony prominence with thin skin and a hollow submalar region. Type IV patients present a combination of malar skeletal hypoplasia and submalar soft tissue atrophy. Type V patients display hollow infraorbital regions about the nasojugal line known as a tear trough deformity. The five basic midfacial contour types benefit maximally from variable preformed alloplastic implants, which include malar, submalar, combined, and tear trough implants. Each implant is preformed and tailored to fit each contour type.

Mandibular Analysis

A combination of photo and cephalometric analysis is the most comprehensive method for evaluation of the mandible. Practically, for cosmetic procedures, most surgeons rely on photographic analysis and patient interview to select the best implant. At a minimum, the analysis should include a thorough evaluation of the patient's anatomy by zones (mentum, body, and angle) to determine the degree of augmentation that is adequate for each region. Chin implants augment projection anteriorly and lateral over the mentum and mandibular body and are more commonly used. Mandible angle implants are placed to give lateral and vertical augmentation to the jaw line over the posterior lateral regions.

No matter which areas are chosen for augmentation, advanced selection of implants and intraoperative confirmation with sizers can be performed to ensure consistently excellent results. Special consideration can be taken in patients with traumatic or postsurgical deformity. These patients benefit maximally from computer-assisted custom implant designs that are specifically tailored to fit each patient's particular deficiency based on a three-dimensional computed tomography analysis. This technology has also gained favor in the subset of patients who suffer midface lipodystrophy from HIV protease inhibitors.

Surgical Technique

Malar Implants

Malar implants can be placed through any of several approaches. The intraoral approach is the most common and has the advantage of leaving no visible scar and can be performed under local anesthesia. Other routes for malar implant placement are subciliary, transconjuctival, or through the incision created for a rhytidectomy or midface lift. In the latter two approaches, the facial nerve must be fastidiously protected and the patient counseled that a prolonged period of facial swelling may result. The subciliary approach, although direct, adds an increased risk of ectropion to the procedure.

Prior to the procedure, the specific areas to be augmented are outlined with a marking pen with the patient sitting upright. After adequate sedation, the oral cavity is prepared with Peridex (3M Corporation, St. Paul, MN) or a similar oral rinse. A mixture of lidocaine and bupivacaine with epinephrine (see Chin Augmentation section) is injected along the line of the mucosal incision as well as along the plane of dissection. This mixture reduces operative bleeding and provides long-lasting anesthesia. The intraoral approach then begins with an upper gingivobuccal sulcus incision and a subperiosteal dissection toward the zygoma. The incision should be placed at least 1 cm above the attached gingiva to allow a simplified closure. The dissection plane should be subperiosteal, and the surgeon should elevate the periosteum off of the anterior and lateral face of the zygoma creating a snug pocket for the implant (**Fig. 9.10**).

The infraorbital nerve is not specifically identified unless dissection in its vicinity is necessary for placement of the implant. Implant sizers may then be used to confirm the proper implant size and position. Extension of the subperiosteal dissection may continue directly over the superior fibers of the masseter muscle to accommodate a submalar, combined, or malar shell type implant. Meticulous hemostasis is necessary in this region as the buccal fat pad and masseter house a rich vascular plexus. The plane of dissection is directly over the muscle body. This will ensure a well-seated implant. After the creation of an adequate pocket, the implant may be secured with either nonabsorbable sutures or screws or simply held in place by a tight pocket of periosteum. Confirmation of implant symmetry and position by standing at the head of the patient and sighting down the face to assess adequate projection is recommended. The patient may also be placed in a seated position on the operative bed to give a better assessment. The incision is then closed in layers after final implant fixation.

Mandibular Angle Implants

Mandibular angle implants can be placed through intraoral or external approaches. For cosmetic purposes, the implant

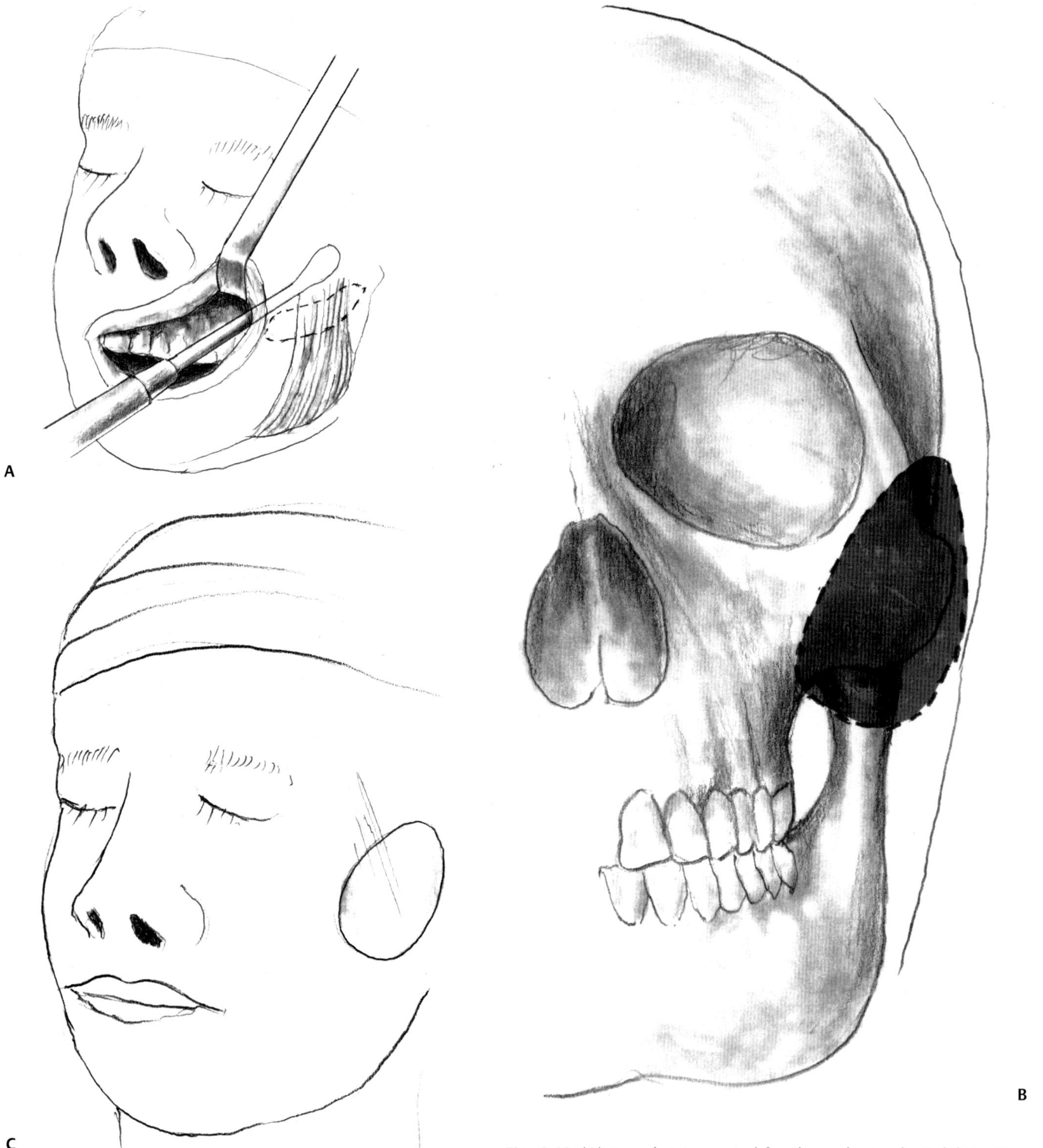

Fig. 9.10 (**A**) A pocket is created for the malar implant. (**B**) Position of implant on facial skeleton. (**C**) Position of implant in face

is usually placed intraorally.[15] The intraoral approach involves a 2-cm vertical vestibular incision through periosteum. Subperiosteal dissection is then carried to the posterolateral border of the mandibular angle under the pterygomasseteric sling. Curved elevators help facilitate the release of attachments along angle and posterior ramus. Care should be taken to stay on bone to create a snug pocket. A well-contoured angle implant is then inserted into the subperiosteal pocket. The pocket is normally sufficient to hold the implant in place, but a screw may be used to secure the implant to the lateral cortex of the mandible (**Fig. 9.11**). After fixation, the wound is copiously irrigated with antibiotic solution. A meticulous layered closure is performed with absorbable suture. A light pressure dressing may be placed over the mandibular angle for stability and to minimize swelling and seroma formation.

Despite the fact that these implants are usually placed through the mouth, the overall risk of infection is low.[16] The use of preoperative and intraoperative antibiotics when planning an alloplastic implant will decrease the risk of infection. Ideally, the implant should remain uncontaminated throughout its placement, with the use of a no-touch technique in which the implant does not come in contact with gloved hands, skin, or oral mucosa. The implant should be soaked in antibiotic solution prior to placement. Rinsing the pocket thoroughly and changing surgical gloves just before placing the implant may serve to decrease the overall bacterial load. Consideration should also be given to the vascular supply of the proposed implant site. Poor vasculature as a result of radiation, surgical scarring, vascular disease, or tobacco use can adversely affect the ability of the surrounding tissue to fight infection.

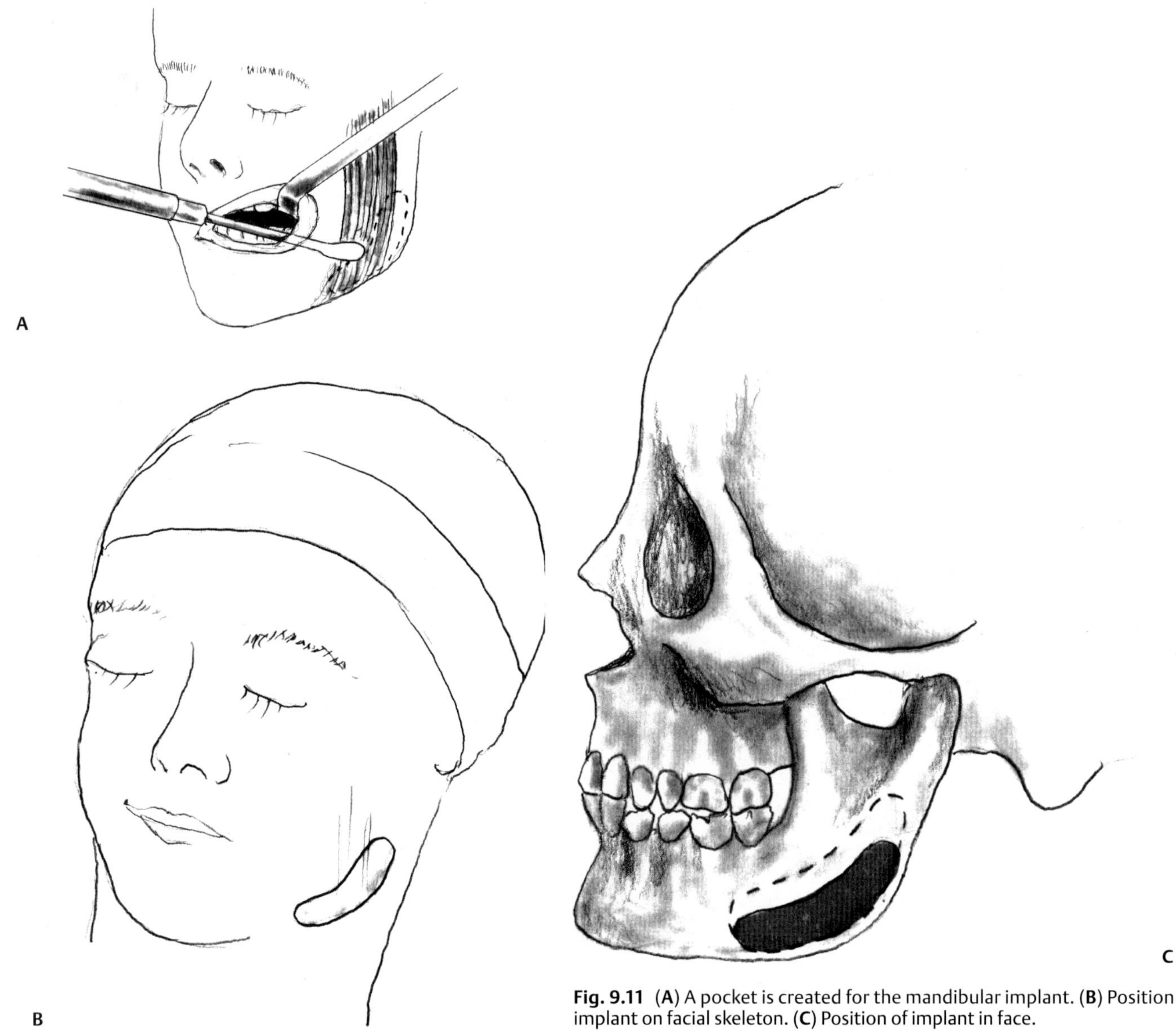

Fig. 9.11 (**A**) A pocket is created for the mandibular implant. (**B**) Position of implant on facial skeleton. (**C**) Position of implant in face.

Complications

Complications from placement of midface and mandibular angle alloplastic implants are rare. They include infection, hematoma, seroma, extrusion, migration, nerve injury, facial asymmetry, and an improperly sized implant. Many of these complications are avoidable with proper surgical planning and technique.

Infection requires prompt recognition and is typically managed by timely removal of the implant and the use of concomitant empiric then culture-directed antibiotic therapy. Replacement of the implant may be contemplated after the infection has resolved.

Hematoma can generally be prevented with meticulous operative hemostasis. Larger hematomas should be drained as they increase the risk of implant infection. The incidence and size of seromas can be minimized by placement of compressive dressings and limiting dissection planes to precise pockets that only accommodate the implants and leave no excess dead space. This technique also prevents implant displacement.

Injury to nerves exiting bony foramina is also a potential risk of facial implant placement. In general, dissection should avoid these areas, and nerves should not be exposed unless it is necessary for correct placement of the implant. Malar implants generally are placed lateral to the infraorbital nerve. Chin implants should be placed below the mental foramen. Angle implants should not expose the inferior alveolar nerve. Paresthesias, when they occur, are usually temporary and resolve within the first year. Anesthesia or dysesthesias may be due to compression by the implant or laceration of the nerve. If the surgeon believes that an implant is compressing a nerve, it should be repositioned or removed.[17]

◆ Conclusion

Alloplastic facial skeletal implants provide the facial plastic surgeon with a multitude of ways to help the patient. Each type of implant material has advantages and disadvantages, and each facial site possesses its own unique challenges and opportunities for facial enhancement. Before employing a synthetic implant, the surgeon must consider if an autologous, homologous, or animal-derived material would better serve the patient's needs. If the answer to this question is no, then the task at hand is to select the best material available for the specific facial site. With proper material selection, preoperative planning, surgical technique, and postoperative care, the surgeon can often deliver a result that will please the patient and repay the surgeon's diligence.

References

1. Stucker F, Shaw G, Ephrat M. Biologic tissue implants. In: Papel I, ed. Facial Plastic and Reconstructive Surgery. 2nd ed. New York, NY: Thieme Medical Publishers; 2002
2. Maas CS, Gnepp DR, Bumpous J. Expanded polytetrafluoroethylene (Gore-Tex soft tissue patch) in facial augmentation. Arch Otolaryngol Head Neck Surg 1993;119:1008–1014
3. Mittleman H, Newman J. Aesthetic mandibular implants. In: Papel I, ed. Facial Plastic and Reconstructive Surgery. 2nd ed. New York, NY: Thieme Medical Publishers; 2002
4. Quatela V, Sabini P. Synthetic implant. In: Papel I, ed. Facial Plastic and Reconstructive Surgery. 2nd ed. New York, NY: Thieme Medical Publishers; 2002
5. Davis PKB, Jones SM. The complications of Silastic implants: experience with 137 consecutive cases. Br J Plast Surg 1971;24:405
6. Godin MS, Waldman SR, Johnson CM. Nasal augmentation using Gore-Tex: a ten-year experience. Arch Facial Plast Surg 1999;1:118–121
7. Godin M, Costa L, Romo T, Truswell W, Wang T, Williams E. Gore-Tex chin implants: a review of 324 cases. Arch Facial Plast Surg 2003;5:224–227
8. Porex Surgical Website. Available at: http://www.porexsurgical.com/english/surgical/smedpor.asp. Accessed December 28, 2006
9. Romo T, Sclafani AP, Sabini P. Use of porous high-density polyethylene in revision rhinoplasty and in the platyrrhine nose. Aesthetic Plast Surg 1998;22:211–221
10. Tardy ME. Rhinoplasty. In: Cummings CW, ed. Otolaryngology-Head and Neck Surgery. St. Louis, MO: CV Mosby; 1986:699–749
11. Adamson PA. Grafts in rhinoplasty. Arch Otolaryngol Head Neck Surg 2000;126:561–562
12. Binder WJ. A comprehensive approach for aesthetic contouring of the midface in rhytidectomy. Facial Plast Surg Clin North Am 1993;1:231–255
13. Bartlett SP, Wornom I III, Whitaker LA. Evaluation of facial skeletal aesthetics and surgical planning. Clin Plast Surg 1991;18:1–9
14. Kent JN, Craig MA. Secondary autogenous and alloplastic reshaping procedures for facial asymmetry. Atlas Oral Maxillofac Surg Clin North Am 1996;4:83–105
15. Terino EO. Implants for male aesthetic surgery. Clin Plast Surg 1991;18:731–749
16. Rubin JP, Yaremchuk MJ. Complications and toxicities of implantable biomaterials used in facial reconstructive and aesthetic surgery: a comprehensive review of the literature. Plast Reconstr Surg 1997;100:1336–1353
17. Lo LJ, Wong F, Chen Y. The position of the inferior alveolar nerve at the mandibular angle: an anatomic consideration for aesthetic mandibular angle reduction. Ann Plast Surg 2004;53:50–55

10

Skin Rejuvenation

Steven J. Pearlman and Monica Tadros

Advances in medicine have fostered a healthier, longer life span. With this, individuals are conscious that their changing outward appearance no longer matches their physical wellness. The concept of aging with grace has been transformed to convey an image of seasoned beauty with youthful preservation. Positive self-image with advancing age and an appreciation for the effects of photoaging on the skin are at the forefront of popular culture. Skin rejuvenation continues to be a rapidly expanding discipline encompassing medicine, technology, and the beauty industry. Our patients seek more youthful skin through ever-improving skin care and laser technology. In the United States, cosmeceuticals represent a \$5.4 billion per year industry that is propelled by a stream of new products offering age-defying and other appearance-enhancing benefits and is predicted to grow 8.5% annually.[1] According to the 2005 survey of the American Academy of Facial Plastic and Reconstructive Surgery, laser skin rejuvenation has increased by 64%, microdermabrasion by 103%, and botulinum toxin use for facial wrinkles has increased 162% since 2001.[2]

Improved surgical techniques have facilitated a more natural, aesthetic appearance in the treatment of the aging face. However, it is important to understand that complete facial rejuvenation must include skin restoration in addition to surgical facial rejuvenation. The three targets for reversing skin aging are (1) skin color and texture, (2) loss of skin elasticity and collagen degradation, and (3) dynamic lines from hyperactive facial muscles acting on the overlying skin. Skin products can now target aged skin with several ingredients that stimulate collagen production, increase epidermal turnover, and reverse photoaging. Skin peels have been used for centuries to restore more youthful skin. Botulinum toxin treatment complements skin care regimens by relaxing facial muscles that cause overlying wrinkles.

Laser skin resurfacing technology has also paralleled the growing quest for more youthful skin. What was the mainstay for cutaneous exfoliation a decade ago—the CO_2 laser—has been eclipsed by less invasive techniques. Several lasers with shorter or even no healing time have been developed. Minimally invasive lasers, otherwise known as nonablative lasers and laser-like devices, when coupled with skin care are slowly approaching results once only achievable with ablative lasers or deep chemical peels. With such a variety in treatments, the cosmetic surgeon must properly evaluate the patient's needs and select an appropriate treatment plan.

Skin type, extent of photoaging, associated dynamic wrinkles, and facial aging must all be taken into account (**Table 10.1**). As with all of medicine, treatment for facial aging starts with proper diagnosis. Therapy can range from home topical products to minimally invasive office procedures to aggressive, ablative resurfacing. Treatment can then be directed at the diagnosed problems and tailored according to the patient's tolerance for minimal to invasive treatment. Comprehensive care for the aging face often encompasses treating patients with several skin care modalities. Combination treatments can then address multiple causes for the aging face for superior results.

◆ Facial Skin Aging

The primary goal of skin rejuvenation is to combat aging, photodamaged skin. Years of exposure to the sun causes significant skin changes and accelerates natural skin aging (**Table 10.2**). Skin changes manifest as facial lines, irregular pigmentation, erythema and telangiectasias, and textural changes. Facial aging is most often equated with the appearance of wrinkles. Wrinkles, rhytides, creases, folds, and furrows come from several causes and are only a part of what makes a face appear older. Aging changes within the

Table 10.1 Five Areas of Facial Aging

1. Inherent changes within the skin
    - (a) Epidermal changes
    - (b) Skin tone and color
    - (c) Skin vasculature
    - (d) Skin lesions
2. Dynamic lines
    - (a) Facial muscles acting on the skin
3. Loss of tissue elasticity
    - (a) Decreased elastin
    - (b) Disarray of collagen bundles
4. Effects of gravity
5. Soft tissue and bone loss
    - (a) Shifting of facial soft tissue

Table 10.2 Skin Changes

1. Wrinkles (rhytides)
2. Coarse skin texture
3. Pigment changes
   (a) Dyschromia, lentigines, sallow color
4. Epidermal skin lesions
   (a) Keratoses to frank skin cancers
5. Vascular changes
   (a) Telangiectasias
   (b) Purpura
6. Large pores

Table 10.3 Histologic Skin Changes Associated with Photodamage

1. Thicker, irregular epidermis
   (a) Irregular stratum corneum
2. Thinner dermis
   (a) Decreased elastin
   (b) Thicker, irregular, disorganized collagen bundles
   (c) Decreased ground substance
3. Reduced appendages and glands
   (a) Drier skin
4. Reduced microcirculation
   (a) Vessels become dilated and tortuous
5. Thinner subcutaneous tissue

skin make wrinkles more prevalent. Wrinkles have been found to have no distinguishing histologic features.[3] They may occur from redundant skin, muscular expression, or loss of skin support. These changes are only minimally affected by resurfacing. Another interpretation divides them into fine wrinkles that are present at rest and may be less evident with facial expression.[4] Medium wrinkles, which we call dynamic wrinkles, are accentuated by facial expression and may have alteration in the elastosis of the surrounding skin. Coarse, deep wrinkles are visible at rest, too. These are accentuated by facial expression, such as nasolabial folds and areas of fat herniation and tissue redundancy. Medium and deep wrinkles may be better treated by other or combined modalities such as facial fillers and surgery.

Aging skin is accelerated by photodamage, resulting in coarser texture, pigment changes, telangiectasias, actinic keratoses, and even epidermal malignancies (**Table 10.3**). The skin ages by thinning of the epidermis and flattening of the junction with the dermis.[5] Photoaged skin (a more common finding in patients seeking resurfacing) actually has a thicker epidermis, but the outer keratin layer is irregular. There is increased water loss from the skin and a decrease in the sebaceous glands lubricating the skin. More abnormal cells accumulate in aged skin, especially if there is chronic sun damage, leading to precancerous and cancerous lesions. Photoaging also causes chronic inflammation within the skin. There is an increase in elastin that clusters into thick bundles with sun damage. Collagen decreases as we age, and the bundles of collagen become looser and lose strength. Capillaries and small blood vessels regress from the skin, reducing blood flow. The more superficial vessels can thicken from sun exposure, also reducing their capacity to nourish the skin. Telangiectasias (spider veins) appear on the surface of the skin, which are too superficial to provide nourishment. Loss of blood supply can also contribute to thinning of the hair and paler skin.

The skin becomes less able to resist stretching with loss of elasticity. When coupled with gravity, muscle pull, and tissue changes beneath, wrinkling occurs. The skin is also less able to resist mechanical damage and heals more slowly from insult. Water loss and breakdown of bonds between the cells reduces the barrier function of the skin. Pore size increases as well. It becomes more evident that maturing skin comprises only two of the five components that contribute to facial aging.

◆ Skin Evaluation and Diagnosis

Analysis of the aging face with proper diagnosis of the dominant causes is necessary for appropriate treatment. Facial aging occurs by five independent yet interactive components: inherent skin changes, dynamic lines, loss of tissue elasticity, effects of gravity, and soft tissue loss. Understanding these changes, how they manifest and what promotes them, is the first step in proper pretreatment analysis (**Fig. 10.1**).

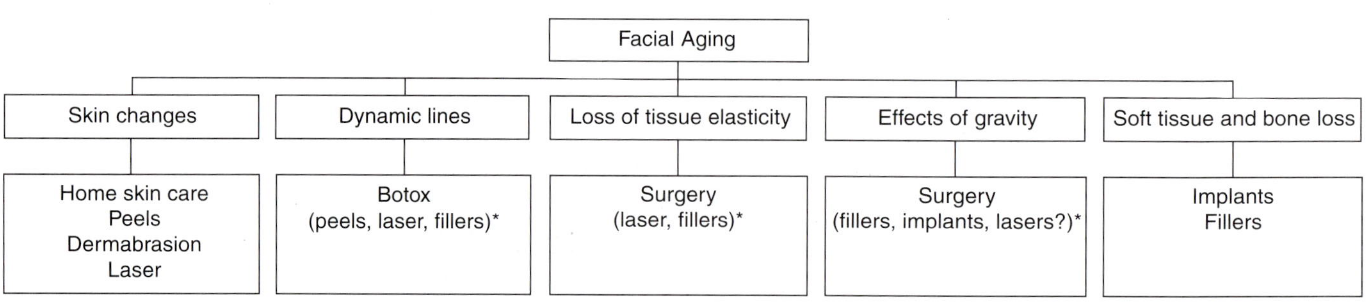

Fig. 10.1 Facial aging: classification of the five causes and treatment for each (alternative treatments are in parentheses; *less effective alternatives).

Table 10.4 Fitzpatrick Classification of Skin Types

Type	Hair Color	Skin Color	Eye Color	Reaction to Sun
I	Red, blonde	Very white or freckled	Blue-green	Burns, never tans
II	Blonde	Light	Blue	Burns, may tan
III	Brown	Medium	Brown (or blue)	Burns then tans
IV	Brown, black	Brown	Brown	Tans, rarely burns
V	Black	Dark brown	Dark	Tans
VI	Black	Black	Dark	Tans

Once the aging components most troublesome for each particular patient can be determined, the best course of therapy can be planned. Home skin care can compliment any treatment offered for facial rejuvenation. However, it may take many months to see demonstrable changes without adjunctive procedures. Lasers and medium to deep skin peels primarily remedy inherent changes within aging and photodamaged skin but can also improve skin elasticity and compliment treatment for the other areas of facial aging. Skin texture, color, vascular changes, and even pore size can all be remedied by lasers. Although fine wrinkles respond to skin peels and ablative lasers, deeper wrinkles and facial folds are best treated by other means. Dynamic folds in the upper face are treated by botulinum toxin and in the lower face by filler injections. Combination therapy targeting multiple causes will provide the best results.

Patient Selection

Patient selection begins with a careful skin history. One must inquire about skin care routines, sun habits, smoking, medications that may increase photosensitivity, and general medical conditions. Included in the history is use of the Fitzpatrick classification of skin types (**Table 10.4**).[6] This classification helps us predict the reaction to photoenergy from laser treatments and medium to deep chemical peels. The Fitzpatrick classification quantifies the amount of inherent melanin in the skin as a primary chromophore. This system is then used in determining appropriateness for ablative treatments as well as laser settings for more predictable results.

The extent of photodamage should be determined by skin inspection. A scale is used to record skin changes to aid in planning and provide a tangible description of the skin. Both Fitzpatrick[7] and Glogau[8] described useful classifications for photodamaged skin (**Tables 10.5 and 10.6**). Proper diagnosis and classification is then used to

Table 10.5 Fitzpatrick Classification of Facial Wrinkles (Perioral and Periorbital)

Class	Score	Wrinkling	Degree of Elastosis
I	1–3	Fine wrinkles	Mild (fine textural changes with subtle skin lines)
II	4–6	Fine to moderate depth, moderate number of lines	Moderate (distinct popular elastosis, individual papules with yellow translucency, dyschromia)
III	7–9	Fine to deep wrinkles, numerous lines, with or without redundant skin	Severe (multipapular and confluent elastosis, thickened yellow and pallid cutis rhomboidalis)

Table 10.6 Glogau Classification of Facial Aging

- Type I: Mild (age, twenties to thirties)
  - No keratoses, little to no wrinkling (even with animation)
  - Minimal or no makeup needed
- Type II: Moderate (age, thirties to forties)
  - Early actinic keratoses, slight yellowish discoloration or brownish cast with increased freckling
  - Early wrinkling (especially with motion)
  - Loss of smoothness
  - Light makeup usually worn (to cover skin color irregularities)
- Type III: Advanced (age, fifties)
  - Obvious visible actinic keratoses
  - Sallow, yellowish skin discoloration (from accumulated degenerated collagen and elastin in the upper dermis) with telangiectasias
  - Wrinkles at rest
  - Heavier makeup always worn to even skin color but can accentuate deeper wrinkles
- Type IV: Severe (age, sixties to seventies)
  - Actinic keratoses and skin cancers (profound accumulation of solar elastin and collagen in the upper dermis)
  - Almost no pink color at all
  - Wrinkling heavy
  - Heavy makeup worn that cakes and does not cover well

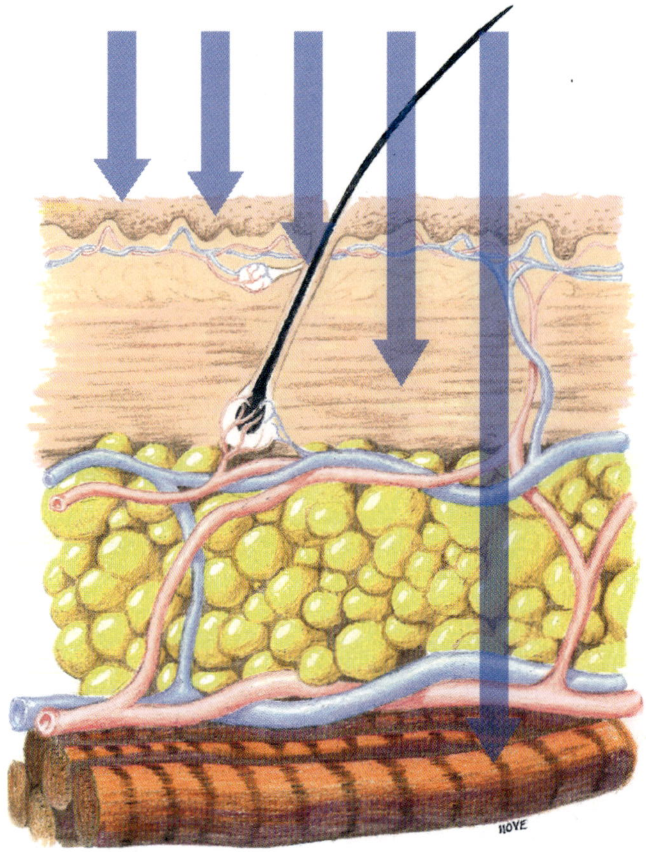

Fig. 10.2 Depth of penetration of skin treatments. Left to right (*arrows*): (1) home skin care treats superficial epidermis; (2) superficial peels and microdermabrasion to deep epidermis; (3) laser and medium-depth peels treat pigment in papillary dermis and vessels in papillary/reticular dermis, superficial collagen; (4) ablative and nonablative lasers and deep chemical peels treat collagen to depth of hair follicles; (5) botulinum toxin and surgery affect full-thickness skin. (From Pearlman SJ, Chernoff WG. Laser resurfacing of the face: analysis and diagnosis. Facial Plast Surg Clin 2003;11:335–347. Reprinted with permission.)

plan treatment. Photographs are taken in the frontal (full face), oblique, and lateral (profile) views with close-ups of any areas of particular interest. Uniform lighting and camera exposures are necessary to document the often-subtle changes in skin tone and texture. Less commonly used diagnostic techniques for pretreatment evaluation include digital photography that allows skin magnification for closer skin inspection, ultraviolet exam, high-resolution dermal diagnostic ultrasound, and three-dimensional microtopography.[9]

Treatment Planning

Facial skin rejuvenation ranges in complexity and depth of penetration from home topical cosmeceuticals to office procedures such as microdermabrasion and medium-depth chemical peels to ablative laser resurfacing and deep chemical peels. Topical skin products rejuvenate, and some exfoliate, the skin. They penetrate the stratum corneum and can reach the superficial papillary dermis. Superficial peels remain within the epidermis or granular layer with a depth of penetration of ~0.06 mm. Medium-depth peels (both laser and chemical peels) extend into the papillary or upper reticular dermis at a depth of ~0.45 mm. Deep peels extend into the midreticular dermis with a depth of ~0.6 mm (**Fig. 10.2**).[10] Although superficial chemical peels do not produce dramatic results, they are safe to use in all skin types. Laser resurfacing and medium-depth and deep chemical peels may be more effective but given their depth of penetration carry an increased risk of pigmentary complications in patients with Fitzpatrick skin types III through VI.[11] Nonablative lasers can penetrate to variable depths in what will later be described as "subsurface" skin rejuvenation (**Fig. 10.3**). Ablative lasers rejuvenate to the papillary-reticular junction with deeper thermal effects.

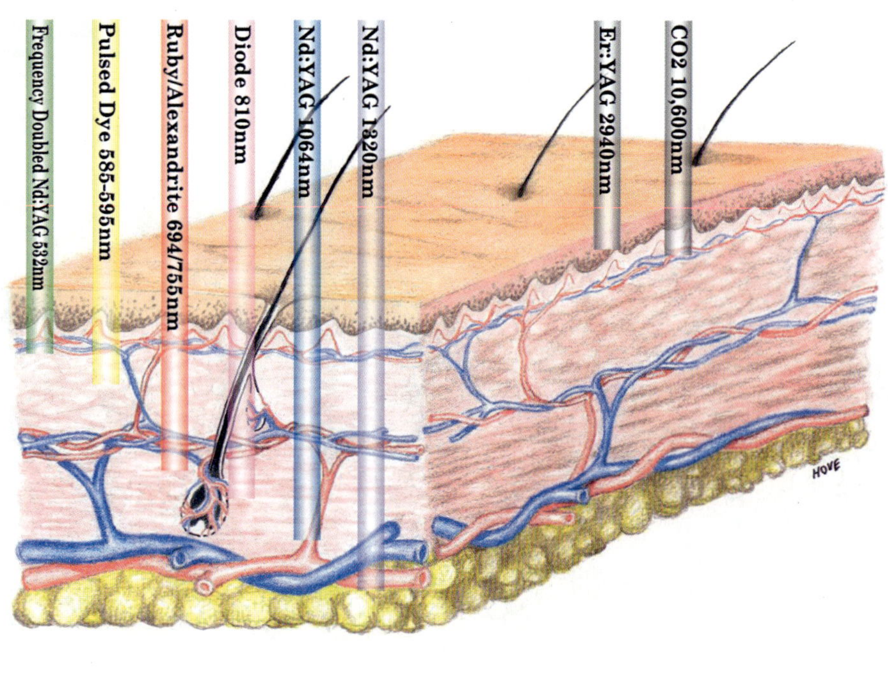

Fig. 10.3 Depth of penetration of (*left*) nonablative and (*right*) ablative lasers. (From Pearlman SJ, Chernoff WG. Laser resurfacing of the face: analysis and diagnosis. Facial Plast Surg Clin 2003;11:335–347. Reprinted with permission.)

◆ Chemical Peels

Superficial

The depth of penetration from superficial peels remains at the level of the epidermis. A light superficial peel removes only the stratum corneum, whereas a full superficial chemical peel destroys the entire epidermis. Progression beyond the epidermis into the papillary dermis constitutes a medium-depth peel, whereas a deep chemical peel results in further penetration into the reticular dermis (**Table 10.7**).[11]

Glycolic acid peels with concentrations in the range 30 to 50% and Jessner's solution are popular superficial chemical peels for the treatment of acne and photoaging that produce deeper epidermal exfoliation. Jessner's solution is composed of 14% resorcinol, 14% salicylic acid, and 14% lactic acid usually formulated in 100 mL ethanol.[12] Trichloroacetic acid (TCA) peels in the range 10 to 30% and salicylic acid at concentrations of 20 to 30% can also be used to achieve a superficial peel.[13,14] The clinical efficacy of these peels is variable and dependent on the clinical scenario and desired outcome. Studies have shown that superficial peeling agents help exfoliate the skin but do not diminish sebum production, one of the main etiologic factors resulting in acne formation.[15] They are safe to use in the majority of skin types, but it is always prudent to initiate treatment with the lowest concentration superficial peel to survey sensitivity in patients with Fitzpatrick skin types IV through VI.

Microdermabrasion

Microdermabrasion was first described in Italy in 1985. Its relative ease, safety, and lack of down-time have fostered its current popularity in the United States. Treatments are so gentle that they are offered in spas and salons without direct medical supervision. Microdermabrasion is a gentle abrasive procedure that uses the assistance of a closed-loop vacuum apparatus to mechanically débride the thickened keratin layer of epidermis. Skin is exfoliated by the projection of a stream of aluminum oxide crystals at a controlled intensity generated by a vacuum compressor. Greater treatment depth is created by increasing the pressure of the jetted crystals, increasing the suction to stretch the skin tautly, and decreasing the speed of each pass.[12] As the suction removes dead epidermal skin cells and stretches the skin, it stimulates blood flow to the skin surface and may result in a transient hyperemia. This improved microcirculation in response to superficial intraepidermal injury presumably stimulates local collagen production by fibroblasts in the papillary dermis and improves lymphatic drainage of the deeper structures.

Microdermabrasion has gained popularity in treating photoaging, dyschromia, acne, mild scarring, and, to a lesser degree, fine wrinkles. Conservative treatments can be performed by microdermabrasion in a series of treatments at weekly intervals until desired results are achieved, followed by monthly maintenance therapy with no down-time. Microdermabrasion is touted to rejuvenate skin, soften fine wrinkles and stretch marks, and treat hyperpigmentation and acne scars. Results from these latter claims are minimal. It is safe to use on all skin types at all ages and has minimal if any recovery time. Adjustments in settings and technique can be tailored to the sensitivity of the individual. If deep erosion of the epidermis is attempted in patients with less sensitive skin, more marked desquamation a few days after treatment should be anticipated.

Clinical improvement after serial treatments is attributable to chronic stimulation of a low-grade reparative process at the level of both the dermis and the epidermis. The stratum corneum is buffed and compacted with flattening of the rete pegs after a single microdermabrasion procedure.[16,17] After serial procedures, comparative histopathologic analysis reveals epidermal and dermal hyperplasia, decreased pigmentation, perivascular inflammation, and hyalinization of the papillary dermis with a small increase in dermal collagen and elastin.[18,19]

The results of microdermabrasion for facial rejuvenation remain subjective and patient dependent, but studies suggest that short-term improvements in texture and skin tone are observed.[16] Because microdermabrasion is effective in exfoliation and refining pore size, it is best considered an adjunct to skin care in patients with sebaceous skin or large pores that frequently plug with keratin debris.

Whereas superficial peels and microdermabrasion both provide epidermal exfoliation, microdermabrasion additionally stimulates fibroblasts and dermal collagen deposition through an unidentified mechanism. The efficacy of superficial peels and microdermabrasion is dependent on patient compliance with routine skin care regimens and the continuation of maintenance procedures. The frequency of maintenance procedures is patient specific but in many cases is required monthly.[15] Concurrent topical therapy may include tretinoins, hydroxyacids, bleaching agents, and sunscreens. For example, mild photoaging can be addressed with microdermabrasion combined with an α-hydroxyacid skin care regimen, and acne scarring or melasma can be optimized with the concurrent use of retinoid therapy.[13]

In an era of widespread availability and technological advancements, the importance of simple skin care adjunct

Table 10.7 Chemical Peels: Depth of Penetration

Superficial	Medium depth	Enhanced medium depth	Deep
30–50% glycolic acid Jessner's solution	70% glycolic acid 35% TCA	Jessner's solution then 35% TCA Solid CO_2 freeze then 35% TCA 70% glycolic acid then 35% TCA	Phenol

procedures cannot be underestimated. Even where more invasive procedures are indicated, final outcomes are improved by taking the time to address skin tone and texture. The safety profile and minimal down-time of superficial peels and microdermabrasion are their most attractive features, but their outcomes are often criticized with regard to facial rejuvenation. The practitioner must appreciate that superficial resurfacing strictly achieves skin rejuvenation by improving tone and texture, which is only one component of complete facial rejuvenation. For this reason, patient selection and informed consent are critical to maintaining satisfaction with superficial procedures.

Darker-skinned individuals have more complaints of pigmentary dyschromia and acne when compared with Caucasians who more commonly complain of photodamage and rhytides. With this variability, the requirements for skin rejuvenation are often different for darker skin types. Darker skin types have thicker skin with increased layers of stratum corneum and a tendency to produce exaggerated responses to cutaneous injury.[13] These patients benefit most from epidermal exfoliation procedures that do not result in dermal penetration or melanocyte activation. Appreciation of this fact highlights the utility of superficial skin resurfacing, especially in this population of patients. Pretreatment with 4% hydroquinone or 20% azelaic acid for 2 weeks is recommended to diminish melanocyte activity and minimize posttreatment hyperpigmentation.[13]

Dermabrasion

Dermabrasion dates back to 1500 BC, when Egyptians first used sandpaper to smooth scars. The use of sandpaper progressed to motorized dermabrasion in 1905 when Kromayer, a German dermatologist, demonstrated that ablation into the reticular dermis could be used to treat various skin conditions without scar formation.[20] Throughout the 20th century, dermabrasion remained the gold standard to which all new deep skin resurfacing modalities were compared.

Dermabrasion removes the epidermis and dermis by use of a rotary abrasive motorized hand-piece. The depth of injury is at the level of the middermis near the junction of the papillary and reticular dermis. Wound healing is lengthy and requires reepithelialization by the remaining dermal adnexal structures. Because scars and keloids lack adnexae, they do not respond as favorably to dermabrasion.[21] Dermabrasion has been used to successfully treat postacne scarring, melasma, rhinophyma, and a variety of lesions including actinic and seborrheic keratoses. Tattoo removal can be addressed with dermabrasion, but given the advent of lasers that treat pigment directly without scarring, dermabrasion has fallen out of favor for this purpose except where cost is a prohibitive factor.[12,20]

Deep

The Baker phenol peel is a deep peel that has been used for decades to reliably improve heavy rhytides (**Figs. 10.4 and 10.5**). The Baker formula phenol may be applied with or without occlusion. Occlusion deepens penetration to the midreticular dermis by the application of waterproof zinc oxide tape as soon as the agent is applied to each subunit. With deeper penetration comes the increased risk of scarring should the reticular dermis be breached.

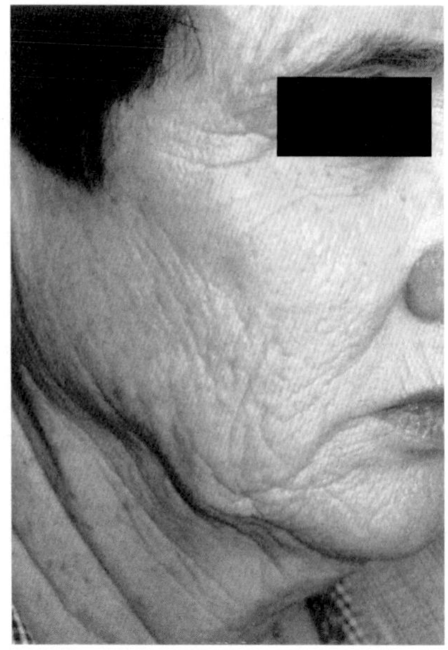

Fig. 10.4 Deep chemical peel with Baker-Gordon formula (before treatment).

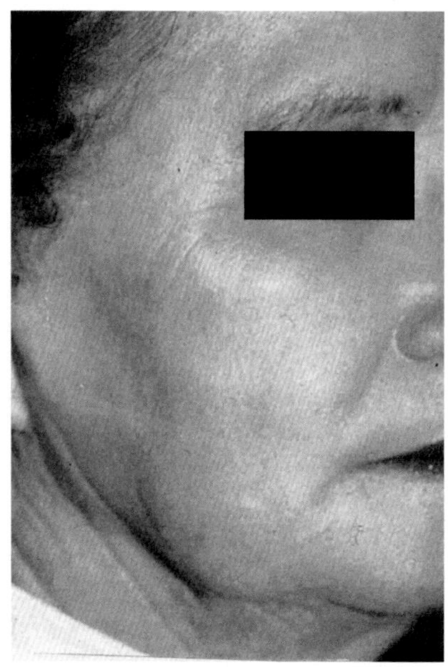

Fig. 10.5 Deep chemical peel with Baker-Gordon formula (after treatment).

In 1961, the Baker-Gordon modification reduced the concentration of phenol from full strength to 55% phenol. Whereas full-strength phenol caused immediate coagulation blocking further penetration by the agent, dilution enabled keratolysis to improve depth of penetration.[11]

The addition of croton oil facilitates deeper penetration of the phenol.

Phenol is absorbed through the skin and causes concentration-dependent toxicity. This procedure requires preoperative hydration and intravenous sedation. Typically, 1 L of fluid is given preoperatively, and 1 L is given during the procedure to dilute serum concentrations. Additional precautions include the use of supplemental oxygen and treatment of facial units at 15-minute intervals extending the time of application of a full face peel to 90 minutes. EKG monitoring for cardiac arrhythmia is performed, and the procedure is stopped if any signs of premature ventricular contractions or premature atrial contractions are encountered. The peel is contraindicated in patients with a history of cardiac disease or hepatic or renal compromise. In the event of an adverse reaction, mineral oil can be used as a diluent of phenol.[11]

With the availability of numerous alternatives, despite its efficacy, phenol has fallen out of favor for most practitioners given its rare but life-threatening complication of cardiac arrhythmia. Stronger concentrations of 50% or greater TCA alone are also less commonly used, given the poor control of injury and high risk of scarring at concentrations of 50% or greater.[22]

Enhanced Medium-Depth

TCA may be used alone in the concentration of 35% to achieve a standard medium-depth peel. Enhanced medium-depth peels are the preferred technique to deepen a medium-depth peel with less risk of complication than with a true deep peel. Pretreatment with other agents such as freeze technique using solid CO_2 followed by 35% TCA,[22] Jessner's solution followed by 35% TCA,[23] or 70% glycolic acid followed by 35% TCA[24] first removes the epidermal barrier with a superficial peel to achieve a stronger, more even medium-depth peel in the same setting. These alternative enhanced 35% TCA peels achieve results comparable with 50% TCA with fewer complications.[11] In the event that an inappropriate concentration of an acidic formulation is used, saline and bicarbonate of soda can be used as a diluent.

Enhanced medium-depth chemical peels are suitable for patients with Glogau type II or III photoaging including pigmentary changes, lentigines, epidermal growths, actinic keratosis, dyschromia, and rhytides. They are safest to use in Fitzpatrick type I or II patients; many type III patients may also qualify depending on their skin type. Thicker skin types in patients reporting a low propensity for scar formation or pigmentary abnormalities are better candidates.[11]

Enhanced medium-depth peels are relatively safe, single-stage procedures with a recovery time of approximately 7 to 10 days. Patients do not require intravenous sedation; mild sedation and pain medication are generally sufficient. Antiviral medications are initiated on the day of resurfacing and are continued until the skin is fully reepithelialized in patients with a history of herpetic infection.[25] The use of prophylactic antibiotics remains controversial. Patients with Fitzpatrick skin types IV through VI are pretreated with 4% hydroquinone or 20% azelaic acid for 2 weeks to diminish melanocyte activity and minimize posttreatment hyperpigmentation.

The technique is as follows: the patient is positioned upright at 30 degrees with his or her eyes closed. Degreasing the skin with cleanser and gauze to débride the stratum corneum is critical to ensure uniform penetration of the agent. Preparation with a cleanser such as Septisol (STERIS Corporation, Mentor, OH) followed by acetone to remove residual oil and debris is recommended for this purpose. A commonly used enhanced medium-depth peel (preferred by the authors) was first described by Monheit[23]: the Jessner's with 35% TCA peel. One or two coats of Jessner's solution are applied with a cotton-tip applicator or small gauze to achieve a very light frost. The patient feels only heat and experiences a mild erythema with this initial application. TCA 35% is then applied using one to four cotton-tip applicators. An immediate burning sensation is experienced upon application; as the frosting is completed, the burning subsides. Depth is titrated by the number of applicators used over a given area and time of application. Anatomic areas should be peeled sequentially from areas of thicker skin to more sensitive areas of thin skin. Application with broad strokes over the forehead, then temple and malar area usually requires four applicators. Two applicators are next used to apply the peel to the subnasal/supralabial area and finally one applicator across the periorbital area. Application in the perioral area should be performed over the lip skin into the vermilion, and feathering should be performed at the hairline, jaw line, and orbital rims. Tears should be dried immediately with dry cotton-tip applicators during the peeling process to prevent uneven dilution of the peel by tears as well as upward migration of the peel solution into the eye.

Upon application, frosting indicates keratocoagulation and completion of the protein denaturation process. Peak frosting occurs after 3 to 4 minutes. If frosting is incomplete or uneven, a thin application of solution should be reapplied in those areas.[26] Because overcoating with TCA will result in a deeper peel, it is prudent to carefully monitor areas of reapplication for the desired level of frosting. Level 1 frosting remains superficial and manifests as erythema with a blotchy frosting. Level 2 frosting is desired in the majority of sensitive regions and manifests as a white-coated frosting with visible erythema. Sensitive eyelid skin and areas over bony prominences with increased scar tendency including the zygomatic arch, jaw line, and chin should be treated until level 2 frosting is achieved. Level 3 frosting is a thick white frosting and indicates denaturation into the papillary dermis. Level 3 frosting should be restricted to areas of thicker skin and heavy actinic damage. Upon adequate frosting, the peel is diluted with cool saline compresses to neutralize its activity.[23]

The postoperative regimen to be followed by patients at home includes application of 0.25% acetic acid soaks followed by a mild emollient cream such as Aquaphor (Aquaphor Corporation, Wilton, CT) or Vaseline (Unilever, Englewood Cliffs, NJ). The acetic acid soaks can be made by diluting 1 tablespoon of white vinegar in 1 pint of warm water and are applied 4 times a day for the first 24 to 48 hours. The patient may shower after 24 hours and use mild cleanser. Marked edema, erythema, and desquamation are anticipated. As desquamation completes in 4 to 5 days, it is replaced with intensified erythema, which gradually subsides by days 7 to 10 to the appearance of mild sunburn.[25]

Wound Healing and Complications

The appearance of the patient after medium and deep peels can be intimidating as wound healing progresses. The four stages of wound healing include inflammation, coagulation, reepithelialization, and fibroplasia. Onset of inflammation is marked by erythema, which progresses to a dusky appearance over the first 12 hours. As coagulation occurs, the epidermis is separated with a significant production of exudate and crusting. As exudate formation begins, it is important to treat the patient with acetic acid soaks for gentle débridement and occlusive ointments such as previously described. The use of acetic acid helps remove necrotic debris and has antibacterial properties. The mild acidic pH is physiologic for healing tissue.

After the first 48 hours, reepithelialization begins and continues for 7 to 10 days. This stage is promulgated by ointments and the prevention of crust accumulation. The final phase of fibroplasia is a maturation phase that continues for up to 4 months with angiogenesis and new collagen formation. Improved texture and rhytides parallels collagen formation, and therefore progressive improvement can be seen for up to 4 months.[21] Frequent postoperative checks are important for surveillance of wound healing. Poor wound healing may be attributable to underlying infection, allergic or contact dermatitis, or other systemic disorders. Such conditions increase the risk of scarring and require prompt evaluation and treatment. Infections should be cultured and treated with oral antibiotics taking into consideration high risk of staphylococcal, streptococcal, coliform (*Escherichia coli*), and pseudomonal infections. In case of a posttreatment dermatitis, the offending agent should be eliminated, if possible, and should improve with corticosteroids therapy.

Persistent erythema beyond 5 days for a superficial peel, 1 month for a medium-depth peel, or 2 to 3 months for deep chemical peels is considered abnormal. Contact sensitization or dermatitis or reactivation of a prior skin disorder are factors to consider. Prompt treatment with topical and systemic steroids is important to prevent scarring. Once scar formation has occurred, intralesional steroid injection, use of silicone sheeting, and laser treatment may help address these scars.[14,21]

Herpes simplex can be exacerbated from any facial skin rejuvenation procedures, but thorough evaluation will help identify those at risk. Patients with prior history should initiate antiviral medication on the day of the procedure and continue for up to 10 days, depending on the depth of dermal resurfacing. Antivirals such as acyclovir and valacyclovir inhibit viral replication in intact epidermal cells. In cases of acute exacerbation after resurfacing procedures, the antiviral medication must be continued until the skin has fully reepithelialized, typically 10 days for medium-depth peels and 2 weeks for deep peels and laser resurfacing.[11] In cases of active herpetic infections, early treatment with antiviral medications usually precludes scarring.

◆ Home Skin Care

Many of us embarked upon chemical peels and laser resurfacing as a method for aggressive facial skin rejuvenation. From that beginning, it became apparent that the skin responds better when prepared by pretreatment with home care regimens. These home care products have been found to sometimes preclude the need for laser therapy. The goals of pretreatment are to reduce the keratinized stratum corneum layer, downregulate melanin metabolism, and create good skin care and sun protection habits in the patients. Skin product regimens include retinoic or α-hydroxyacid, a bleaching agent, and sunscreens. Pretreatment has been shown to enhance reepithelialization after ablative resurfacing[5] and to reduce adverse reactions in intense pulsed light (IPL) treatments.[27]

As a first step, all patients are placed on a carefully controlled skin care regimen. This will not only help prepare the skin for resurfacing but also recruit patients into taking part in their skin care. Patients may not be appropriate candidates for ablative resurfacing and the involved posttreatment skin care if they cannot comply with regular product application.

There has been a tremendous onslaught of products in the marketplace that have little scientific validity but are backed by multimillion-dollar marketing packages. Patients should be educated on label examination of products and the value of determining what the act of concentration of product ingredients are. The use of a glycolic acid base with a minimum of 10 to 20% glycolic acid and/or a retinoid product should be recommended to patients. This at-home regimen should also be kept as simple as possible to ensure patient compliance.

A typical skin care regimen includes a 10 to 20% glycolic acid facial, 10 to 20% glycolic acid toner, and a lipid-based serum. As the skin is a fatty bilayer, water-based moisturizers are not absorbed but rather evaporate. Numerous companies now formulate lipid-based serums that are high in vitamins A, C, and E and hyaluronic acids. These known antioxidants, when absorbed into the dermis, are beneficial to fibroblastic stimulation and the ongoing revitalization of the collagen matrix. Vitamin A derivative (Retin-A [Ortho Dermatological, Skillman, NJ], Renova [Ortho-McNeil Pharmaceuticals, Inc., Titusville, NJ], Kinerase [Valeant Pharmaceuticals International, Viejo, CA]) or related-activity products have also been shown to be beneficial to fibroblastic stimulation. Several additional fibroblast/collagen stimulating products are available but are beyond the scope of this chapter. The combination of these with lipid-based moisturizers to balance their drying effect should be proposed to the patient.[28]

Proper sun protection is critical not only to prevent skin cancer but also to improve the blending process for skin hyperpigmentation. SPF 15 sun block is recommended for daily use. An SPF of at least 30 should be used if exposed to direct sun or participating in any activities that may have prolonged sun exposure. The sun should be avoided completely for at least 3 to 4 weeks after nonablative treatments directed at melanin and hemoglobin chromophores and for at least 3 months after ablative resurfacing.

The majority of patients presenting with pigment variation can be helped using a combination of products that have been shown to block the melanocytic conversion of tyrosine to melanin. An accepted regimen is the synergistic application of glycolic acid, hydroquinone 4 to 8%, and retinoic acid.[5] Patients should be advised that when used alone (without laser), a fair trial of this regimen is daily use for at least 6 months. These products may also improve the ultimate result and reduce short-term reactions to lasers. The melanin downregulation is useful for both nonablative and ablative lasers. The recommended period of pretreatment is at least 3 weeks for Fitzpatrick type III patients and is more important for more highly pigmented skin.

◆ Laser Skin Rejuvenation

Laser is an acronym for light amplification by the stimulated emission of radiation. Albert Einstein first postulated the use of stimulated emission producing photon energy in 1916. Medical applications of lasers did not begin until the 1960s. Two decades later, the CO_2 laser was found to be able to vaporize skin in specific layers when used in a superpulsed or rapid scanning mode.[29] The principle that allows precise ablation is selective photothermolysis. Lasers produce energy in a single wavelength that is absorbed by specific color or type of tissue called a chromophore. For the CO_2 and erbium lasers, the chromophore is water.

Selective photothermolysis is the ablation of tissue with minimum damage to surrounding structures by rapidly heating the target tissue. Heating and cooling is so fast that the adjacent tissue is minimally damaged. The high content of water in the skin absorbs the CO_2 and erbium laser energy causing rapid heating and vaporization of the superficial layers of the skin, eliminating or minimizing dermal injury and scarring. The erbium laser is absorbed 12 to 18 times more efficiently than is the CO_2 laser allowing more superficial absorption with less penetration.[6] This allows even less collateral damage. Over the past decade, technology has concentrated on improving delivery of the laser energy by increasing precision of the depth of layers being ablated and further minimizing deeper collateral damage. Precise depth of injury can be predicted with both lasers.

Traditional ablative treatments for aging skin have relied on tissue ablation, epidermal and dermal wounding, and subsequent collagen remodeling.[30,31] Raw skin, oozing, and redness, significant healing time, and intensive patient wound care predictably accompany use of ablative lasers such as the CO_2 and erbium:YAG (Er:YAG), similar to that seen with deep chemical peels.[32,33] Complications of CO_2 laser, although uncommon, may include hyperpigmentation, prolonged erythema, infection, scarring, and hypopigmentation.[29] Side effects and complications of the Er:YAG laser are similar to those of the CO_2 laser but tend to be less severe and frequent.[6] Although procedures accompanied by these predictable side effects may be necessary for moderate to severely aged or photodamaged skin, the remainder of the patient population can benefit significantly from less invasive techniques.

Ablative Laser Skin Resurfacing

The CO_2 laser vaporizes the most superficial layer of skin by heating it to more than 100°C.[34] After this ablation of the superficial epidermis, the next layer undergoes tissue necrosis from heating to temperatures ranging from 70°C to 100°C. Deep to that are tissue effects on collagen. Collagen is partially denatured between 37°C and 70°C; there also may be some "tightening" of the collagen. With the first pass of the CO_2 laser, ~20 to 60 μm of skin is vaporized with standard laser settings.[35] There are significantly deeper thermal effects on collagen. Subsequent passes ablate less tissue but increase tissue tightening by deeper collagen effects. Wound healing continues for several months after laser treatment and includes collagen remodeling and new collagen production. This new collagen layer is more uniform and gives the overlying skin surface a smoother appearance (**Figs. 10.6 and 10.7**).

The erbium laser vaporizes the epidermis more efficiently with a very narrow zone of thermal necrosis. This is because the erbium laser is absorbed significantly more efficiently by water in the skin than is the CO_2 laser. Erbium remains more superficial and has fewer long-term effects on the collagen. This is due to a thermal necrosis zone of 30 to 50 μm compared with up to 200 μm for CO_2.[36] Therefore,

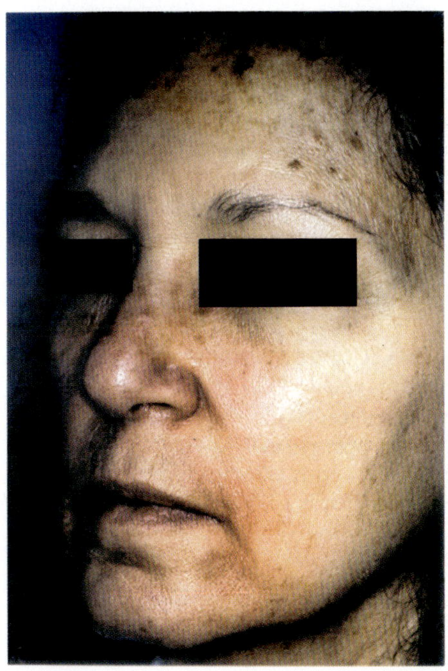

Fig. 10.6 CO_2 laser resurfacing (before treatment).

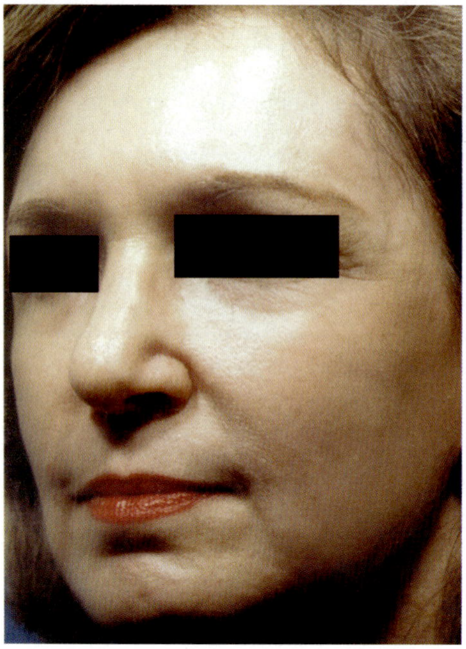

Fig. 10.7 CO_2 laser resurfacing (after treatment).

more rapid healing occurs after erbium resurfacing, which might make it a more attractive alternative. The erbium laser can be used to the same depth as the CO_2 laser but with equivalent postoperative healing and less margin of safety.[37] Because of minimal heat effects, however, long-term results of ablative resurfacing for deep wrinkles are superior for CO_2 laser than for erbium laser. Erbium laser is a safer, more precise laser for ablative resurfacing. The best patients for erbium laser have superficial photodamage and wrinkles. For longer-lasting treatment of deeper rhytides, the CO_2 laser is a better choice but with longer healing and more treatment risk.

Newer applications of these ablative lasers have shortened healing time and reportedly reduced potential complications. Sequentially treating with the erbium laser after CO_2 laser passes removes the region of thermal injury with similar results to CO_2 laser resurfacing.[36] Newer variable-pulse erbium lasers can produce more thermal damage providing greater collagen tightening.[35] This laser reportedly still has reduced healing time when compared with the CO_2 laser. Lastly, single-pass CO_2 laser treatment can be effective for superficial photodamage and skin aging.[38] Generally, it has been the authors' contention that the results of ablative resurfacing are directly proportional to the healing time. Faster healing means less smooth skin, less energy, less collagen remodeling, less erythema with subsequently less rhytide softening.

For patients with severely photodamaged skin, ablative resurfacing is the best treatment. Significant improvement can be achieved in a single treatment. Texture, tone, and mild to moderate wrinkles can all be improved. Epidermal lesions, mild to moderate acne scars, actinic keratoses, and recurrent skin cancers can all be treated. However, healing is prolonged, and hypopigmentation is a common side effect. The best candidates are Glogau types III and IV and Fitzpatrick wrinkle scale type III. Patients with less photodamage may be candidates if they desire a single treatment, with the trade-off of protracted healing.

After ablative resurfacing, the skin may appear hypopigmented. This may be a true destruction of melanocytes in the skin by the laser or restoration of its true natural color. Relative to the rest of the exposed body, unexposed skin appears pale. During the consultation, patients are asked to hold the inside of their upper arms to their face to demonstrate the relative color difference. This is especially important if regional treatment of the perioral or periorbital areas is being considered for rejuvenation. Those areas will become smoother and lighter than the surrounding facial skin. Once the face is treated, the neck may need treatment as well. This can be accomplished with very careful erbium or CO_2 laser treatment, blending with light chemical peels or nonablative laser treatment.

Patients need to be prepared with skin products prior to treatment as practice for the intense commitment for posttreatment care. Resurfacing is performed under local anesthesia for small areas and regional anesthesia with sedation or general anesthesia for full-face rejuvenation. Treatment parameters are well described[5,32,34] and are beyond the scope of this publication. Posttreatment care includes an occlusive biologic dressing, antibiotics, and antiviral and analgesic medications. The skin will take from 5 to 7 days to reepithelialize. The face will be red for a few weeks and may remain pink for 3 to 6 months. Reepithelialization and healing is more rapid for erbium and single-pass CO_2 laser treatments. Patients are instructed preoperatively that they may need to wear makeup daily for up to 6 months.

Laser resurfacing has almost replaced older modalities such as dermabrasion and medium or deep chemical peeling for skin rejuvenation[39] for most practitioners. Numerous physicians still prefer the more traditional methods, but more laser procedures are performed than are deep peels. The laser appears to produce a more precise, predictable peel depth for physicians not highly skilled in mechanical dermabrasion or chemical peeling.

Nonablative Laser Skin Resurfacing

Nonablative remodeling rejuvenates skin without superficial epidermolysis by attacking tissue beneath the surface (**Fig. 10.8**). Laser energy penetrates through the epidermis without absorption and associated damage. This process reduces or eliminates posttreatment erythema caused by ablative treatments. A direct dermal wound with new collagen formation effacing wrinkles and acne scarring is the goal. Nonablative remodeling may be more appropriately termed *subsurface remodeling*.[39] Some nonablative lasers also target other aging changes including irregular pigmentation, abnormal blood vessels, and telangiectasias (**Table 10.8**).

After the introduction of the CO_2 and erbium lasers for skin rejuvenation in the 1990s, there was a large increase in patients seeking skin resurfacing. However, healing time

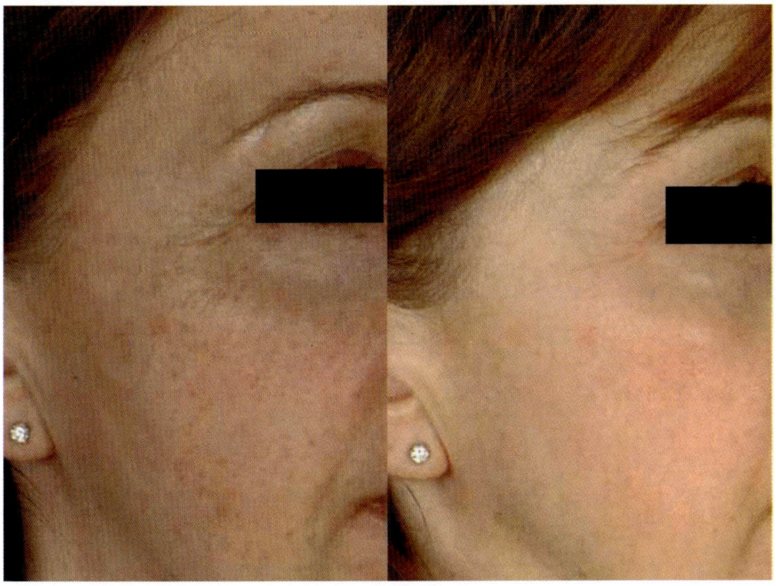

Fig. 10.8 Nonablative treatment: IPL and long-pulse 1064-nm Nd:YAG laser (**A**) before and (**B**) after five treatments. (Courtesy of Dr. Gregory Waslen.)

did not improve above that of deep peels and dermabrasion. Many patients were found to be unwilling to tolerate the healing time necessary for improved skin texture, tone, and color. There was also concern about potential permanent pigment problems with deep resurfacing.[29] More Asian, Mediterranean, and African-American patients also presented for skin rejuvenation. In response to these dilemmas, nonablative lasers have markedly increased in popularity.

Numerous lasers and "laser-like" devices (to be categorized as lasers for simplicity) began to be developed for nonablative skin rejuvenation (**Table 10.9**). The goal of these newer devices is to treat the dermis without the surface ablation. The concept of nonablative remodeling came from skin changes witnessed in conjunction with hair removal, vascular, and pigment lasers that target subepidermal chromophores. Additionally, the collagen deposition that occurs over the months after ablative lasers led investigators to find ways to stimulate collagen production. Ideally, a controlled injury would be inflicted in the dermis without affecting the overlying epidermis. The newly stimulated collagen would tighten and smooth the skin from under the surface without the side effects of prolonged erythema, pigment alteration, and risks of scarring and infection associated with surface ablation.[40]

Table 10.8 Skin Changes Treatable by Laser Resurfacing

Nonablative Lasers	Ablative (CO_2 and Erbium) Resurfacing
Photodamage (mild)	Photodamage (moderate to severe)
Skin texture (mild)	Skin texture (moderate to severe)
Uneven pigmentation	Uneven pigmentation
Fine wrinkles	Fine and medium wrinkles
Benign vascular lesions	Early redundant skin
Telangiectasias	Actinic keratoses
Rosacea and erythema	History of superficial skin cancers
Mild acne scars (?)	Traumatic and mild to moderate acne scars
Large pores	Benign epidermal lesions
	Dermal lesions

Nonablative lasers achieve subsurface remodeling by several different modalities.[41] Selective epidermal cooling uses cryogen spray or contact cooling to protect the epidermis. Longer wavelengths promote deeper penetration. Multiple rapid laser pulses at lower fluences reduce superficial heat accumulation. Lastly, deeper focus of the laser energy aids epidermal preservation. Nonablative lasers can be divided into two types: infrared lasers that stimulate collagen remodeling, targeting fine lines and skin texture; and visible light lasers for collagen remodeling and treating pigment and vascular changes. Minimally invasive or nonablative lasers are used for skin color correction, treating red and brown changes in the skin. Improvement can be made in photodamaged skin with uneven pigmentation. Included in the color correction is reduction of telangiectasias, rosacea, and vascular lesions. IPL, pulsed dye, and diode lasers are best suited for color and general skin tone improvement.

Skin texture and fine wrinkles can be improved as well as mild acne scars and reduction of large pores by replenishing collagen. The collagen systems act in two manners by either stimulating fibroblasts specifically to create new collagen or by causing a subthreshold injury to the endothelial cells, which subsequently are responsible for cytokine and growth factor release causing neocollagenesis. For collagen reorganization smoothing rhytides, neodymium:YAG (Nd: YAG) lasers are superior with some improvement after IPL treatments.

Glogau and Fitzpatrick aging skin types I and II with some Glogau type III patients are candidates for nonablative skin remodeling. Severely photodamaged patients with advanced wrinkles are better candidates for ablative resurfacing. However, when combined with microdermabrasion, skin care, botulinum toxin, and repeated treatments, more advanced photodamaged skin can be improved.

Nonablative systems such as IPL can be safely used on nonfacial areas. Patients often present with photodamage

Table 10.9 Types of Systems (Lasers and Other Devices) for Rejuvenation

Laser	Wavelength (nm)	Target Tissue	Special Notes
Nonablative			
KTP	532	Endothelial cells	
Intense pulsed light	550–1200	Endothelial cells, melanocytes	Multiple cutoff filters for wavelength selection
Pulsed dye	585, 595	Microvessels	"Subpurpuric" doses
Diode	980	Melanocytes	Thermal hand-piece
Nd:YAG	1064	Melanocytes	Long pulse or Q-switched
Nd:YAG	1320	Fibroblasts	Thermal feedback sensor, dynamic cooling
Erbium:glass	1540	Fibroblasts	
Diode	1450	Fibroblasts	Epidermal cooling
Ablative			
Er:YAG	2940	H_2O in cells	Ablative
CO_2	10,600	H_2O in cells	Ablative
Coblation	Radiofrequency	H_2O in cells	Bipolar cautery

and vascular changes such as poikiloderma of the neck and upper chest.[42] Only the most experienced laser specialists should be treating the neck with ablative lasers.[5,43] Conservative settings are used to reduce demarcation previously seen with full-face ablative resurfacing. Alternative treatment is with nonablative laser treatment. Nonablative treatment of the neck is also used primarily with or without facial treatments for photodamage.[27] Even areas such as the hands are amenable to nonablative rejuvenation for skin color correction and texture improvement.

Minimal to No Down-time with Nonablative Lasers

Most of these systems are designed as minimally invasive. Minimally invasive means there is no patient down-time. Down-time is one of the most sought after indications for patients seeking laser skin rejuvenation. Patients typically return to normal activities the evening of or next day after treatment. There is mild to moderate discomfort, equated with the snapping of a rubber band. Topical anesthetic cream helps to reduce this sensation. Many of the newer lasers have built in cooling devices that significantly reduce treatment discomfort.

Some edema and erythema may last for a few days but can usually be covered by makeup. Each system has specific parameters for number and duration of treatment. Most nonablative lasers are used in a series of up to five treatments spaced 3 to 4 weeks apart. Quarterly to semiannual maintenance treatments are then recommended. Skin care maintenance also includes ongoing use of skin products and superficial peels and/or microdermabrasion for the epidermis.

1320-nm Nd:YAG Laser

The first nonablative laser was called the Cool Touch (CoolTouch Corp., Roseville, CA), which coupled a cryogen spray with a surface thermal sensor and 1320-nm Nd:YAG laser. Dynamic cooling protects the epidermis from thermal injury as the laser is delivered deeper to stimulate collagen. In one study,[44] mild improvement in rhytides was seen in just over 60% of patients and best results for mild to moderate wrinkles. The author of that study recommended concurrent botulinum toxin and/or facial fillers for severe rhytides. A multicenter study also demonstrated small but statistically significant long-term improvement in severe rhytides only.[45] Updates to this laser (Cool Touch II and III) have yielded better results for acne scarring and a lower incidence of treatment discomfort.[46]

1064-nm Nd:YAG Laser

In early studies, a 1064-nm Q-switched Nd:YAG laser was demonstrated to yield improvement in skin texture and elasticity as well as rhytide reduction.[47] However, there was persistent erythema in some patients. Newer long-pulse 1064-nm Nd:YAG lasers have been demonstrated to produce statistically significant improvement in fine wrinkles, coarse wrinkles, skin laxity, and overall skin appearance.[48] When combined with a long-pulse 532-nm potassium titanyl phosphate (KTP) laser, results were superior to either laser alone along with minor improvement in erythema and dyschromias.[35]

585-nm Pulsed Dye Laser

The pulsed dye laser has traditionally been used for vascular anomalies. The 585-nm yellow light is absorbed preferentially by superficial blood vessels leaving the surrounding tissue relatively uninjured. It has also been found to improve skin texture and hypertrophic scars by changes in elastin and possibly dermal collagen.[49] Initial patients had purpura, as commonly occurred with the pulsed dye laser. However, another study with the N-Lite (ICN Photonics, Costa Mesa, CA) version of this laser reduced the joules and produced increased collagen production in 84% of patients with an improved "wrinkle value" without purpura.[50] This laser targets the oxyhemoglobin and deoxyhemoglobin in the superficial blood vessels affecting adjacent collagen at levels that do not injure the vessels.

Intense Pulsed Light

Intense pulsed light (IPL) uses a broad spectrum of light that can be adjusted through filters and computer-controlled parameters to customize the light energy to the target within the skin (such as brown spots, red blood vessels, hair follicles, and collagen). IPL is a noncoherent (thus not categorized as a laser) high-energy broadband-pulsed flashlamp that emits light in the range of 500 to 1200 nm.[31] Absorption filters are selected to block wavelengths of light below the selected number. Spot size and energy also affect depth of penetration. Wavelengths can be selected from 515 to 1064 nm. The primary chromophores are hemoglobin with peak absorption between 577 to 585 nm and melanin with a range of 500 to 850 nm. Lower-wavelength cutoff filters are used for more superficial melanin. The higher filters penetrate to melanin in the hair shafts. Therefore, appropriate filters can be selected to target superficial vessels and superficial and deep melanin. Dermal collagen can be reached with 640- and 755-nm cutoff filters.[27] The 1064-nm Nd:YAG laser attachment affects larger blood vessels, deeper collagen, and may improve wrinkles.

IPL yielded improvement in at least some facial rhytides in 83% of patients.[31] However, photodamaged skin is more than just wrinkles. Fine wrinkling, irregular pigmentation, skin texture, pore size, telangiectasias, and facial erythema all were found to improve in a majority of patients.[51] There was also an 88% satisfaction rate for patients in this study. The IPL thus far has been a more useful nonablative device for the broad range of facial skin aging. For rhytides alone, the 1064-nm Nd:YAG laser was found to be superior.[52]

Fractional Resurfacing

Fractional resurfacing attempts to combine the concept of superior results from ablative resurfacing with the reduced adverse effects of nonablative lasers. Using an erbium laser, microscopic zones of thermal injury are created.[53] The skin heals within less than 24 hours because normal skin remains between treatment spots. Side effects also appear to be less severe than with ablative resurfacing. Improvement has been demonstrated in skin texture, tone, dyschromias, and scars. A similar device called ActiveFx (Lumenis Corp., Santa Clara, CA; direct communication) is under investigation that uses a CO_2 laser to create the microthermal zones.

Other Lasers and Laser-like Devices

There are several additional laser and laser-like devices that target the dermis and attempt to tighten facial tissue. Radiofrequency devices may cause skin tightening and can create measurable brow elevation.[46] These devices are undergoing constant improvement. Because they do not specifically address photoaging, they are beyond the scope of this chapter.

Ethnic Considerations

A careful history is very important for laser skin rejuvenation. Fitzpatrick described the most universally used system for determining skin type (**Table 10.4**). Fanous modified the Fitzpatrick classification to reflect the racial origins of patients seeking resurfacing.[54] These run from north to south along the central axis of Europe to Africa. They parallel the Fitzpatrick classification but are based on color and coarseness of features. The six types are Nordic, European, Mediterranean, Indo-Pakistani, African, and Asian. The goal for both systems of classification is to quantify the amount of inherent melanin in the skin, as a primary chromophore, skin thickness, and texture. These classifications determine how the skin reacts to thermal energy. Accurate patient evaluation is paramount for obtaining the best results with the smallest incidence of complications. Misdiagnosis is one of the most common causes for complications and prolonged healing time.

Complications

When considering laser skin rejuvenation or deep chemical peels, it is important to remember that the skin is an organ that reacts to damage by an inflammatory response and subsequent healing. Wound healing and the posttreatment course for ablative laser resurfacing is similar to deep chemical peels and has been previously described in this chapter. Complications for all laser treatments are greater when treating patients with Fitzpatrick classification skin type IV and higher. Hyperpigmentation is the most common complication for these patients. Ablative treatment for patients with higher Fitzpatrick types is better achieved with the erbium laser for the reduced depth of penetration and reduced effect on melanin.[39]

The incidence of complications from nonablative laser treatments is extremely low. When they occur, they more resemble treatment with an ablative laser. Patients usually heal without long-term sequelae. The superficial nature and low fluences used significantly reduces this risk. The most common short-term side effects are blistering of the skin and erythema after treatment. This may lead to postinflammatory changes with temporary hyperpigmentation or hypopigmentation. However, these conditions resolve over time. To reduce the reaction to laser treatments, pretreatment with the skin care regimen outlined above prepares the skin and downregulates the melanocytes.

Prolonged side effects from nonablative lasers are unexpected by both patients and physicians because these lasers are represented as minimally invasive. Alterations in treatment parameters have reduced these complications. Treatment of higher Fitzpatrick types has an increased incidence of side effects after nonablative laser therapy. Improper assignment of a skin type can lead to treatment parameters that are too aggressive for a given patient and have been the most common cause for prolonged side effects. It is even more important for patients with Fitzpatrick skin type IV and higher to strictly adhere to the pretreatment skin care regimen.

We suggest that treatment should be initiated conservatively especially because it is performed in a series. Until the laser surgeon becomes familiar with the system being used, the first treatment should be set for a fluence that is at least 10% lower than the manufacturer's recommendations and/or increase the delay between pulses. Patients will understand that for nonablative lasers, this conservative approach will keep treatment truly noninvasive.

◆ Botulinum Toxin

The earliest signs of aging include wrinkles that develop as hyperdynamic lines caused by repetitive movement of underlying muscles. Fibrous attachments to the skin cause accentuation of hyperdynamic lines with animation. With advancing age, the loss of skin elasticity leads to skin redundancy manifesting as deep furrows present during both animation and at rest.

Dynamic facial wrinkles are caused by muscular contraction with normal facial animation. Dramatic improvements in fine lines and wrinkles of the face are noted within hours to days of injection into the belly of a muscle. Injection of botulinum toxin works locally to inhibit muscle contraction by selective chemical denervation preventing the presynaptic release of neurotransmitters at the neuromuscular junction of nicotinic acetylcholine receptors. Time of onset to muscle relaxation depends on the concentration of available neurotransmitter prior to inhibition and may take up to 5 days.[55] Theoretically, maximal results are seen weeks after injection, which is attributable to disuse muscle atrophy.

The therapeutic utility of botulinum toxin was first discovered in treatment of ophthalmic and subsequent neuromuscular disorders of the head and neck with a proven safety profile. In 1992, Drs. Jean and Alastair Carruthers published the first article on the cosmetic effectiveness of botulinum toxin for the treatment of glabellar frown lines,[55] and since then the cosmetic usage of botulinum toxin has surpassed its functional applications.

Botulinum toxin A (BTX-A; Botox; Allergan Inc., Santa Barbara, CA) is commercially available in vials of 100 units that are stored frozen at −5°C until they are reconstituted. Botox should be reconstituted with 0.9% saline to the desired concentration, drawn up in a tuberculin syringe, and injected with a 30- or 32-gauge needle. Using a short 30-gauge mesotherapy or tuberculin needle may offer more control during serial punctures. Dosing should be thought of in terms of units rather than volume. There is no known variability of efficacy at different dilutions when equivalent dosing is used; however, more dilute concentrations are associated with a greater degree of diffusion, and males typically require more concentrated injections than do females to achieve the same effects.[55] Single-strength dilution is typically performed with dilution of 100 units in 4 mL saline to a final concentration of 2.5 units per 0.1 mL. Double-strength dilution is performed by reconstituting 100 units in 2 mL saline to a final concentration of 5 units per 0.1 mL. The shelf-life of Botox after reconstitution is controversial. Botox has U.S. Food and Drug Administration (FDA) approval for use within 4 hours, because of the need to reconstitute the agent and concerns for sterility. Several controlled studies suggest that potency may remain for up to 4 weeks with no change in efficacy when refrigerated after use.[56]

Botox can be combined with dermal fillers, chemical peels, laser resurfacing, or microdermabrasion to maximize skin rejuvenation. Botulinum toxin is contraindicated in patients with neuromuscular disorders such as myasthenia gravis, Eaton-Lambert syndrome, and amyotrophic lateral sclerosis because its effects might be potentiated in this population. Aminoglycoside antibiotic is also known to possibly alter sensitivity to botulinum toxin and should be avoided until after therapy is completed. Although there are no teratogenic effects reported, treatment of pregnant or nursing women is not advisable.[57]

Resistance to Botox is no longer a problem. Older formulations of high-molecular-weight Botox were more prone to a neurotoxin dose-linked resistance secondary to the formation of blocking antibody. Since then, the Botox formulation is one fifth the molecular weight with a more active form of the same protein. In more than 5 million injections, resistance has never occurred at the lose dose required for cosmetic purposes. All incidences of reported resistance are in patients treated with frequent doses of 100 units to 200 units for neurogenic disorders. In the rare case of resistance, Myobloc (Solstice Neurosciences, Inc., Malvern, PA) (BTX-B) may be used as an alternative as there is no known cross-reactivity between these subtypes.[55] Although the potency of BTX-A is ~100 times that of BTX-B, BTX-B is available in vials of 2500, 5000, and 10,000 units for injection. Myobloc is also FDA approved to be used within 4 hours of reconstitution for purposes of sterility; however, studies demonstrate even greater stability with efficacy of up to 21 months when refrigerated.[58]

Technique of Treatment

A thorough understanding of facial anatomy is imperative to successfully treat the face and avoid complications. The face can be divided into upper, middle, and lower thirds. Botox injections are most commonly performed on the upper one third of the face, although treatment of the lower one third of the face and neck can be rewarding. Treatment of the middle one third of the face in an attempt to flatten the nasolabial fold can greatly affect the smile resulting in a diminished ability to raise the central upper lip. Treatment of this area is rarely indicated except in cases of facial synkinesis or facial paralysis. Following are only suggested patterns for injection. However, each patient must be individually examined and his or her specific pattern of facial muscle contraction mapped and noted for treatment. The authors actually use dots on the skin with an eyebrow pencil to mark areas of maximal muscle contraction for botulinum toxin treatment. This pencil is easily cleaned off after treatment. Observation of skilled physicians coupled with a comprehensive course in botulinum toxin treatment is imperative for consistent results.

Evaluation of the upper one third of the face includes analysis of the forehead, brows, and periorbital areas. Deep vertical glabellar creases convey an angry, frowning appearance and can be addressed by injecting the corrugator supercilii muscles. The frontalis superiorly and procerus muscles extending inferiorly to the nasion may contribute to the horizontal creases of the glabellar region. In a small population, the medial aspect of the superior fibers of orbicularis oculi muscles may contribute to deep furrows where the lateral glabellar region meets the medial brow.[29] It is prudent to address brow position and asymmetry with patients before injection. Appreciation of traction and countertraction of opposing depressors and elevator muscles will allow the physician to maintain or correct brow position as needed.

To treat the glabellar rhytides (**Figs. 10.9 and 10.10**), a range of 5 to 10 units of Botox should be injected into each corrugator muscle. The muscle bulk and degree of hyperactivity is appreciated by asking the patient to squint or frown. The extent of frontalis and procerus muscle involvement is also appreciated by asking the patient to raise his or her eyebrows. Typically, 3 to 4 units injected in the central glabellar area will adequately treat the procerus muscle.[59] The remaining horizontal furrows are treated by injecting the frontalis muscle along the length of the remaining wrinkles injecting ~2.5 units across the central forehead in at least six sites between the lowest and highest furrow or just below the furrow in cases of a single wrinkle. Additional sites can be injected depending on the location of furrows.

One of the original patterns for treatment of horizontal brow lines was by injection in a V-shaped formation. This best treats wrinkles that are only prominent centrally without involvement of the temporal portion of the frontalis muscle. The physician must appreciate that injection in this configuration will result in central paralysis and lateral compensation manifesting as a temporal lift. This may be advantageous in certain patients desiring a lateral brow lift. Afterward, however, this V-shaped formation may result in an exaggerated lateral brow elevation in patients with hyperactive temporal frontalis muscle activity. The manifestation of this "sinister" appearance is unacceptable and can be avoided by continuing the injection into the lateral frontalis muscle to depress the lateral brow (**Figs. 10.11 and 10.12**).[60]

Patients with naturally low-set brows and significant frontalis muscle rhytides may not be candidates for Botox because frontalis injection will accentuate brow ptosis by paralyzing the brow elevators. Although laterally the orbicularis oculi muscles act as brow depressors and may be injected to compensate, medially low injection of the corrugator

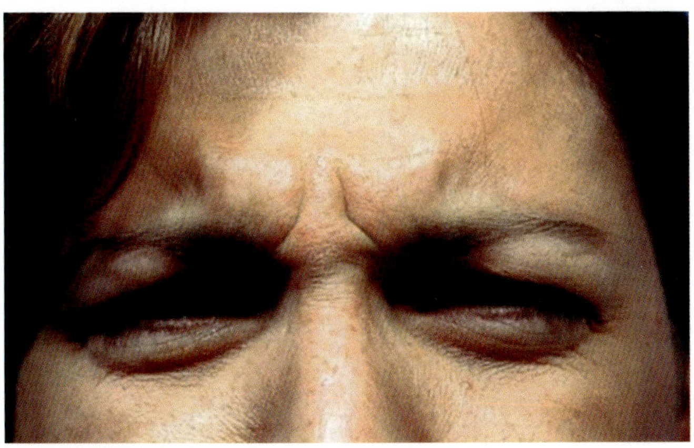

Fig. 10.9 Botulinum toxin treatment of glabellar wrinkles (before treatment).

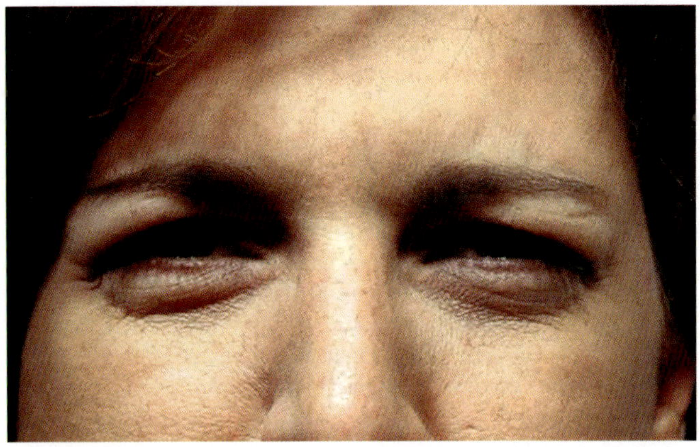

Fig. 10.10 Botulinum toxin treatment of glabellar wrinkles (after treatment).

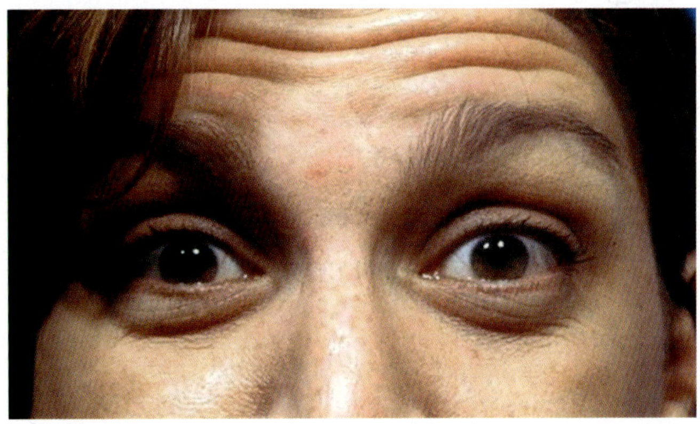

Fig. 10.11 Botulinum toxin treatment of horizontal brow wrinkles (before treatment).

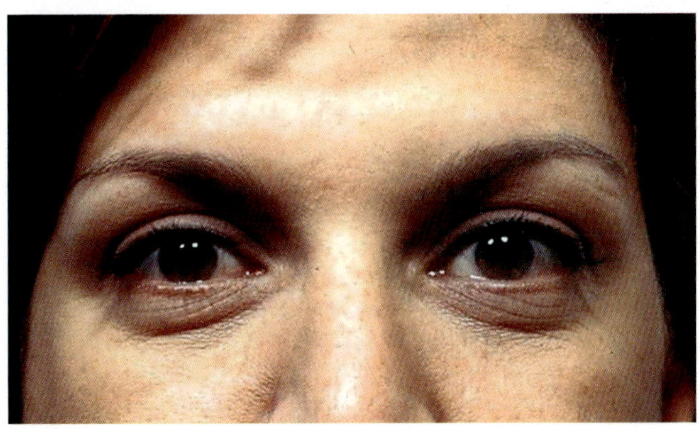

Fig. 10.12 Botulinum toxin treatment of horizontal brow wrinkles (after treatment).

supercilii, depressor supercilii, and procerus muscles will unlikely provide sufficient compensation. In all patients, care must also be taken to remain at least 1 cm above the brow when lateral to midpupillary line to prevent lateral brow ptosis and diffusion to the levator palpebrae superioris muscle resulting in the rare complication of eyelid ptosis.[60]

The characteristic crow's-feet are wrinkles that extend radially along the lateral course of the orbicularis oculi muscle. Injection in this area requires a small amount of agent to produce marked improvement. Finesse in injection is most important to avoid complications in this area. Patients should be evaluated for the integrity of lower lid tone using a snap test. Improper injection of the orbicularis oculi muscle can result in ectropion and should be avoided in patients with lower lid laxity. The delicate periorbital tissue is surrounded by many small veins that can result in significant ecchymosis if violated. Careful injection entry, use of loupe magnification, and icing before and after injection are best to avoid this complication. If bleeding or hematoma formation is noted on needle injection, immediate pressure and ice will usually stop progression. All periorbital injections should be kept superficial within the dermis to avoid diffusion through the orbital septum into the ocular muscles resulting in the rare complication of diplopia. One to 2 units injected between lines at three to five sites is usually sufficient per side.[61] Advanced injections may be used to address subciliary lines, but such injections should be performed only by experienced users. Whereas Botox may erase these subciliary lines, paralysis of the orbicularis oculi muscle in this region may accentuate unwanted skin redundancy and herniated periorbital fat.[61]

The lower third of the face and neck can also benefit from Botox therapy. The downward angulations at the corner of the mouth can be softened with a single conservative injection of 2 to 4 units into the belly of the depressor anguli oris muscle. The depressor anguli oris is a triangular-shaped muscle whose apex inserts adjacent to the oral commissure.[56] Injection must be precise and remain lateral to the oral commissure and closer to the muscle origin ~1 cm above the body of the mandible. The bulk of the muscle can be appreciated when patients are instructed to grit their teeth. Identification and avoidance of the more medial depressor labii inferioris muscle are critical to avoid lower lip weakness and protrusion.[55]

The perioral lip fine lines that extend radially from the vermilion border opposite the course of the orbicularis muscle are a challenging problem. Because of their fine nature, the majority of fillers are too thick to address these lines smoothly. Extremely conservative perioral injection of Botox can soften these rhytides. A symmetric injection of 1 unit per site not to exceed 4 units per lip is advised. Perioral injection will weaken the patient's ability to fully purse his or her lips. Preinjection asymmetries must be pointed out to the patient and recognized by the physician as treatment can accentuate these asymmetries. Potential complications of this treatment include lip weakness and asymmetry, drooling, and impaired mastication and articulation. Patient selection is critical, and treatment should be avoided in singers and wind instrument musicians.[57]

The appearance of peau d'orange of the mentum can also be improved with 4 to 8 units injected into the inferior, medial aspect of the chin. Again, staying more medial will help avoid inadvertent injection of the depressor labii inferioris, which can result in unacceptable complications of lip asymmetry and drooling. Platysmal banding in the neck can also be identified by instructing the patient to grit his or her teeth. Typically, two injection sites along the length of each band with a total of 30 to 50 units over ~8 to 10 sites is effective in treating this zone. Although dysphagia is an uncommon complication, restricting injection to 1 cm above the thyroid cartilage and not exceeding the above dosage should avoid this risk.[57]

◆ Combination Skin Therapy

Aging of the facial skin results from several causes. To appropriately select a treatment regimen, each patient should be evaluated in terms of cutaneous, dynamic muscle and structural aging. Priorities can then be established regarding treatment. Frequently, more than one condition exists. Treatment plans can then be arranged to address each of the patient's concerns. In this chapter, we covered skin rejuvenation, which addresses two to three of the five areas of facial aging: inherent changes within the skin, dynamic facial lines, and possibly improvement of skin elasticity. Pictured in **Figs. 10.13** and **10.14** is an example of a patient treated with botulinum toxin, microdermabrasion,

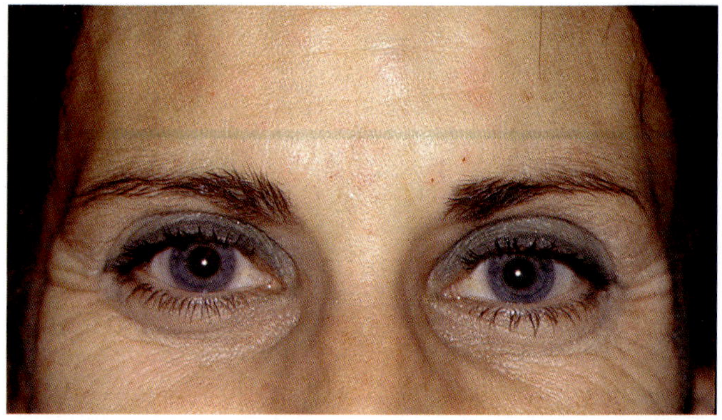

Fig. 10.13 Combination treatment: microdermabrasion, home skin care, and botulinum toxin (before treatment).

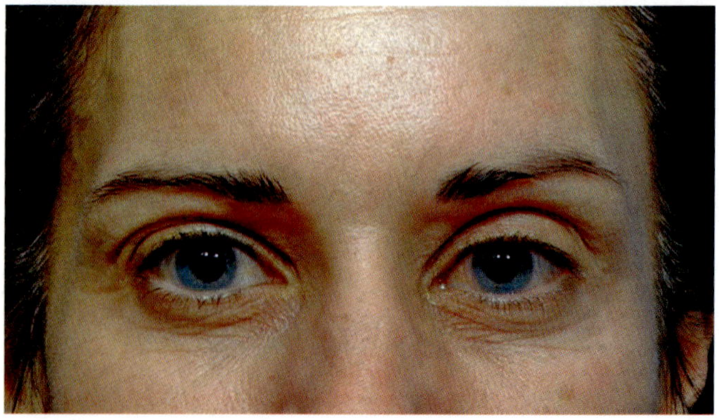

Fig. 10.14 Combination treatment: microdermabrasion, home skin care, and botulinum toxin 1 year after treatment.

and light chemical peels for skin texture and color as well as home skin care, including sun protection. Frequently, we have found that coupling skin rejuvenation with facial fillers has allowed patients to delay surgery for years. Having all these treatments available in a facial plastic surgery practice will help the physician provide comprehensive care for the aging face.

◆ Conclusion

Facial rejuvenation utilizes a number of modern techniques to restore youthful skin. Analysis should include all aspects of facial aging: inherent changes within the skin, dynamic facial lines, loss of tissue elasticity, effects of gravity, and soft tissue loss. Included in the preoperative evaluation is a careful history outlining the principal concerns each patient has regarding their priority for skin rejuvenation among those five conditions and confirmation by physical exam.

Skin treatment begins with home skin care products and progresses to chemical peels that range from superficial to deep peels. Nonablative laser skin rejuvenation can also generate significant results when treating the skin, especially texture and color changes. Deeper wrinkles may require more aggressive treatment by ablative laser resurfacing or deep chemical peels. Botulinum Toxin addresses hyperdynamic facial lines. Often, one category of treatment is not sufficient as most remedies for the aging face have synergistic effects.

Understanding the role and use of each of these tools will allow comprehensive facial rejuvenation.

References

1. The Freedom Group, Inc. Cosmeceuticals to 2010, Study 214. Cincinnati, OH: October 2006
2. American Academy of Facial Plastic and Reconstructive Surgery. Annual survey. Alexandria, VA: American Academy of Facial Plastic and Reconstructive Surgery; 2005
3. Zimbler MS, Kokoska MS, Thomas JR. Anatomy and physiology of facial aging. Facial Plast Surg Clin North Am 2001;9:179–187
4. Prystowsky JH, Siegel DM. Anatomy of facial lines and wrinkles In: Blitzer AB, Binder WJ, Boyd JB, Carruthers A. eds. Management of Facial Lines and Wrinkles. Philadelphia, PA: Lippincott Williams & Williams; 2000:1–7
5. Pearlman SJ, Chernoff GW, Freeman MS. Laser skin resurfacing. In: Blitzer AB, Binder WJ, Boyd JB, Carruthers A. eds. Management of Facial Lines and Wrinkles. Philadelphia, PA: Lippincott Williams & Williams; 2000:81–99
6. Fitzpatrick TB. The validity and practicality of sun-reactive skin types I through IV. Arch Dermatol 1988;124:869–871
7. Lemperle G, Holmes RE, Cohen SR, Lemperle SM. A classification of facial wrinkles. Plast Reconstr Surg 2001;108:1735–1752
8. Glogau RG. Chemical peeling and aging skin. J Geriatr Dermatol 1994;2:30–35
9. Friedman PM, Skover GR, Payone G. 3D in-vivo optical skin imaging for topographical quantitative assessment of non-ablative laser technology. Dermatol Surg 2002;28:199–204
10. Matarasso SL, Glogau RG. Chemical face peels. Dermatol Clin 1991;9: 131–150
11. Monheit GD. Medium-depth combination peels. Dermatol Ther 2000; 13:183–191
12. Hirsch RJ, Dayan SH, Shah RA. Superficial skin resurfacing. Facial Plast Surg Clin North Am 2004;12:311–321
13. Grimes PE. Agents for ethnic skin peeling. Dermatol Ther 2000;13: 159–164
14. Roberts WE. Chemical peeling in ethnic/dark skin. Dermatol Ther 2000;17:196–205
15. Lee SH, Huh CH, Park KC, et al. Effects of repetitive superficial chemical peels on facial sebum secretion in acne patients. J Eur Acad Derm 2006;20:964–968
16. Hernandez-Perez E, Ibiett EV. Gross and microscopic findings in patients undergoing microdermabrasion for facial rejuvenation. Dermatol Surg 2001;27:637–640
17. Rubin MG, Greenbaum SS. Histologic effects of aluminum oxide microabrasion on facial skin. J Aesth Derm Cosm Surg 2000;1:237–239
18. Shim EK, Barnette D, Hughes K, et al. Microdermabrasion: a clinical and histopathologic study. Dermatol Surg 2001;27:524–530
19. Freedman BM, Rueda-Pedraza E, Waddell SP. The epidermal and dermal changes associated with microdermabrasion. Dermatol Surg 2001; 27:1031–1033
20. Lawrence N, Mandy S, Yarborough J, et al. History of dermabrasion. Dermatol Surg 2000;26:95–101
21. Le Pillouer PA, Casanova D. Scarring process after induced dermabrasion. Wound Repair Regen 2002;10:113–115
22. Brody HJ. Trichloroacetic acid application in chemical peeling, operative techniques. Plast Reconstr Surg 1995;2:127–128
23. Monheit GD. Combination medium-depth peeling: the Jessner's & TCA peel. Facial Plast Surg 1996;12:117–124
24. Coleman WP III, Futrell JM. The glycolic acid trichloroacetic acid peel. J Dermatol Surg Oncol 1994;20:76–80
25. Roenigk HH. Treatment of the aging face. Dermatol Ther 2000;13: 141–153
26. Nguyen TH, Rooney JA. Trichloroacetic acid peels. Dermatol Ther 2000;13:173–182
27. Mulholland RS, Bitter PH. Photorejuvenation: FotoFacial, Laser Laxity vectors & WrinkleLite therapy. 3rd ed. Toronto, Canada: Beautiful Solutions Ltd.; 2002
28. Glaser DA, Rogers C. Topical and systemic therapies for the aging face. Facial Plast Surg Clin North Am 2001;9:189–196
29. Nanni CA, Alster TS. Complications of carbon dioxide laser resurfacing. Dermatol Surg 1998;24:315–320
30. Goldberg DJ. New collagen formation after dermal remodeling with and intense pulsed light source. J Cutan Laser Ther 2000;2:59–61
31. Goldberg DJ, Kutler KB. Nonablative treatment of rhytids with intense pulsed light. Lasers Surg Med 2000;26:196–200
32. Weinstein C. Carbon dioxide laser resurfacing. Clin Plast Surg 1998; 25:109–130
33. Jacobson D, Bass LS, VanderKam V, Achauer BM. Carbon dioxide and ER:YAG laser resurfacing results. Clin Plast Surg 2000;27:241–250
34. Fitzpatrick RE. CO_2 laser resurfacing. Derm Clin 2001;19:443–451
35. Rostan EF. Laser treatment of photodamaged skin. Facial Plast Surg 2005;21:99–109
36. Caniglia RJ. Erbium:YAG laser skin resurfacing. Facial Plast Surg Clin North Am 2004;12:373–377
37. Adrian RM. Pulsed carbon dioxide and erbium:YAG laser resurfacing: a comparative clinical and histologic study. J Cutan Laser Ther 1999; 1:29–35
38. Khosh MM, Larrabee WF, Smoller B. Safety and efficacy of high fluence CO_2 laser skin resurfacing with a single pass. J Cutan Laser Ther 1999; 1:37–40

39. Alster TS, Lupton JR. Erbium:YAG cutaneous laser resurfacing. Dermatol Clin 2001;19:453–466

40. Trelles MA, Allones I, Luna R. Facial rejuvenation with a nonablative 1320 nm Nd:YAG laser: a preliminary clinical and histological evaluation. Dermatol Surg 2001;27:111–116

41. Kelly KM, Majoraon B, Nelson JS. Nonablative laser and light rejuvenation: the newest approach to photodamaged skin. Arch Facial Plast Surg 2001;3:230–235

42. Goldman MP, Weiss RA. Treatment of poikiloderma of Civatte on the neck with an intense pulsed light source. Plast Reconstr Surg 2001; 107:1376–1381

43. Goldman MP. CO_2 laser resurfacing of the face and neck. Facial Plast Surg Clin North Am 2001;9:283–290

44. Newman J. Nonablative laser skin tightening. Facial Plast Surg Clin North Am 2001;9:343–349

45. Kelly KM, Nelson JS, Lask GP, Geronemus RG, Bernstein LJ. Cryogen spray cooling in combination with nonablative laser treatment of facial rhytids. Arch Dermatol 1999;135:691–694

46. Kim KH, Geronemus MD. Nonablative laser and light therapies for skin rejuvenation. Arch Facial Plast Surg 2004;6:398–409

47. Goldberg DJ. Nonablative resurfacing. Clin Plast Surg 2000;27:287–292

48. Dayan SH, Vartanian J, Menaker G, Mobley SR, Dayan AN. Nonablative laser resurfacing using the long-pulse (1064-nm) Nd:YAG laser. Arch Facial Plast Surg 2003;5:310–315

49. Zelickson BD, Kilmer SL, Bernstein E, et al. Pulsed dye laser therapy for sun damaged skin. Lasers Surg Med 1999;25:229–236

50. Bjerring P, Clement M, Heickenorff L, Egevist H, Kiernan M. Selective non-ablative wrinkle reduction by laser. J Cutan Laser Ther 2000; 2:9–15

51. Bitter PH. Noninvasive rejuvenation of photodamaged skin using serial, full-face intense pulsed light treatments. Dermatol Surg 2000;26: 835–843

52. Goldberg DJ, Samady JA. Intense pulsed light and Nd:YAG laser non-ablative treatment of facial rhytids. Lasers Surg Med 2001; 28:141–144

53. Geronemus RG. Fractional photothermolysis: current and future applications. Lasers Surg Med 2006;38:169–176

54. Fanous N. TCA peel for Asians: a new classification and a modified approach. Facial Plast Surg Clin North Am 1996;4:1195–1200

55. Carruthers A, Carruthers J. Upper face treatment. In: Carruthers A, Carruthers J, eds. Botulinum Toxin. Philadelphia, PA: Elsevier; 2005: 31–44

56. Carruthers A, Carruthers J. Clinical indications and injection technique for the cosmetic use of botulinum exotoxin A. Dermatol Surg 1998; 24:1189–1194

57. Dayan SH, Bassichis BA. Evaluation of the patient for cosmetic Botox injections. Facial Plast Surg Clin North Am 2003;11:349–358

58. Rohrer TE, Beer K. Background to botulinum toxin. In: Carruthers A, Carruthers J, eds. Botulinum Toxin. Philadelphia, PA: Elsevier; 2005:9–17

59. Bassichis BA, Thomas JR. The use of Botox to treat glabellar rhytids. Facial Plast Surg Clin North Am 2003;11:453–456

60. Chen AH, Frankel AS. Altering brow contour with botulinum toxin. Facial Plast Surg Clin North Am 2003;11:457–464

61. Flynn TC, Carruthers JA, Carruthers A, et al. Botulinum A toxin in the lower eyelid: dose-finding study. Dermatol Surg 2003;29: 943–949

11

Soft Tissue Fillers

Corey S. Maas, Kevin H. Ende, and David A. Lewis

The portfolio of products available for surgeons in the soft tissue filler market has grown rapidly over the past several years. Clinical indications have expanded beyond just simply treating nasolabial folds and lip augmentation. Today, fillers are used for all types of facial contouring and fine line management. Market awareness has increased dramatically with the advent of Restylane (Medicis Aesthetics, Scottsdale, AZ) and successful advertising and marketing campaigns. Additionally, there is a huge demand from the baby boomer generation, who want minimally invasive treatments to improve the changes associated with aging, including the development of rhytides and the loss of facial contour.

When studied carefully, it is an interesting dilemma for surgeons. The return on investment for performing injectable soft tissue augmentation and/or neuromodulators in terms of time spent with patients is dramatically better than with surgical procedures, even in the cosmetic arena. These procedures in addition provide an entrée for patients for relationship building with the surgeon that may lead to future surgical procedures. The real dilemma that has occurred in recent years relates to whether or not busy cosmetic surgeons should use nurse or physician-assistant injectors as an adjunct to their surgical practice and as physician extenders. Using these providers represents a double-edged sword in current practice, as they diminish the ability of the surgeon to develop an intimate relationship with patients, which relationship may ultimately result in surgical cases. The key to success with the plethora of products available is being able to position them well within your practice. As providers, we need to be able to explain to our patients why we use certain products for certain areas, and this may include several different products for a single patient.[1] We must understand each product's benefits and limitations and be able to successfully explain these to our patients.

◆ Injectable Fillers: The Quest for Durability and Predictability

For purpose of classification, we have placed the available soft tissue fillers into a handful of basic categories. These include injectable biological materials, injectable synthesized bioactive materials, and injectable synthetic materials.

The techniques employed using these various materials include serial puncture, linear threading, fanning, and, of course, cross-hatching, with the latter two being primarily used for facial contouring (**Fig. 11.1**). The long-held thought that all fillers should be injected intradermally has now been challenged by many clinicians who use the hyaluronic acid (HA) fillers subdermally. Some other products, such as Sculptra (Dermik Laboratories, Bridgewater, NJ) which will be discussed later, are injected even deeper. Clearly, most collagen products and, in particular CosmoDerm (Allergan Inc., Irvine, CA) are excellent products for intradermal use in the augmentation and correction of fine lines.

Tissue-Derived Biologics

Among the biologic products that are tissue derived include:

1. Autologous fat
2. Zyplast (Allergan, Inc.)
3. Resoplast (bovine collagen; Rofil Medical International, Breda, Holland)
4. Evolence (porcine collagen; Colbar Inc., Tel Aviv, Israel)
5. Hylaform and Hylaform Plus (HAs derived from cock combs; Genzyme Corporation, Cambridge, MA)
6. Fascian (Fascia Biosystems, Beverly Hills, CA) or heterologous particles of fascia
7. Cymetra (LifeCell Corporation, Branchburg, NJ)
8. AlloDerm (heterologous sheets of dermis; Lifecell Corporation) and Surgasis (porcine sheets of product)

These products in general are effective and soft to palpation but have definite half-lives in vivo. Most of the biologic fillers as described are derived from animal tissues. These include bovine collagen from cowhide, Dermalogen (Collagenesis Corporation, Beverly, MA) and AlloDerm, as well as others from human tissue, and Hylaform, which is derived from the combs of roosters. These are carefully synthesized and purified and placed in sterile syringes for immediate use off the shelf.[2]

Among the more interesting of the recent developments is a porcine collagen called Evolence (**Fig. 11.2**). This product has recently been acquired by Johnson & Johnson, which is developing an aesthetic care unit. Clinical trials are under

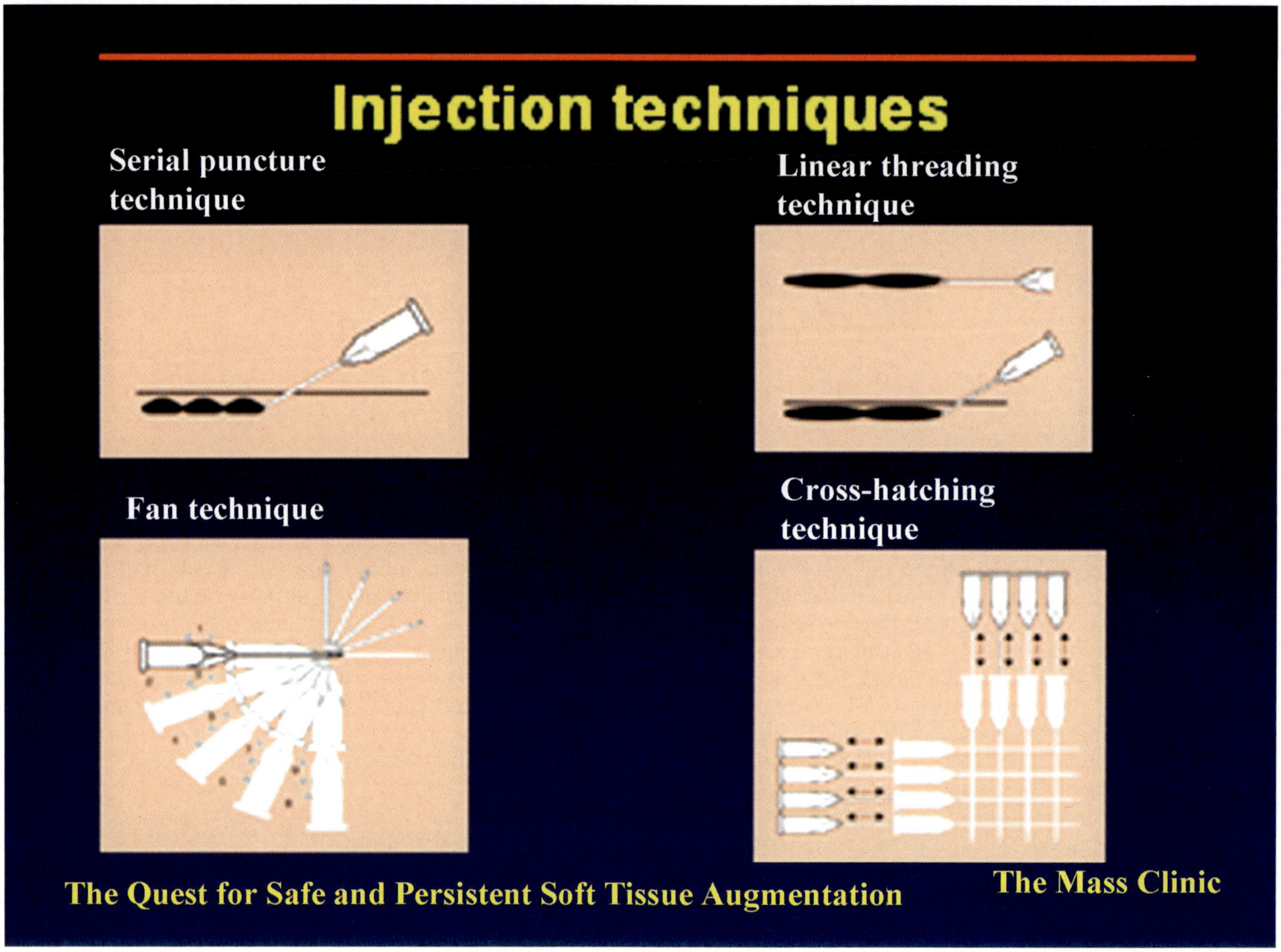

Fig. 11.1 Various injection techniques for soft tissue augmentation.

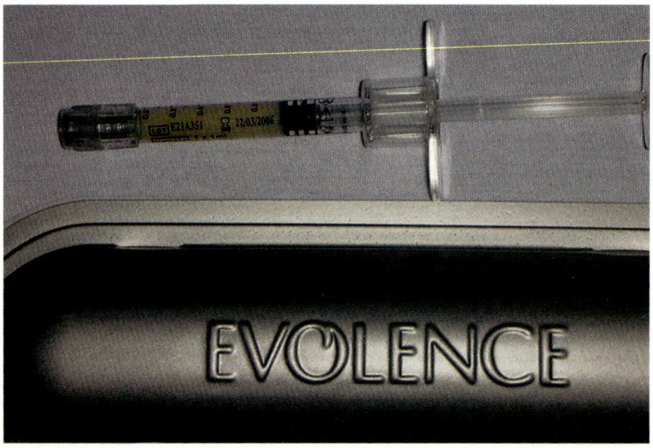

Fig. 11.2 New collagen product Evolence promises up to 12 months' duration.

way in the United States, and the product promises 1-year duration with deep dermal or subcutaneous placement.

AlloDerm and Surgasis are products that are derived from acellular dermis, Surgasis being from porcine dermis and AlloDerm being human derived. These require rehydration prior to implantation, and whereas their effectiveness was once touted as being permanent, most believe now that these products last from 6 to 12 months before reabsorption occurs. Autologous fat transfer is very popular and appropriate, in particular for facial contouring cases. In our experience, fat has limited value in lip, nasolabial fold, and tear trough deformities due to its unpredictable nature of reabsorption. With that said, autologous fat transfer remains one of the standards of care as it is quite easy to harvest fat from areas of fat excess, to centrifuge and/or wash the fat carefully, and to carefully prepare it for easy injection with a small-bore needle in cases of facial contouring.[3] Most of the data associated with autologous fat suggest that it requires

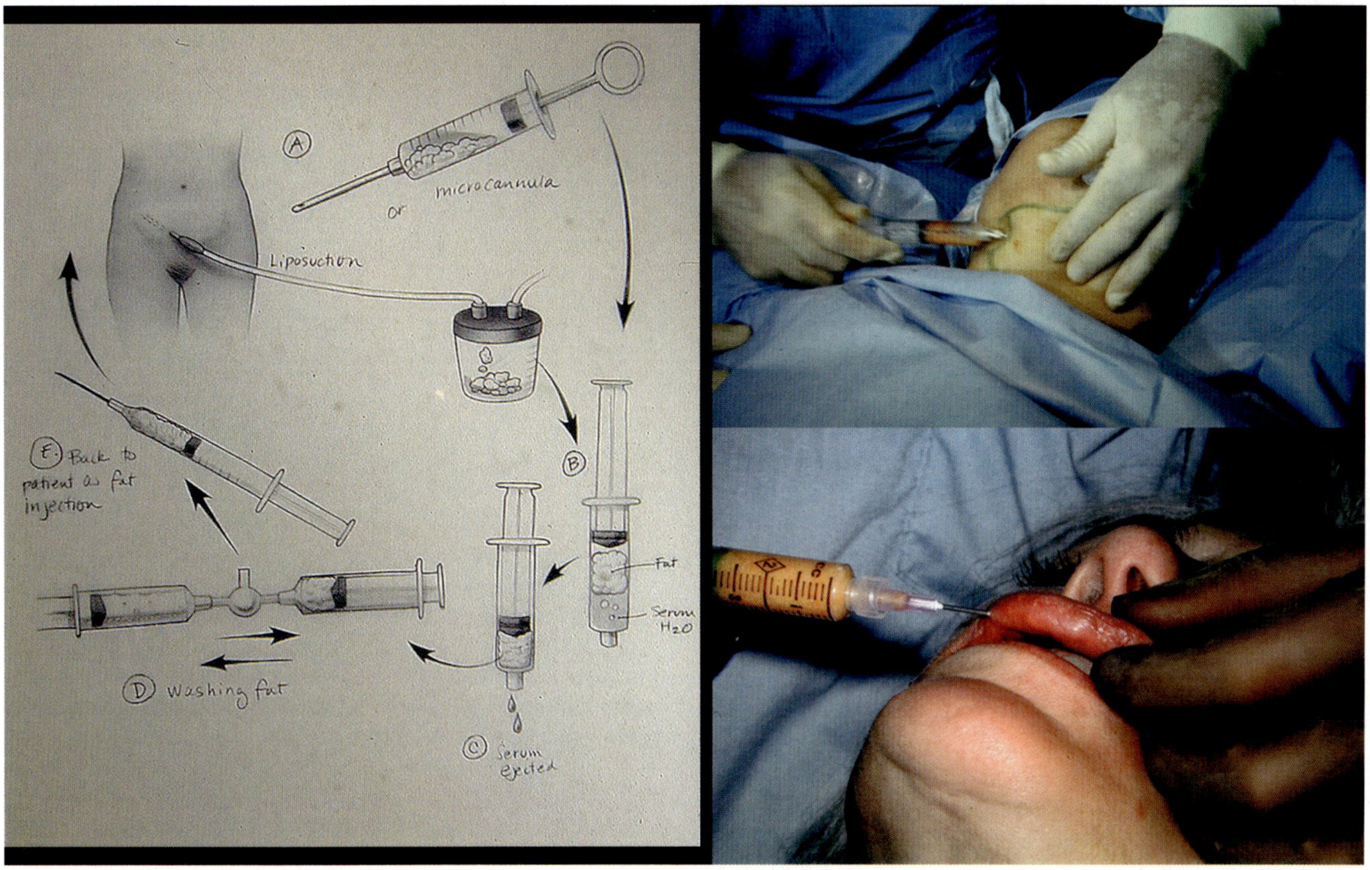

A B C

Fig. 11.3 (**A**) Autologous fat transfer technique. Fat is harvested using a microcannula. It is then processed and washed to purify the fat. Various sizes of microcannulas are used for injection using linear threading techniques for soft tissue augmentation. (**B**) Fat harvest can be done during submental liposuction. (**C**) Fat transfer to the lips.

very careful handling and limited trauma to have long-term success. In general, extensive local nerve blocks are performed prior to fat transfer with gentle handling of the fat, and the best chance of success with fat transfer employs fine streaks or beads of fat applied in the deep subcutaneous tissue close to muscle (**Fig. 11.3**). One to 4 weeks of recovery are required for this because of the extensive swelling seen with fat transfer, and probably the best one can expect is 25 to 50% correction for intermediate- and long-term results.

Each of these biological products has its advantages and disadvantages. In general, the main advantages include that they are injectable, they require limited anesthesia, and they are generally well accepted by patients, as they are soft and natural feeling. With the exception of fat transfer, these products have a very short recovery period. The disadvantages, particularly in the animal-derived products, include the possibility of hypersensitivity reactions, which, for example, occur in 1 to 4% of patients injected with bovine or porcine collagen.[4] These products generally have a temporary effect due to reabsorption, which can be a disadvantage as they require repeat injections; however, this can also be looked at as somewhat of an advantage as it negates the long-term risk of granuloma formation or infections that can be associated with permanent and synthetic injectable materials.[5,6]

Synthesized Bioactive Products

The synthesized bioactive products that are currently available include CosmoDerm and CosmoPlast, which are recombinant human collagen products; Radiesse, which is composed of calcium hydroxylapatite; Restylane, which is recombinant HA; Captique, which is recombinant HA; Sculptra, which is polylactic acid; and Juvéderm, which is homogeneous HA.

All these products are effective, soft, and reliable, although sometimes they can result in modest amounts of inflammation that typically will last 1 or 2 days. Human collagen is provided in the form of CosmoDerm and CosmoPlast, which are manufactured using recombinant technology and have similar handling characteristics to the previously known Zyplast and Zyderm products.[4,7] This requires no skin testing, and in our practice CosmoDerm remains the product of choice for intradermal injection to treat fine lines.

These products are tissue-engineered from human dermal fibroblast cells. They are allowed to multiply on a collagen scaffold and the collagen is then harvested, placed in syringes, and refrigerated until used. Another benefit to collagen is that it appears to enhance platelet aggregation, which may decrease bruising. Additionally, it contains lidocaine, which negates the need for local nerve blocks and reduces pain. In addition, there may be some benefit in local reduction in eosinophil degranulation, which theoretically results in decreased swelling, making it the injectable filler with the least amount of down-time.[8] The biggest disadvantage to most of the collagen products is that they only last for 2 to 3 months.[9,10]

The shorter-duration hyaluronic acid products that are available include Hylaform and Captique. Hylaform, as previously mentioned, is derived from rooster combs, whereas Captique is a 5.5 mg/dL concentration of human bioactive synthesized HA. HA is a naturally occurring substance that is one of the most abundant glycosaminoglycans in the dermis. It is a linear polysaccharide made up of alternating units of glucuronic acid and glucosamine.[11] It is identical in all species, which makes it unique in that it reduces the risk of inflammatory reactions after injections. Most of these products contain some degree of free HA in addition to modified and/or cross-linked HA, which allows the product to be manufactured as a liquid, a gel, or a nearly solid filler.[12]

Varying hydration levels of the HA fillers have an impact on their performance overall. Where Hylaform Plus and Captique have concentrations, as mentioned, of 5.5 mg/dL HA, Restylane has 20 mg HA, and Juvéderm has 24 mg HA cross-linked per milliliter of water. These properties make them extremely hydrophilic, which results in more swelling upon injection of the product, as tissue fluids get absorbed by the higher-concentration product.

Our clinical experience with Hylaform and Captique suggests that they last about as long as Zyplast, which is for most patients around 3 months, that it is certainly a safe product, and that there appear to be no long-range issues with Hylaform or Captique. The flow characteristics are quite good for both products, but it is difficult to find a place to position these products in practice given the performance of CosmoDerm and CosmoPlast and the alternative HAs Juvéderm and Restylane.

Restylane has had a huge impact on the fillers market since its recent introduction. In its first year, it more than doubled the soft tissue filler market, as it offered a substantial increase in durability and duration of effect. Restylane is a synthesized bioactive HA that is provided in a 20 mg/dL gel-particle suspension, 20% of which is uncross-linked HA packaged in a 1-cc syringe (**Fig. 11.4**).

In a randomized, double-blind, multicenter comparison of the efficacy and tolerability of Restylane versus Zyplast for the correction of nasolabial folds, Restylane showed in both wrinkle severity rating scale and global aesthetic improvement scale assessments at 6 months that HA gel was superior to collagen products in the majority of patients.[13] The technique of HA injection has been described as deep dermal. Our preference for this application is a subcutaneous injection with linear threading and fanning techniques being primary for the nasolabial fold and facial contouring and linear threading for labial augmentation.[14,15] The product is quite viscous and requires significant plunger-pressure, and due to the discomfort associated with the product, we recommend local nerve blocks prior to injection. Juvéderm is another synthesized bioactive HA that is provided in 24 mg/dL solution in a presterilized syringe containing 0.8 mL active product. Juvéderm is considerably easier to inject and softer than is Restylane. We have found that it has some advantages in some applications and disadvantages in others. The majority of clinical data available in describing Juvéderm demonstrates similar performance characteristic to that of Restylane with the average duration of effect being in the 6-month area. In particular, these data from the U.S. Food and Drug Administration (FDA) trials were generated from the nasolabial fold region where long-term results were clearly demonstrated in these patients. The softness of Juvéderm allows less injection pressure and molding pressure when providing injections making it an excellent choice for augmentation of the tear trough and the nasolabial fold (**Figs. 11.5 and 11.6**). In contrast, in our practice, we find that the firmer nature of Restylane makes it ideal for labial augmentation.

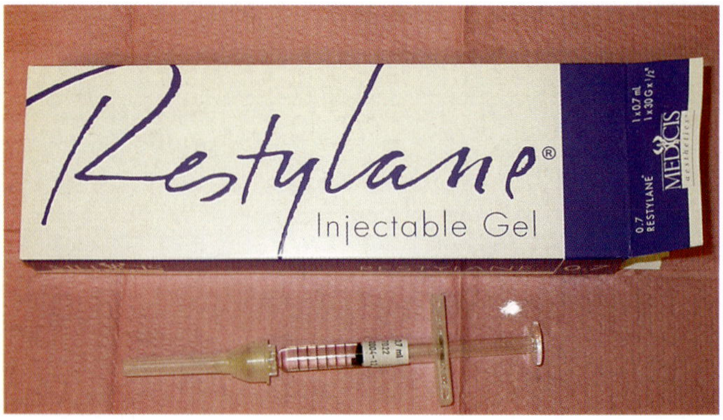

Fig. 11.4 Restylane.

In general, the biosynthesized HA products have some significant advantages in that they are easily injectable, they have very low hypersensitivity profiles, they are reversible, they are absorbable over time, they are soft and natural feeling, and they are relatively long lasting. Their disadvantages include that they may be considerably thicker and more difficult to inject than are the collagen products, there is slightly more swelling and bruising, and they, in our opinion, require injectable anesthetic and/or local nerve blocks for patient comfort reasons.

Synthesized Bioactive Agents

Sculptra or New-Fill

Sculptra was recently introduced by the Dermix Company. It is an injectable poly-L-lactic acid product, which is provided as a powder for reconstitution.[16] The product itself is very similar to Vicryl (Ethicon, Inc., Somerville, NJ) sutures, and there is a minimal 6-year experience in Europe with this product. The basic principle behind its use is that is stimulates an inflammatory response with the attendant deposition of soft tissues over time. The treatment is approved only for use for HIV

A
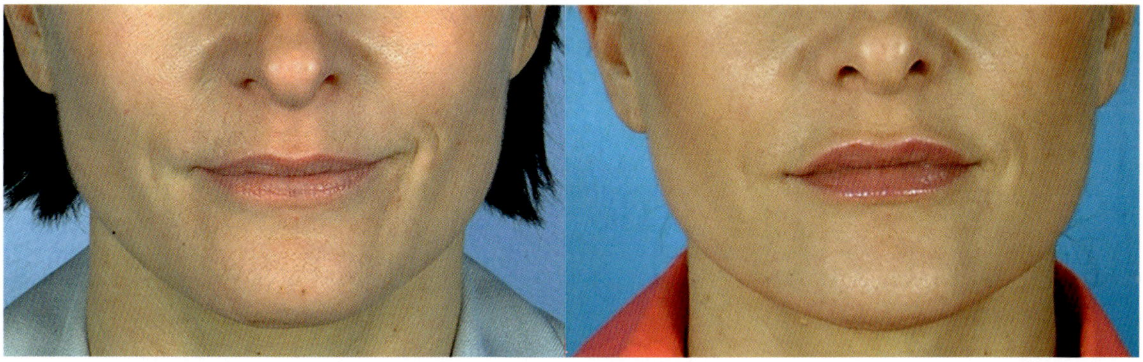
B

Fig. 11.5 (**A, B**) Restylane for lip augmentation.

lipoatrophy, although the company is seeking cosmetic indications currently (**Fig. 11.7**). Three to five treatments are required over a 12- to 18-month period with the patient seeing initial swelling and improvement followed by subsequent diminution of most of the initial augmentation, which ultimately results in gradual restoration of volume due to the granulomatous inflammatory response.

Its use in cosmetic surgery has gained some traction in the United States whereas it has been diminishing generally in Europe with the advent and availability of other products that give immediate results. The Sculptra technique ideally requires the rehydration of the product or reconstitution at least 6 to 12 hours before the procedure to ensure that there is no clogging of needles, and deep placement in the subdermal tissue is appropriate in fanning or cross-hatching techniques. Subcutaneous nodules can occur as a result of uneven dispersion of the product, and in particular, this product should be avoided in thin-skinned areas where a subcutaneous nodule might become quite evident. A study published in the dermatologic surgery literature demonstrated satisfactory results in overall patient satisfaction on a long-term follow-up of 18 months, with 79% of patients requiring an average of three visits to receive the desired enhancement, and 21% requested additional treatment sessions beyond the initial three sessions to achieve the desired degree of augmentation.[16] The preliminary studies for Sculptra all revolve around its use in lipodystrophy. Its role in other types of volume replacement is yet to be determined, but the most significant limiting factor preventing its widespread popularity is the absence of an immediate improvement.

Radiesse

Radiesse is a calcium hydroxylapatite product that is manufactured synthetically. It is a very thin paste, which comes ready to inject in a 1.3-cc syringe. FDA trials for nasolabial fold augmentation were completed, and the data have been very promising suggesting a statistical preference over the control product and durability up to 12 months. Unpublished data from a European control trial against a long-acting HA filler demonstrated superiority both for the patient and physician in palpability and longevity when applied in the nasolabial fold area. The company recommends using cross-hatching or

A
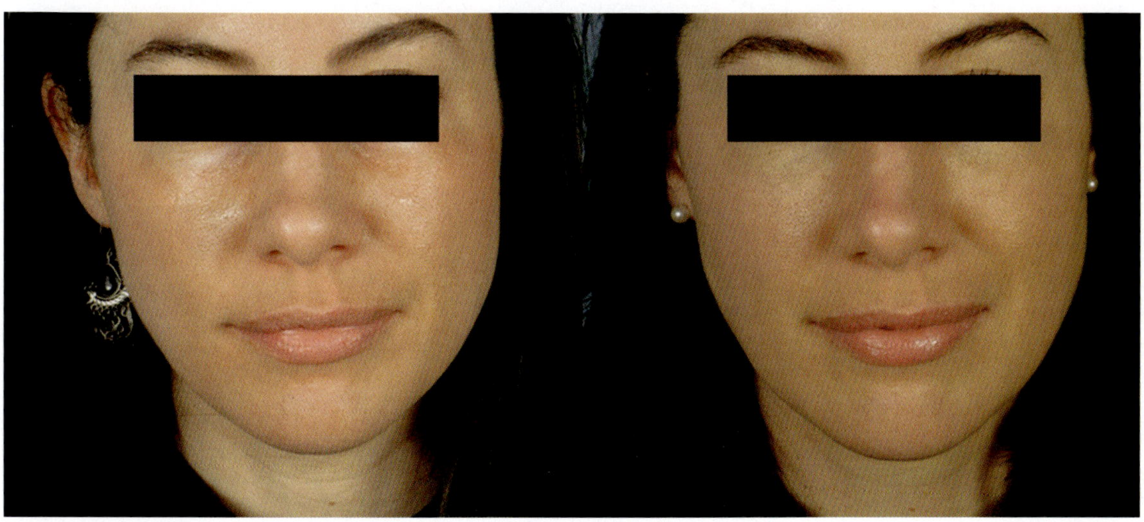
B

Fig. 11.6 (**A, B**) Restylane for nasojugal folds.

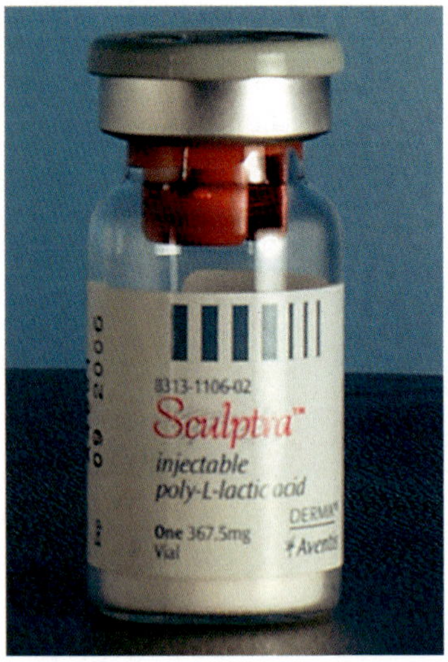

Fig. 11.7 Sculptra, for treatment of patients with HIV lipoastrophy.

fanning techniques to distribute the product using even beads into the subcutaneous tissues to provide augmentation and contouring for the face (**Fig. 11.8**). The product should not be used in the lips as nodule formations can occur. In general, Radiesse offers a great deal of promise for facial contouring and nasolabial fold augmentation. Although it is probably suboptimal in thin-skinned areas, such as the tear trough region, in the labiomandibular sulcus, the submalar region, and the nasolabial fold, this may well prove to be the soft tissue filler of choice in many patients who want longer results with a soft and natural feel.

Synthetic Injectables

The list of synthetic injectables available worldwide has grown to greater than 40. In the United States, we are limited to basically two synthetic injectable products, which include injectable liquid silicone, which is not approved

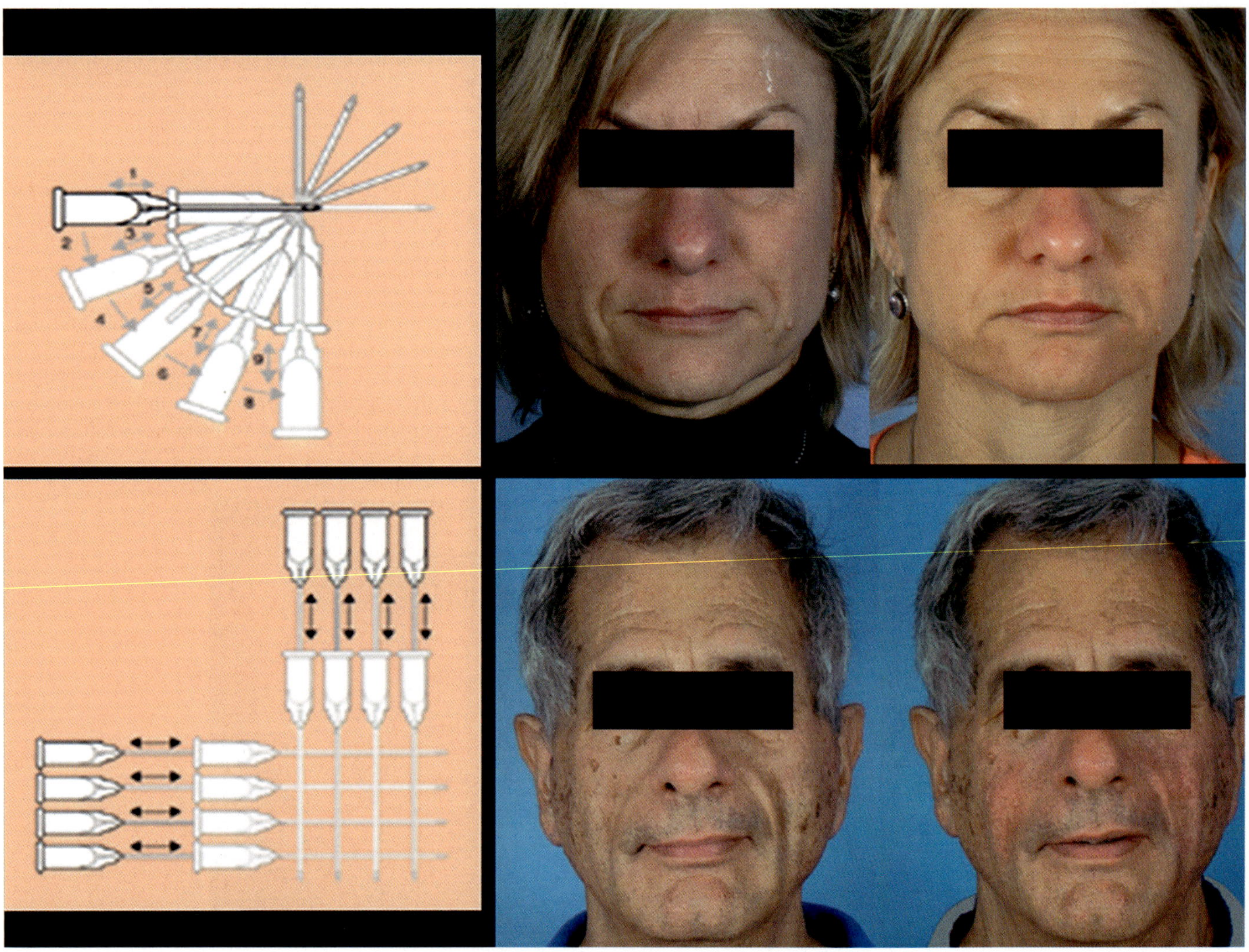

A B C

Fig. 11.8 (**A**) Injection techniques for Radiesse injection. (**B**) Radiesse in the nasolabial folds. (**C**) Radiesse for lipodystrophy.

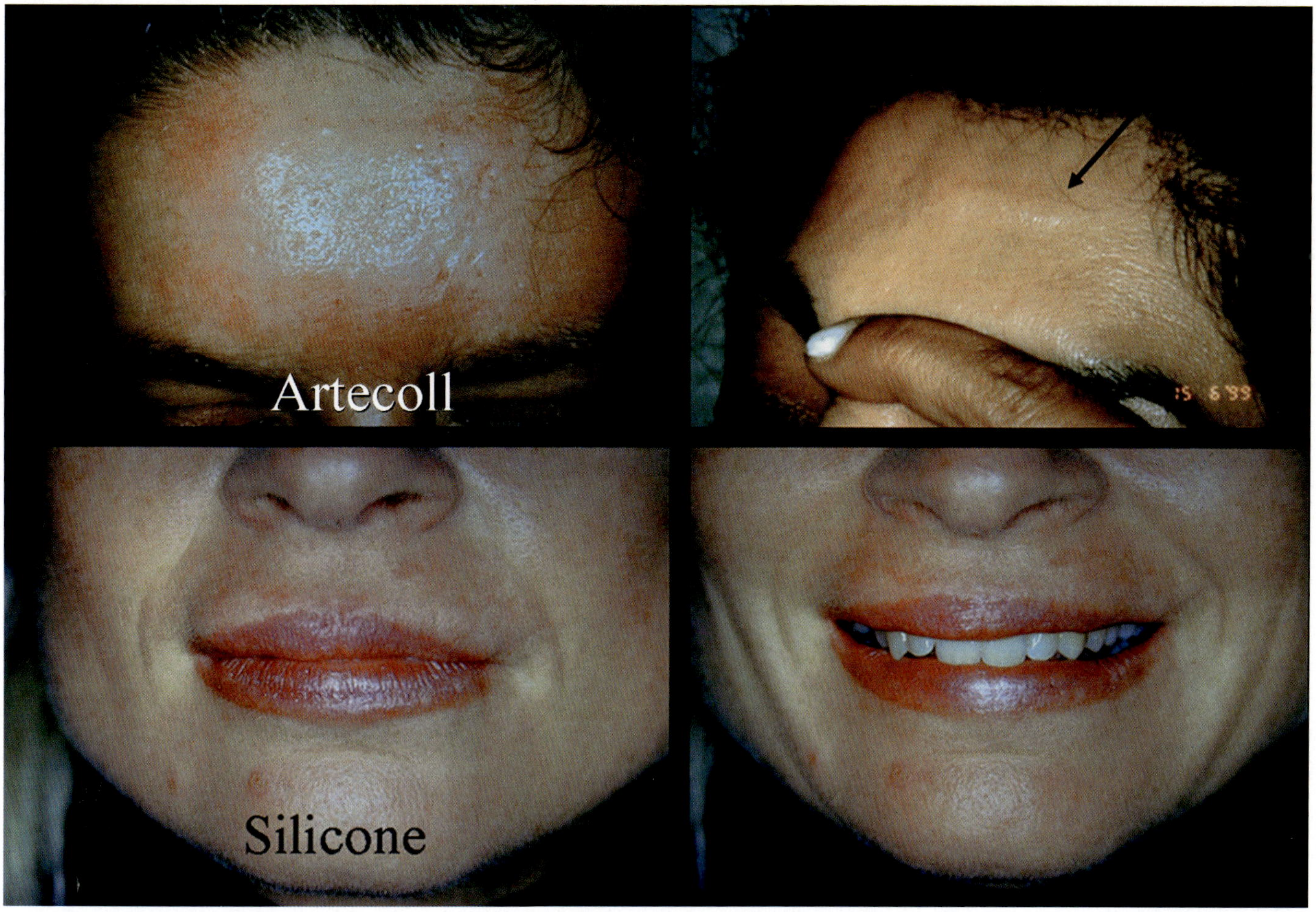

A B C D

Fig. 11.9 (**A**) Artecoll injection showing early erythema. (**B**) Same patient shown in (**A**) now with nodule formation (*arrow*). (**C, D**) Silicone injection to lips with resultant nodularity and irregularity.

specifically for cosmetic use but for intraocular use in orbital reconstruction, and Artefill (Artes Medical, Inc., San Diego, CA) medical, which has been recently approved for cosmetic soft tissue augmentation.[17,18]

Artefill consists of methyl methacrylate microspheres of 30 to 40 μm in diameter. Recent advances in the product have resulted in an increase in absolute surface smoothness seen by electron microscopy, which presumably reduces the electrical charge that was previously produced during the manufacturing process, and thereby reduces the risk of the inflammatory and granulomatous responses that were occasionally seen with the earlier Artecoll product used in Europe. It is supplied in sterile packages and is intended for subcutaneous injection. The company recommends serial injection be performed to ensure a gradual build up of the product and to avoid overaugmentation secondary to overinjection and/or a granulomatous and fibrous tissue response.

Silicone injection has been well described in the literature by Barnett and others. Many surgeons and authors have described its use in great success over many years of duration and insist that it is completely safe in patients for soft tissue augmentation.[19,20] It is given via a microdroplet technique.[21]

One must keep in mind that potential complications with synthetic injectable agents, as they are permanent, include the permanent risk of inflammatory granulomatous nodularity and/or infection[22–24] (**Fig. 11.9**). In addition, the aging face certainly changes over time, and it will be interesting to trace patients over the long-term to see if the correction generated by injection of these products is maintained as tissues become deflated and move under the effects of gravity in aging. In addition, these synthetic injectable agents must be precisely placed, as they can result in fullness in areas that are undesired, which can result in permanent cosmetic morbidity.[25]

Finally, synthetic injectables do offer some measurable risk of long-term complications including chronic granulomas, fibrosis, and/or chronic infection in which treatment would require wide local tissue excision. These risks must be discussed at length with the patients prior to the use of such products.

◆ Treatment Strategies

With the plethora of products we have mentioned, one must develop a comprehensive strategy for patients when using these products. It is our suggestion that this be done on an anatomic and individual basis rather than selecting one product that might be good for all patients.

In general, for nasolabial fold augmentation, we offer Radiesse, Restylane, and Juvéderm. Similarly, at the area of the labiomandibular groove and submalar augmentation with facial aging and lipoatrophy that is attendant with facial aging, these same products offer the benefit of longer correction and fullness. Of these, Radiesse lasts the longest, and because of its longevity, it has the potential to become the most popular product of the three in areas of thicker skin. We recommend Juvéderm in areas of thin skin, such as the tear trough or nasojugal fold.

For the finer lines associated with the perilabial area, in the so-called smoker's or radial lines, our preference remains CosmoDerm, as this can be placed carefully in the upper layers of the dermis without being identified through the skin surface with the blueish line apparent with most of the clear HA products. A wide area can be treated with serial-point injection, and near complete smoothness or correction can be achieved.

For labial augmentation, our preference remains Restylane, as it provides a degree of structural integrity to the lip border. It is slightly more difficult to inject than is Juvéderm, but the structural benefits in terms of re-creating the natural lip border are certainly beneficial. Alternatively, CosmoPlast can be used, which offers an immediate correction with short down-time, less chance of bruising, and no requirement for injection with a local anesthetic. Juvéderm certainly remains a good choice for this area as well.

In summary, our treatment strategies have evolved with the development of several new products that are available. Our general strategy includes an increasing use of fillers for subcutaneous volume enhancement, and the primary products that we are using are Radiesse, Restylane, Juvéderm, and CosmoDerm. New options may become available in the immediate future, in particular Evolence, the porcine collagen product, which promises to have a longer duration of effect than do other forms of collagen and HA products. As the choices increase, we must continue to evolve our strategies for management of the aging patient and remain open-minded about both the products and the newer applications for these products.

References

1. Ashinoff R. Overview: soft tissue augmentation. Clin Plast Surg 2000;27:479–487
2. Lowe NJ, Maxwell CA, Lowe P, Duick MG, Shah K. Hyaluronic acid skin fillers: adverse reactions and skin testing. J Am Acad Dermatol 2001;45:930–933
3. Peer LA. Loss of weight and volume in human fat grafts. Plast Reconstr Surg 1950;5:217
4. Skouge JW, Diwan RV. Soft tissue augmentation with injectable collagen. In: Papel ID, Nachlas NE, eds. Facial Plastic and Reconstructive Surgery. St. Louis, MO: Mosby-Year Book; 1992:208
5. Maas CS, Papel ID, Greene D, Stoker DA. Complications of injectable synthetic polymers in facial augmentation. Dermatol Surg 1997;23: 871–877
6. Newcomer VD, Graham JH, Schaffert RR, Kaplan L. Sclerosing lipogranuloma resulting from exogenous lipids. AMA Arch Derm 1956;73: 361–372
7. Cheng JT, Perkins SW, Hamilton MM. Collagen and injectable fillers. Otolaryngol Clin North Am 2002;35:73–85, vi.
8. West TB, Alster TS. Autologous human collagen and dermal fibroblasts for soft tissue augmentation. Dermatol Surg 1998;24:510–512
9. Bailin PL, Bailin MD. Collagen implantation: clinical applications and lesion selection. J Dermatol Surg Oncol 1988;14:21–26
10. Castrow FF II, Krull EA. Injectable collagen implant–update. J Am Acad Dermatol 1983;9:889–893
11. Maas CS. Characteristics of implant materials. Arch Facial Plast Surg 2000;2:67
12. Duranti F, Salti G, Bovani B, Calandra M, Rosati ML. Injectable hyaluronic acid gel for soft tissue augmentation. A clinical and histological study. Dermatol Surg 1998;24:1317–1325
13. Narins RS, Brandt F, Leyden J, Lorenc ZP, Rubin M, Smith S. A randomized, double-blind, multicenter comparison of the efficacy and tolerability of Restylane versus Zyplast for the correction of nasolabial folds. Dermatol Surg 2003;29:588–595
14. Krauss MC. Recent advances in soft tissue augmentation. Semin Cutan Med Surg 1999;18:119–128
15. Boss WK Jr, Marko O. Isologen. In: Klein AW, ed. Tissue Augmentation in Clinical Practice: Procedures and Techniques. New York, NY: Marcel Dekker; 1998:335–347
16. Burgess CM, Quiroga RM. Assessment of the safety and efficacy of poly-L-lactic acid for the treatmentof HIV-associated facial lipoatrophy. J Am Acad Dermatol 2005;52:233–239
17. Clark DP, Hanke W, Swanson N. Dermal implants: safety of products injected for soft tissue augmentation. J Am Acad Dermatol 1989;21: 992–998
18. Narins RS, Bowman PH. Injectable skin fillers. Clin Plast Surg 2005;32:151–162
19. Orentreich DS, Orentreich N. Injectable fluid silicone. In: Roengk RK, Roenigk HH Jr, eds. Dermatologic Surgery: Principles and Practice. New York, NY: Marcel Dekker; 1989:1349–1395
20. Webster RC, Fuleihan NS, Gaunt JM, et al. Injectable silicone for small augmentations: twenty-year experience in humans. Am J Cosm Surg 1984;1:1–7
21. Pollack SV. Silicone, fibril, collagen implantation for facial lines and wrinkles. J Dermatol Surg Oncol 1990;16:957–961
22. Ben-Hur N, Neuman Z. Siliconoma: another cutaneous response to dimethylpolysiloxane experimental study in mice. Plast Reconstr Surg 1965;36:629–631
23. Achauer BM. A serious complication following medical-grade silicone injection of the face. Plast Reconstr Surg 1983;71:251–253
24. Rapaport MJ, Vinnik C, Zarem H. Injectable silicone: cause of facial nodules, cellulitis, ulceration, and migration. Aesthetic Plast Surg 1996;20:267–276
25. Spira M, Rosen T. Injectable soft tissue substitutes. Clin Plast Surg 1993;20:181–188

12

Complementary Fat Grafting

Samuel M. Lam, Mark J. Glasgold, and Robert A. Glasgold

Volume loss has become increasingly recognized as a vital component to the aging process.[1–3] Facial lifting procedures and skin resurfacing alone cannot address all aspects of aging. Autologous fat transfer has assumed an integral and important role in the authors' respective practices as part of a comprehensive strategy toward facial rejuvenation. A metaphor that can help the surgeon and the prospective patient understand the utility of facial fat grafting is the grape, raisin, and pea. In youth, we are full and ripe grapes. As we age, the volume depletion turns us into raisins. Why then should we cut and pull that raisin, transforming it into a pea, which does not resemble a grape at all? Instead, we should reinflate that raisin back into a youthful grape. Obviously, this reductionist philosophy is not meant to imply a monolithic perspective on the aging process. The title of this chapter, "Complementary Fat Grafting," emphasizes the complementary nature of fat grafting to traditional lifting procedures to attain optimal aesthetic outcomes. Overfilling the face to manage pseudoherniation of fat in the lower eyelid or a ptotic jaw line may lead to unnecessarily long recovery times and, worse yet, unfavorable results. Judicious combination of fat grafting with conservative blepharoplasty and/or a facelift in the appropriate clinical circumstance can yield superior outcomes (**Fig. 12.1**).

A useful adjunct for understanding the importance of volume restoration with autologous fat transfer is to review with the patients photographs of themselves when they were younger. Youthful photographs of the patient can help formulate a surgical plan to achieve a natural-appearing result. These photographs can also help a prospective patient truly understand the dynamic role that volume loss has played in the process of facial aging. The two predominant features that

A 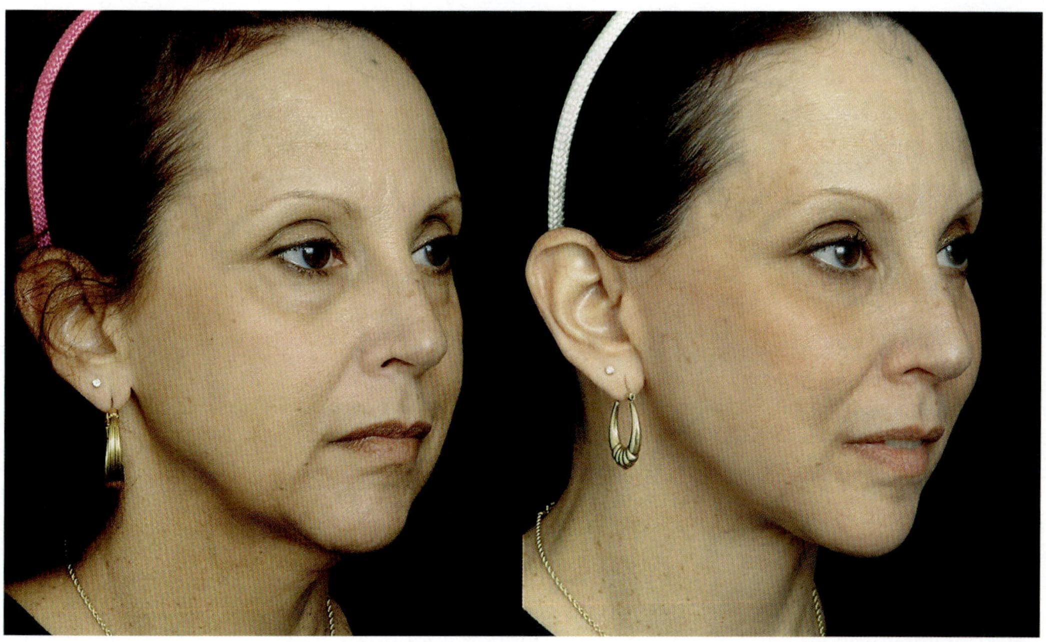 B

Fig. 12.1 (**A**) Preoperative photo. (**B**) Postoperative photo after fat transfer to the inferior orbital rim and midface, in conjunction with a lower lid transconjunctival blepharoplasty and facelift.

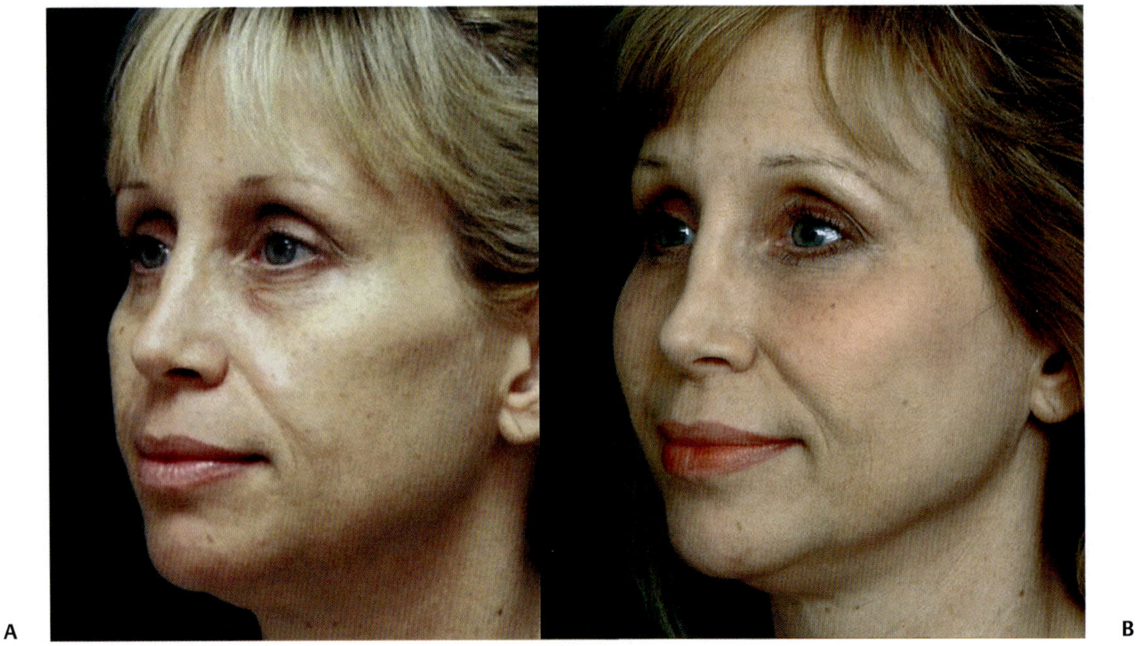

Fig. 12.2 (A) Preoperative and (B) postoperative photos demonstrate how a full periorbital frame is obtained through conservative blepharoplasty in conjunction with periorbital and midface fat transfer.

will become obvious to the patient and surgeon when reviewing old photographs are the presence of a youthful fullness that frames the eyes and the volume and shape that is characteristic of a youthful face. Alternatively, if such photos are unavailable, then it is also useful to review photos of young individuals to help the patient understand what constitutes a youthful appearance and to establish the appropriate surgical goals for that individual.

Traditional blepharoplasty that hollows the orbit through aggressive removal of fat and skin will generally result in a skeletonized eye, making it look surgically "done," not younger. Adding fat to the periorbital region returns the fuller, volumetric frame that circumscribes and defines youthful eyes (**Fig. 12.2**). The approach we take is to combine the fat transfer procedure with a conservative lower lid transconjunctival blepharoplasty. Rejuvenation of the upper lid will generally consist of a skin-only blepharoplasty with fat transfer to the superior orbital rim and, if very sunken, the upper lid. Brow lifting is generally avoided in most of our patients as it further hollows out the eye. Examination of young individuals will reveal that most do not have the high-set brows with a sculpted superior orbital rim that is typically seen after a brow lift.[4] With aging, the brow does not typically descend, it in fact begins to deflate and thereby appears to sag. Reinflation of the brow with fat grafting oftentimes can help restore a patient back to the way he or she used to look.

A youthful face has a characteristic heart shape, with highlights that fall along the prominence of the cheeks and the chin to create this ideal, triangular-shaped face. With advancing age, the cheeks and chin as well as other areas deflate and the jowls gradually become more prominent, transforming that ideal triangle into more of a square or rectangular shape. This change in shape not only is unflattering but also imparts a more masculinized appearance to the female face. For men who desire fat grafting, the anterior cheek should not be overly inflated, as it is a hallmark of youthful femininity. By contrast, the lateral cheek may be more suitably enhanced in the male patient to maintain a more masculine countenance. Besides reaugmenting the apices of the triangle with facial fat grafting, the jowls can be lifted via a facelift to complete the transformation back toward a youthful triangular facial configuration (**Fig. 12.3**). Brow lifting is rarely indicated in our volumetric approach as it tends to lengthen the female face, which accents the aging, squared-off appearance. Framing the eye with fat grafting and restoring the shape back into a youthful triangle are the two major objectives in facial rejuvenation.

In our experience, the two areas that have not been ideal for autologous fat transfer are the lips and the deep facial lines and folds. The amount of adipocyte survival tends to be less in these hyperdynamic areas. Lip enhancement with fat grafting involves a protracted and deforming recuperation. Augmentation of the nasolabial and labiomandibular folds proves to be disappointing in achieving a perceived and durable benefit. In patients undergoing facial fat transfer we will generally transfer fat into these folds so that the augmented malar and chin regions blend favorably along these lines but not in fact to actually efface these lines or folds. Other dermal fillers are preferred to achieve a perceivable benefit for lip enhancement and attenuation of facial lines and folds.

One of the critical questions raised regarding fat transfer is the durability of the result. Our experience is that the

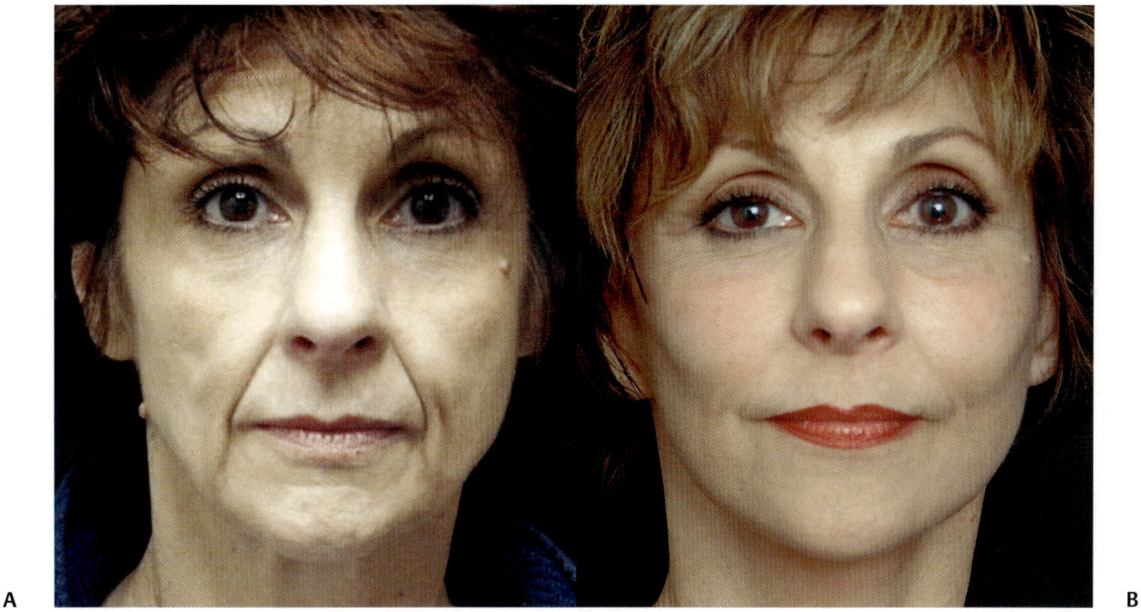

Fig. 12.3 (A) Preoperatively, this patient had an aging appearance, with a squaring off of her facial shape due to volume loss in the midface and the presence of jowls. (B) A more youthful heart shape is created through the combination of fat transfer to the periorbital area and cheeks and a facelift.

amount of fat that survives the transfer is variable, but there is always some degree of viable fat that will persist for many years. We counsel prospective patients that the variable fat graft survival means it will often take two and possibly three transfers to achieve the desired result. Once that result is achieved, it is for all intents a permanent effect.

◆ Operative Technique

Anesthesia Considerations

Autologous fat transfer can be undertaken with almost any level of anesthesia (i.e., from straight local to general anesthesia). We prefer light conscious sedation for patient comfort and to facilitate patient repositioning, if needed, for fat harvesting.

For recipient-site anesthesia, the three primary entry sites used on each side are anesthetized, and a regional nerve block is administered with 1% lidocaine and 1:100,000 epinephrine (**Fig. 12.4**). A standard 18-gauge needle is used to create the three entry sites for fat injection. The local anesthetic is then infiltrated through the entry sites into the areas to be augmented with fat using a blunt fat-infiltrating cannula (Tulip Medical Inc., San Diego, CA). The blunt cannula minimizes tissue trauma and related ecchymosis (**Fig. 12.5**).

The donor area where fat will be harvested from is anesthetized with a mixture containing 5 mL 1% lidocaine and 1:100,000 epinephrine and 15 mL normal saline attached to a 7-inch, 22-gauge spinal needle. Half of the solution is

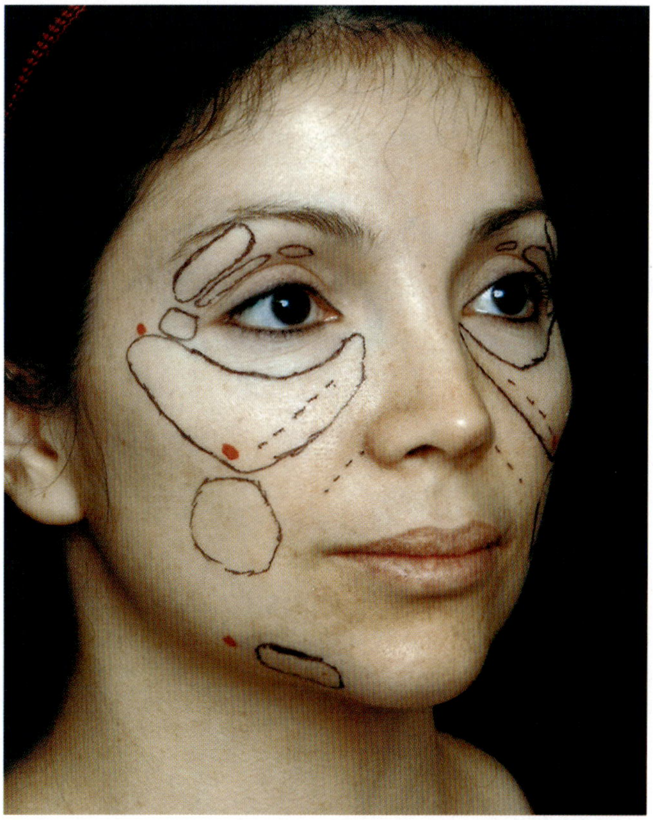

Fig. 12.4 Preoperative patient markings. The black outlined areas represent the planned sites for fat infiltration. The three red dots indicate the three cannula entry points for fat infiltration: lateral canthus, midcheek, jaw line.

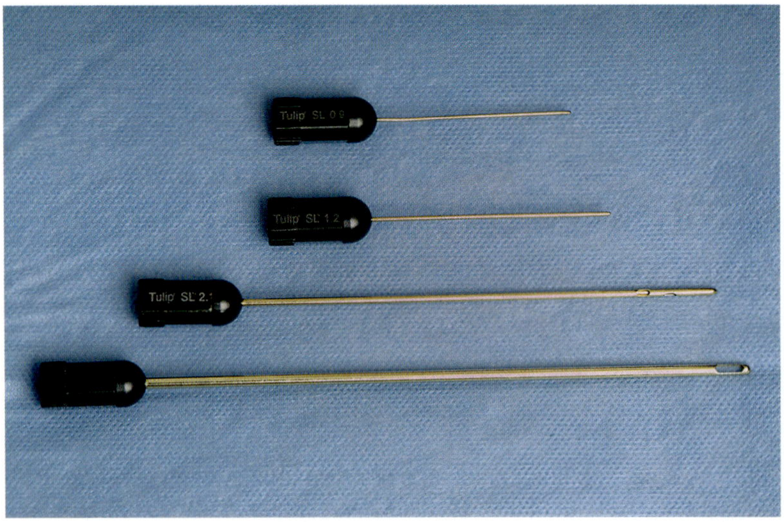

Fig. 12.5 The Glasgold Fat Transfer Set from Tulip Medical Inc. (*from top to bottom*): 0.9 mm × 4 cm blunt spoon-tip infiltration cannula; 1.2 mm × 6 cm blunt spoon-tip infiltration cannula; 2 mm × 12 cm multiport harvesting cannula; 3 mm × 15 cm bullet-tip harvesting cannula.

placed at the superficial aspect of the fat pad (in the superficial subcutaneous plane) with the remainder being placed at the deep aspect of the fat pad. If the procedure is being done without sedation, then a higher concentration of anesthetic is used by mixing 10 mL 1% lidocaine with 1:100,000 epinephrine and 10 mL normal saline.

Donor-Site Harvesting

Selection of the donor site is principally dependent on where that patient stores the most adipose reserves. Physical examination can help determine the ideal body site. However, simply asking the patient where they tend to have the most abundant amount of fat will help narrow down the ideal harvesting site. The lower abdomen and inner thigh are ideal harvesting sites for most individuals, as no patient repositioning is necessary for harvesting.

Fat harvesting is done using a 3-mm bullet-tipped harvesting cannula attached to a 10-cc Luer-Lok (BD, Franklin Lakes, NJ) syringe (**Fig. 12.5**). A stab incision is made using a 16-gauge Nokor needle (or no. 11 Bard-Parker blade) in a discreet location (e.g., the inferior aspect of the umbilicus for abdominal harvesting or the inguinal line for inner-thigh harvesting). The harvesting cannula is inserted through the stab-incision site for harvesting. All harvesting is performed with hand suction using ~1 to 2 cc of negative pressure until 10 cc is collected. Generally speaking, each 10 cc collected translates into ~5 cc of usable fat with the remainder consisting of a mixture of lysed fat cells, blood, and lidocaine. When harvesting, the surgeon should always be mindful of where the cannula tip resides and to remain in the central aspect of the adipose bed to maximize adipose yield as well as to minimize patient discomfort caused by the cannula tip abrading the dermis above or the fascia below. It is also important to ensure that the cannula traverses the entire donor site so as not to overharvest one area and thereby create a contour irregularity. The surgeon's nondominant hand is used only to stabilize the harvest site, not to pinch the fat pad, which could predispose to uneven harvesting and result in a postoperative donor site contour problem.

Fat Processing

Once the 10-cc syringes are filled with fat, a plug is placed onto the Luer-Lok end of the syringe. The plunger is then removed from the end of the syringe, and a cap is placed onto the open end. The cap and plug for the syringes are designed specifically for this purpose (available through Miller Medical Inc., Mesa, AZ); the tiny plastic Luer-Lok cap that comes prepackaged with each syringe should never be used for centrifugation, as it will invariably leak. Each syringe is then inserted sterilely into the centrifuge in a balanced distribution for processing. Centrifuges can be designed so that individual sterile sleeves (Miller Medical Inc.) or a central sterile rotary element (Byron Medical Inc., Tucson, AZ) is inserted to maintain a sterile environment. Generally, the fat can be spun for approximately 2 to 3 minutes at 2000 to 3000 rpm.[5] After centrifugation, the syringes are removed sterilely, and the supranatant and infranatant are decanted (**Fig. 12.6**). The supranatant consisting of lysed fatty cells should always be poured off from the non–Luer-Lok side first. Then, the plug from the Luer-Lok side is unscrewed to permit the bloody infranatant to drain out. (If the infranatant is poured out first, the column of fat will lose vacuum and inadvertently tumble out of the syringe.) At this point, an uncut 4 × 4 gauze or cotton neuropaddie is inserted into the non–Luer-Lok side of each syringe to wick away any remaining supranatant for a period of 5 to 10 minutes.[5]

The processed fat is then poured from the open plunger side (non–Luer-Lok side) of the 10-cc Luer-Lok syringe into the open plunger side of an empty 20-cc Luer-Lok syringe to facilitate preparation of the 1-cc infiltration syringes. The plunger is then placed back into the 20-cc syringe taking care not to spill or eject fat from the syringe. A transfer hub

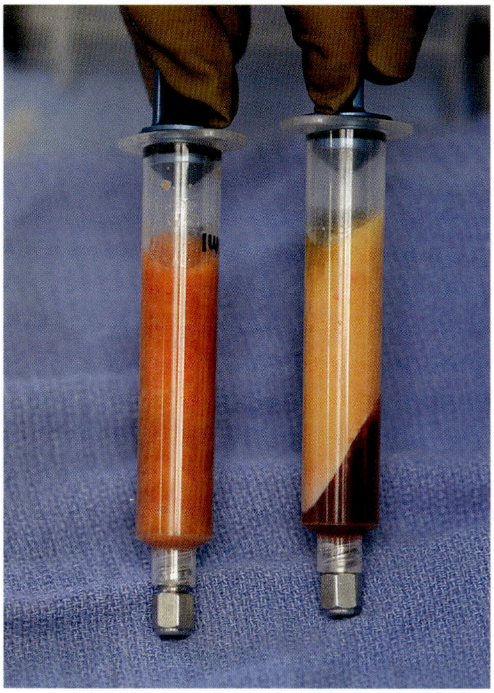

Fig. 12.6 (*Left*) The fat is shown prior to centrifugation. (*Right*) The centrifuged fat shows the infranatant, containing blood and lidocaine, at the bottom and the supranatant, containing lysed adipocytes, at the top.

(Miller Medical Inc.) is used to transfer fat from the 20-cc syringe into the individual 1-cc Luer-Lok syringes that will be used for fat infiltration. The plunger in the 1-cc syringe is gently pulled back as the fat is being injected into the syringe until the plunger is completely removed so as to remove the air bubble at the end. The plunger is then reinserted into the 1-cc syringe and is ready for injection. All fat injections are done using either a 1.2-mm or 0.9-mm spoon-tipped cannula (Tulip Medical Inc.). We recommend using the 0.9-mm cannula for periorbital injections and using the 1.2-mm cannula for all other areas (**Fig. 12.5**).

◆ Injection Technique

Inferior Orbital Rim

The inferior orbital rim remains the most challenging area to achieve safe and reproducible results. The most important technique-related issue for achieving good and consistently safe results is to augment the inferior orbital rim only from a midcheek entry point, with the cannula passing perpendicular to the bony rim. The inferior orbital rim should not be augmented from a lateral-based entry point. From entry point, the surgeon inserts the infiltrating cannula superiorly toward the inferior orbital rim so that the cannula tip resides in an immediate supraperiosteal plane. The nondominant index finger is used to protect the globe and to guide placement of the fat along the rim (**Fig. 12.7**). Only 0.03 to 0.05 cc fat

A

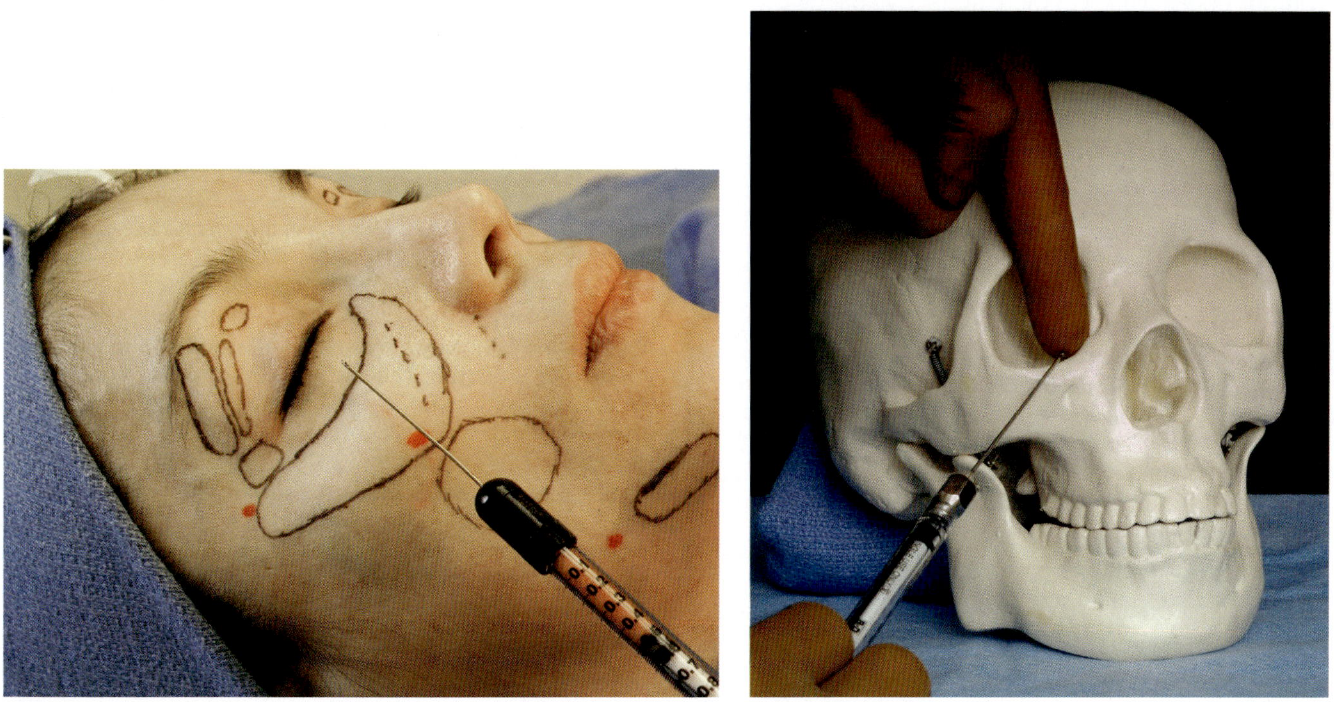

B

Fig. 12.7 Fat infiltration along the inferior orbital rim. (**A**) Fat is injected into the inferior orbital rim from the midcheek entry point. (**B**) Demonstrating the use of the nondominant index finger to protect the globe and to guide placement of the fat.

should be placed along the inferior orbital rim with each pass of the cannula. A total of 1 cc fat can be distributed across the medial half of the inferior orbital rim and another 1 cc fat can be placed along the lateral half of the inferior orbital rim. An additional 1 cc fat can be spread across the entire inferior orbital rim, as needed for patients with a greater degree of volume loss at the inferior orbital rim. As overfilling is a difficult problem to correct, however, it is always advisable to use more conservative volumes, especially along the inferior orbital rim. The admonition that "hitting a double" is much preferred to trying to "hit a home run" should be followed.

Nasojugal Groove

The nasojugal groove is defined as the bony/soft-tissue triangular depression that is circumscribed by the medial inferior orbital rim superiorly and the nasal sidewall medially. A volume of 1 to 2 cc fat can be placed into the nasojugal groove from entry point B into the deeper soft-tissue layer with 0.1 cc per pass.

Brow and Upper Eyelid

The upper eyelid–brow complex represents a continuum that is centered over the lateral bony contour of the superior orbital rim. The brow and upper eyelid are injected from a lateral canthal entry point (point A). Placement of fat into the brow should be undertaken along a plane of minimal resistance, just superficial to the periosteum. In general, 2 cc fat is placed in the brow with 0.1 cc per pass. Correction of a hollow upper eyelid is a more difficult maneuver, associated with a greater likelihood for perceived contour problems and prolonged edema, and thus should be done by an experienced fat transfer surgeon. Injections of fat to the upper eyelid should be placed just deep to the orbicularis oculi muscle with 0.03 to 0.05 cc per pass and using small total volumes.

Anterior Cheek

The focus of the anterior check is the linear malar depression, which runs from the medial inferior orbital rim downward in an inferolateral direction and corresponds with the malar septum deep to it.[6] From entry port A, 2 to 3 cc fat is injected, with placement of 0.1 cc per pass. Fat should be infiltrated in multiple levels from the supraperiosteal deep all the way up to subcutaneous fat superficially. The bulk of the volume is concentrated at, and anterior to, the malar depression.

Lateral Cheek

The lateral cheek represents a continuum with the anterior cheek and is situated over the lateral zygomatic arch. A total of 2 to 3 cc fat is injected, placing 0.1 cc per pass. As with the anterior cheek, the fat is placed in multiple levels with the bulk of the volume being concentrated superficial to the zygomatic arch. Additional fat can be placed in the submalar region, depending on the particular patient's needs.

Buccal

The buccal region resides immediately inferior to the malar eminence and is often very hollow in athletic, gaunt individuals or those with more advanced signs of aging. Placement of fat can be easily and quickly accomplished through entry points A and/or B. The fat is infiltrated into the subcutaneous plane, placing 0.1 cc fat per pass. The total volumes used will vary greatly depending on the degree of volume loss and may range from 2 to 5 cc fat. When significant cheek augmentation is being performed, the buccal area may begin to appear relatively hollow, requiring fat grafting to restore an adequate transition between the two adjacent territories. If a concurrent facelift is planned, care should be taken not to undermine areas where buccal fat has been infiltrated.

Precanine Fossa and Nasolabial Fold

As mentioned in the introductory section of this chapter, fat grafting into the precanine fossa and nasolabial fold is not undertaken with the goal of effacing this fold but to provide improved contour transition from the newly augmented cheek to the upper lip. From entry point B, the precanine fossa–nasolabial fold is approached from a perpendicular direction placing 0.1 cc fat per pass, using a total of 2 to 3 cc on each side. The fat should be placed in multiple levels from the deep supraperiosteal up to the subcutaneous fat.

Prejowl Sulcus

The prejowl sulcus refers to the volume-deficient area immediately anterior to the jowl. The soft-tissue depression of the prejowl sulcus should be thought of as a three-dimensional cylinder that extends from the anterior or lateral face of the mandible and wraps around to the inferior aspect of the mandible. Fat should be injected along the anterior/lateral face of the mandible, the inferior aspect of the mandible, as well as the transition between the two. The injections are done from entry point C in multiple planes (from deep to superficial) placing 0.1 cc per pass. A total of 3 to 5 cc fat can be placed on each side. Augmenting the prejowl sulcus can improve any facelift result and may be all that is needed in the younger patient with minimal jowling to achieve a straight jaw line.

◆ Postoperative Care

As there are no incisions on the body or the face, there is no need for any suturing. No dressings need be applied after the procedure. Patients are advised to apply ice intermittently to the fat transfer sites over the first 48 to 72 hours to minimize ecchymosis and edema. Routine head elevation is also beneficial, especially during the first week after surgery. The patient is reminded that exercise and activities that require bending over and lifting may exacerbate edema during the first several weeks after surgery. Additionally, dietary restriction of salt can help minimize unnecessary swelling.

◆ Complications

Significant complications that are encountered after fat grafting are rare; more commonly we deal with contour irregularities. Infection and hematoma occur in less than 1% of cases. Fat embolism is even more rare and results when fat is injected into a facial vein.[7] This can lead to skin necrosis or blindness and is invariably associated with use of an injection gun technique, which is absolutely contraindicated. Most contour complications that occur with fat transfer are centered in the periorbital region, a very sensitive area that must be treated meticulously. In the periorbital region, particularly the inferior orbital rim, we believe a conservative approach with undercorrection will avoid most problems. In addition, the inferior orbital rim should only be injected from a perpendicular approach.[1]

◆ Conclusion

Autologous fat transfer addresses one of the principal mechanisms of the aging process, that is, soft tissue and volume loss. Viewing fat transfer as a complement to traditional lifting procedures, we perceive management of the aging face as best achieved through a judicious combination of multiple approaches and methods. Fat grafting and volume restoration represent an entirely new aesthetic paradigm for the aging face, which we predict will continue to be more widely accepted and soon be the centerpiece in an overall strategy for facial rejuvenation.

References

1. Lam SM, Glasgold MJ, Glasgold RA. Complementary Fat Grafting. Philadelphia, PA: Lippincott Williams & Wilkins; 2006
2. Coleman SR. Facial augmentation with structural fat grafting. Clin Plast Surg 2006;33:567–577
3. Tzikas TL. Lipografting: autologous fat grafting for total facial rejuvenation. Facial Plast Surg 2004;20:135–143
4. Schreiber JE, Singh NK, Klatsky SA. Beauty lies in the “eyebrow” of the beholder: a public survey of eyebrow aesthetics. Aesthetic Surg J 2005;25:348–352
5. Shiffman MA, Mirrafati S. Fat transfer techniques: the effect of harvest and transfer methods on adipocyte viability and review of the literature. Dermatol Surg 2001;27:819–826
6. Mendelson BC, Muzaffar AR, Adams WP. Surgical anatomy of the midcheek and malar mounds. Plast Reconstr Surg 2002;110:885–896
7. Coleman SR. Structural Fat Grafting. St. Louis, MO: Quality Medical Publishing; 2004.

13

Rejuvenation of the Aging African Face

Anthony E. Brissett and Jose P. Zevallos

Persons of African descent represent the most rapidly growing group of patients seeking cosmetic surgery within the United States. When considering surgical rejuvenation procedures, it is imperative that the facial plastic surgeon recognize the unique characteristics of the aging African face. Because of the photoprotective effects of melanin, persons of African descent experience cutaneous photoaging to a much lesser degree than do Caucasians with similar ultraviolet light exposure. The brow and forehead regions demonstrate minimal signs of aging in Africans compared with those of Caucasians. The periorbital and midface regions represent the most prominent and earliest regions of facial aging in blacks, as a result of the unique skeletal morphology found in this population. Additionally, the effects of thicker skin and subcutaneous tissues on a hypoplastic underlying support system make Africans susceptible to develop the signs of lower face aging. A thorough understanding of the distinctive characteristics of facial aging within the African population allows the facial plastic surgeon the ability to tailor one's surgical management, thus improving outcomes and increasing patient satisfaction.

Over the past several years, there has been a marked increase in the number of African-American patients seeking facial plastic surgery. According to the American Society of Plastic Surgeons, African Americans are one of the most rapidly growing groups of patients seeking cosmetic surgery in the United States. In 2006, African Americans accounted for more than 780,000 cosmetic procedures performed.[1]

The effects of aging on the face are complex and include a multitude of factors such as exposure to ultraviolet radiation, nutrition, and medical comorbidities. When one considers facial rejuvenation in persons of African descent, it is critical to have a thorough understanding of how the aging process may differ from the traditionally described features of facial aging.[2–4]

The African-American population represents a diverse cultural group composed of multiple ethnicities; therefore, generalization about facial structure and the impact of aging is difficult. There are key features of the African face, however, that distinguish it from the faces of other racial or ethnic groups. The purpose of this chapter is to draw attention to the facial features unique to persons of African descent and describe how they change and evolve with age, highlighting important differences from the traditionally described models of facial aging.

◆ Cutaneous Changes Associated with Aging

Anatomic and Physiologic Features of African Skin

The hallmark feature of black skin is the quantity and epidermal distribution of melanin. Melanin has been shown to protect the skin by absorbing and deflecting UV radiation. Racial differences in skin color are determined by variations in the number, size, and aggregation of melanosomes within melanocytes. Whereas it has been established that all races have a similar number of melanocytes, black skin is characterized by having large, nonaggregated melanosomes dispersed throughout the entire epidermis. In contrast, Caucasian skin has aggregated, compact groupings of melanosomes that tend to be found only in the stratum basale. The larger, individually dispersed melanosomes found in African skin have a higher melanin content and are able to absorb more UV energy than do less aggregated, smaller melanosomes in Caucasians.[5]

In addition to differences in pigmentation, important structural variations exist in black skin that impact upon facial aging. The stratum corneum in persons of African descent tends to be thicker than in Caucasians and has increased lipid content.[5] There are also marked differences in the epidermis between black and white skin that become more pronounced over time. Facial skin in older Caucasians has been noted to have numerous areas of focal atrophy and necrosis when compared with facial skin of persons of African descent exposed to similar amounts of UV radiation.[6] The most significant difference between African-American and Caucasian skin lies at the level of the dermis. African-American facial skin has a thicker and more compact dermis, as well as an increased number of active, multinucleated fibroblasts. Additionally, the collagen fiber bundles are smaller and more compact and run more parallel with the epidermis.[6] This preserves the structural integrity of soft tissues in blacks and accounts for the youthful appearance of skin into late life (**Table 13.1**).

Table 13.1 Key Characteristics (and Their Implications) of the Skin of Persons of African Descent

Characteristics	Implications
Epidermis	
Increased melanin content	Less pronounced photoaging
Dermis	
Multinucleated, large fibroblasts	Skin elasticity is preserved Increased incidence of keloid formation
Hair	
Angulated hair follicles/spiral hair type	Pseudofolliculitis
Fewer elastic fibers anchoring follicles to dermis	Increased incidence of alopecias

Photoaging and Its Effects on African Skin

Exposure to solar UV radiation is the main environmental factor that contributes to premature aging of skin. UV radiation results in a decreased production of type I collagen by interfering in the procollagen production pathway. An increased rate of collagen breakdown accounts for a deficit in the structural organization and integrity of the dermal extracellular matrix. The accumulation of damaged, imperfectly organized collagen over years of exposure to UV radiation translates into the clinical findings associated with facial aging, such as fine wrinkles, rhytides, and thinner skin.[7]

Because of the photoprotective effects of melanin, persons of African descent experience photoaging to a much lesser degree than do Caucasians. It has been demonstrated that black skin shows only minor changes with long-term exposure to sunlight compared with profound alterations noted in white skin.[6] The clinical features of photoaging in black skin include fine wrinkling and mottled pigmentation. Unlike Caucasians, the signs of photoaging tend to become apparent in the fifth and sixth decades of life.[8,9]

◆ Structural Changes in the Aging African Face

Because of the minimal impact of photoaging on African-American skin, the signs of aging in the African face are primarily a manifestation of changes to the deep structures of the face, including the superficial musculoaponeurotic system (SMAS), muscular layers, fatty tissues, and underlying facial skeleton. In this section, we will review the structural changes associated with facial aging in persons of African descent and examine the upper, middle, and lower thirds of the face in detail.

Forehead and Brow

A common concern of patients seeking surgical facial rejuvenation is aging of the upper face. Brow ptosis, periocular rhytides, fine and deep rhytides in the forehead and glabella, and loss of elasticity of the upper third of the face are common characteristics of aging. Brow ptosis results from increased skin laxity, gravity, and the repeated downward contractile activity of the orbicularis oculi muscle and glabellar muscles.[4] In addition, there is an elongation of the upper third of the face as the hairline recedes and the brow moves downward over the supraorbital rim.

The age-related changes associated with the eyebrows and upper face are primarily related to alterations in skin laxity. The loss of the skin's structural integrity, as well as pull from the underlying facial mimetic muscles, results in the formation of forehead and glabellar wrinkles. Elasticity of black skin is well preserved into later in life, and thus aging of the upper face tends to be less pronounced in this population. Fine wrinkling, including periorbital rhytides, is less common in persons of African descent when compared with that in other ethnic groups.[10] Additionally, eyebrow ptosis occurs to lesser degree in black patients and has been reported to occur up to a decade later than in their Caucasian counterparts.[3]

Frontal and temporal alopecia are very common in black males and can be seen as early as the fourth decade of life. Temporal alopecia has also been noted in more than 50% of females, beginning at age 30 and peaking at age 50 to 60.[2] Traction alopecia is an important consideration in the black patient and typically results from styling the hair in tight braids in addition to the use of chemical hair straighteners. Over time, repeated, progressive traction results in follicular inflammation and atrophy causing hair to release from its follicular roots. Traction alopecia is found primarily in African-American females but has been increasingly reported in African-American males. The use of chemical straighteners, bleaches, and dyes disrupts the hair's keratin structure and reduces its tensile strength allowing it to become fragile and susceptible to breakage (**Fig. 13.1**).[11,12]

Periorbital Region and Midface

For many men and women, the periorbital region is among the first to show signs of aging and often represents some of the most pronounced structural changes associated with facial aging in persons of African descent. A smooth transition between the infraorbital region and the midface is a critical component of the youthful face that is often lost with aging. The midface region is roughly triangular in shape, the boundaries of which are the malar eminence and anterior border of the masseter laterally, the inferior orbital rim superiorly, and the nasolabial fold medially.

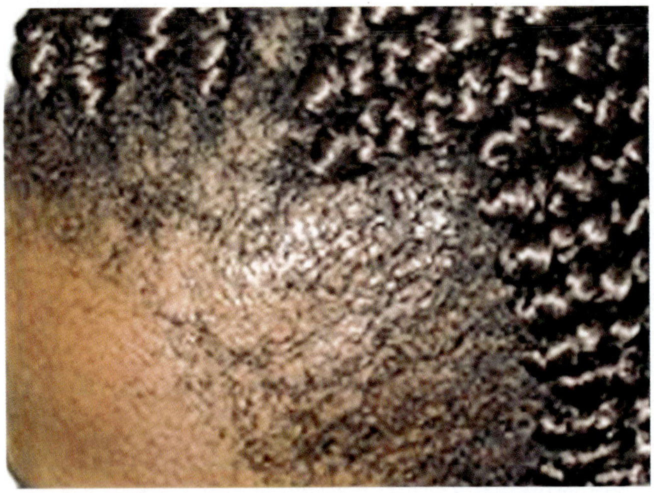

Fig. 13.1 Traction alopecia: progressive traction leads to follicular inflammation and release of hair follicles from their roots. (From Springer K, Brown M, Stulberg DL. Common hair loss disorders. Am Fam Physician 2003;68:93–102. Reprinted with permission.)

Typical findings of aging within the midfacial region include redundancy of the soft tissue envelope, increased laxity of the upper and lower eyelids, pseudoherniation of orbital fat, and descent of the melolabial fat pads.[4] Descent of the malar fat pad results in downward displacement of the eyelid-cheek junction and a double convexity of the midface (**Fig. 13.2**).[13]

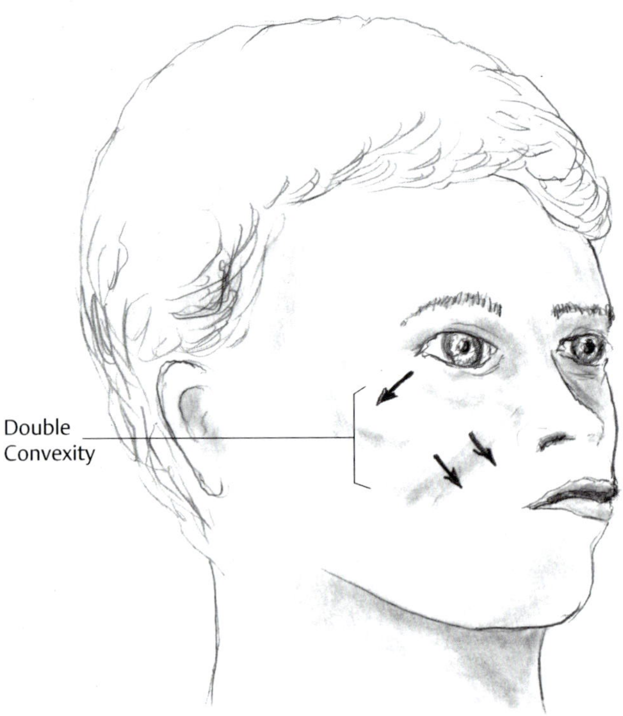

Fig. 13.2 The structural changes related to midfacial aging. Descent of the malar fat pad results in downward displacement of the eyelid-cheek junction and a double convexity of the midface. (From Friedman O. Changes associated with the aging face. Facial Plast Surg Clin North Am 2005;13:371–382. Adapted with permission.)

The periorbital and midface area represents the most prominent and earliest regions of aging in the African face. Unlike the aging process in the upper face, aging within the periorbital area is often exaggerated in the African-American population. Upper eyelid fullness unrelated to brow ptosis is common and is due in part to the relatively low position of the upper eyelid crease in persons of African descent. Medial fat pad pseudoherniation in addition to ptosis of the lacrimal gland also contributes to upper eyelid fullness.[3]

In addition to the soft tissue changes described above, the skeletal morphology of the orbit and maxilla in African Americans may contribute to signs of premature midfacial aging. African Americans tend to demonstrate increased ocular protrusion, a finding that is often present at birth (**Fig. 13.3**). Underprojection of the midface and malar hypoplasia is frequently seen in blacks and can result in midface concavity. Exopthalomopotric measurements between Caucasian and African-American adults demonstrate that African-American men have the highest mean protrusion, followed by African-American women, Caucasian men, and lastly Caucasian women.[14] As a result of this relative proptosis, Africans Americans are more prone to exhibit a negative corneal vector relationship with a resultant increase in scleral show and infraorbital shadowing.[3]

African-American patients presenting with the combination of ocular protrusion and midfacial hypoplasia tend to display more prominent eyes with exaggerated lower eyelid pseudoherniation and are more prone to premature descent of the melolabial mounds.[13] When these facial features are coupled with the increased weight of a thicker dermis and denser subcutaneous, signs of midface aging become more pronounced (**Fig. 13.4**).[3]

Deepening of the nasolabial fold tends to occur more commonly and to a greater degree among African Americans. This takes place as the malar fat descends from its position adjacent to the infraorbital rim and settles along the nasolabial fold. In addition, it is common for selective hypertrophy of the malar fat pad to occur in African Americans, thus contributing to deepening of the nasolabial fold (**Fig. 13.5**).[15]

Lower Third of the Face and Neck

In individuals of any ethnicity, the lower third of the face and neck are prone to develop the stigmata of facial aging. The changes associated with aging are primarily related to skin laxity, soft tissue accumulation, and ptosis of underlying structures. Resorption of the mandible, submental fat accumulation, platysmal banding, and thinning of subcutaneous tissue is also seen. Fat and soft tissue descent along the mandibular line obscures the fine bony definition of the mandible. Jowling may result from accumulation of fat in the neck and subcutaneous tissue, ptosis of the skin, submandibular gland, and SMAS, as well as thinning of the mandible. The anterior neck is also subject to the signs of aging, including loss of the acute cervicomental angle that is characteristic of youth. This results from dehiscence and excess laxity of the platysma, allowing subplatysmal soft

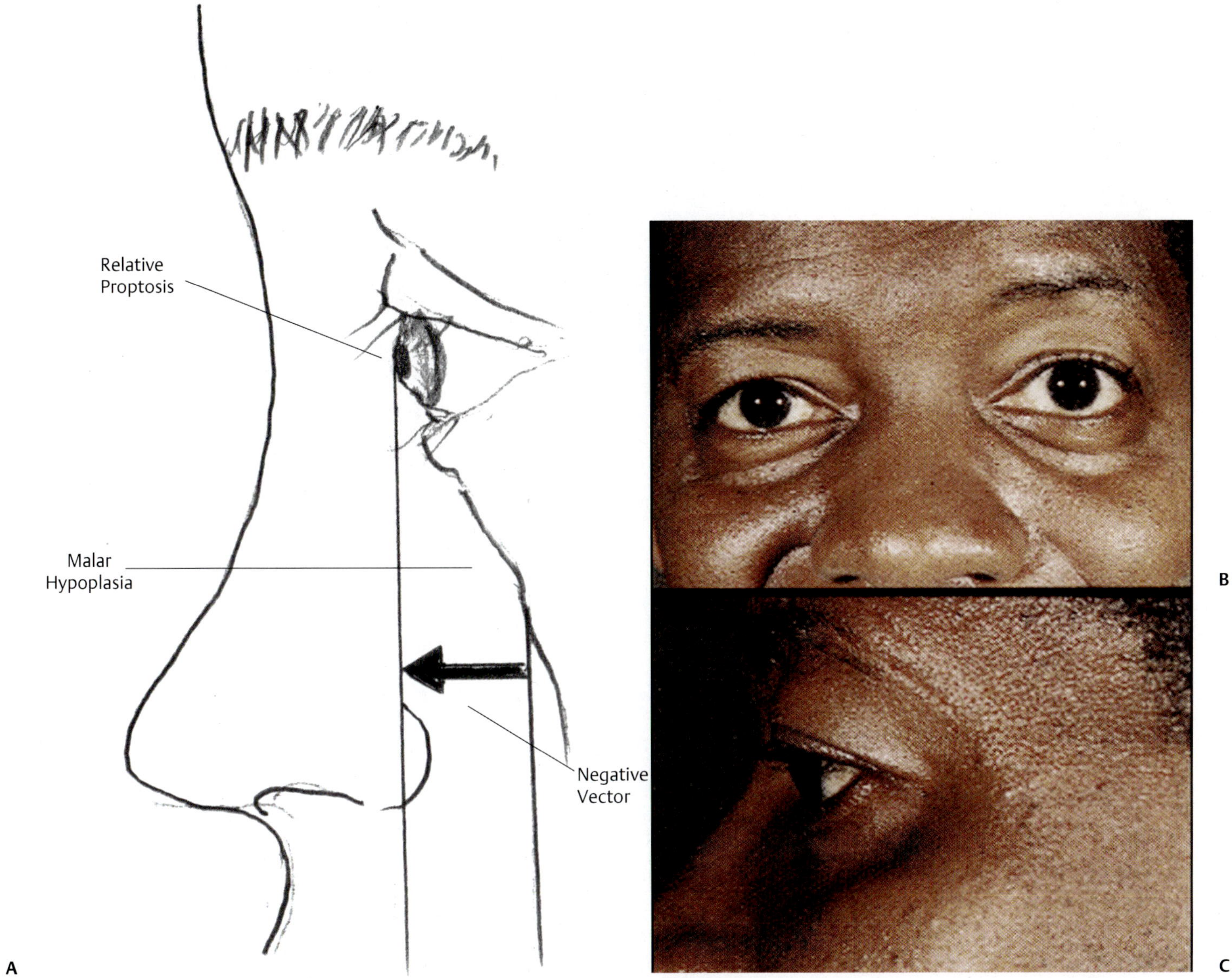

Fig. 13.3 (**A**) Relative proptosis. A negative vector is more common in the African American. (**B**) Frontal view of negative vector relationship. (**C**) Lateral view of negative vector relationship. (Parts B and C from Matory WE. Ethnic Considerations in Facial Aesthetic Surgery. Philadelphia, PA: Lippincott-Raven; 1998:156, Fig. 9. Reprinted with permission.)

tissue and fat to descend and accumulate in the submandibular and submental regions.[4] Fat ptosis, decrease in mandibular height and projection, and excess submental fat also contribute to chin ptosis commonly seen in elderly people.

As was noted in the middle third of the face, the signs of aging of the lower face are primarily related to changes in the soft tissue envelope, underlying fat, and skeletal structures. The effects of thick skin and subcutaneous tissues on a weakened underlying support system make persons of African descent more susceptible to develop the signs of lower-face aging. Jowling, submental and lower facial fatty fullness, and platysmal banding are common features of the aging African-American face.[2]

As aging progresses in the perioral region, there is a decrease in lip volume and thus exposure along the vermilion border. Descent of the lateral commissures and decreased show of the maxillary dentition are also demonstrative of aging within this area. The development of perioral rhytides radiating circumferentially and extending to the nose superiorly and labiomental sulcus inferiorly is a common feature.[4]

African Americans tend to maintain lip fullness and volume minimizing process of aging upon the lips. In contrast with Caucasians, one of the common features associated

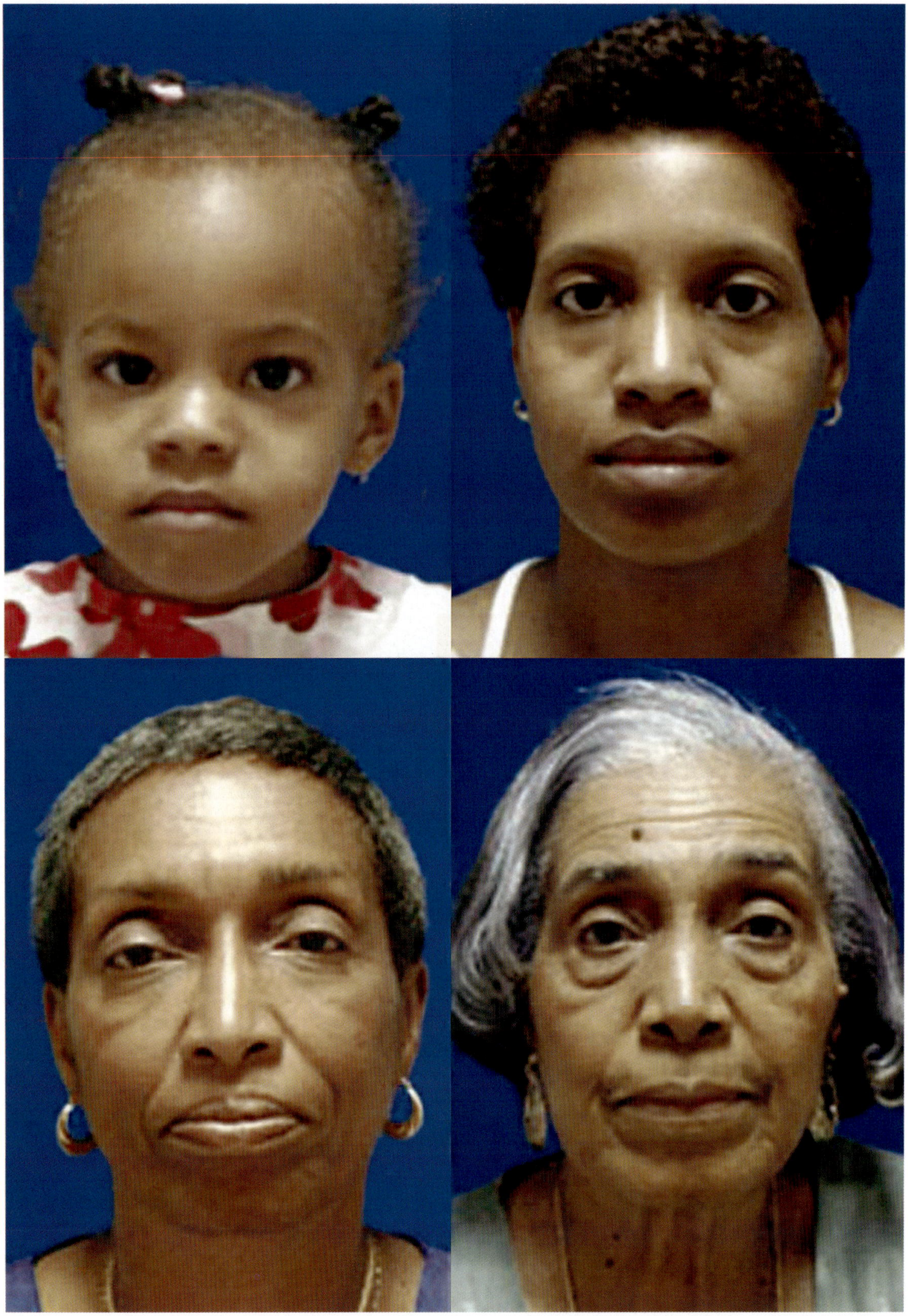

A B C D

Fig. 13.4 (A–D) Progression of facial aging in an African-American family across four generations: ages 2, 34, 56, and 80. Note the pronounced nature of eye and midfacial aging in contrast with a relatively preserved jaw line with the absence of jowling. (From Harris MO. The aging face in patients of color: minimally invasive surgical facial rejuvenation—a targeted approach. Dermatol Ther 2004;17:206–211. Reprinted with permission.)

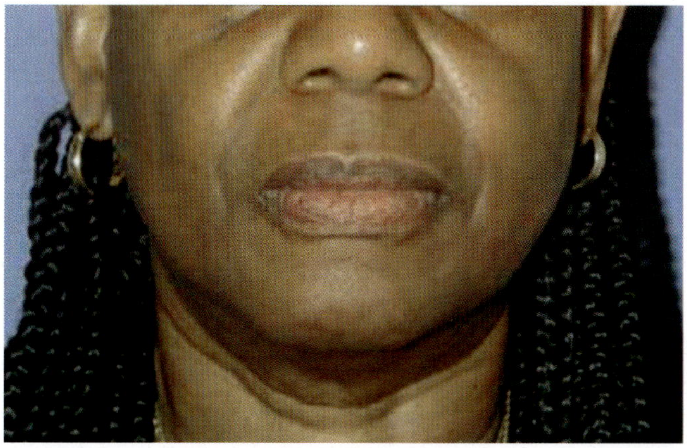

Fig. 13.5 Descent and hypertrophy of the malar fat leads to deepening of the nasolabial fold. (From Harris MO. The aging face in patients of color: minimally invasive surgical facial rejuvenation—a targeted approach. Dermatol Ther 2004;17:206–211, Fig. 3. Reprinted with permission.)

with aging in persons of African descent is increased labial prominence, anterior projection, and pink vermilion show. A feature of lower-face aging that is less common in African Americans is the development of perioral rhytides and radial lip lines. These rhytides develop from a loss of skin integrity caused by a combination of photoaging and repetitive contracture of the orbicularis oris muscle, as well as a decline in the volume of subcutaneous fat. As African-American skin is less susceptible to the effects of UV light, and the lips are more likely to maintain their volume, the African-American lips are less likely to show the signs of aging over time.

Nose

There are several characteristic changes associated with the aging nose, including a loss of relative or absolute nasal tip projection, greater columellar show, exaggeration of a dorsal hump, and increased sebaceous tissue at the nasal tip. Additionally, a decline in skin elasticity and loss of structural support mechanisms often occur overtime.[4]

The platyrrhine nose is characterized by less bone and cartilage support when compared with the leptorrhine nose. Thicker skin and more prominent subcutaneous fibrofatty tissue are often present, creating an amorphous nasal tip with less definition.[16] In addition, the nasal dorsum is frequently convex and the nasolabial angle acute in many persons of African descent.[17] Based on the structural differences previously described, the effects of aging on the black nose are frequently less pronounced when compared with the Caucasian nose.

◆ Conclusion

This chapter reviews the structural and aesthetic features of the African-American face and the changes associated with aging. Although significant variability exists, there are key structural features that are found to varying degrees in the majority of this population. Several anthropometric studies have revealed that the midface and orbital regions are the areas where these differences are most pronounced. As a result of these differences, facial aging in persons of African descent differs from the traditionally described models of facial aging.

This chapter demonstrates that the areas most susceptible to aging in the African face are the midface and periorbital regions. Within the midface, the signs of aging are related to changes in underlying muscle, fat, and skeletal structures. In addition, inherent structural features, including relative proptosis and malar hypoplasia, play a significant role. Persons of African descent are less susceptible to signs of aging in the upper face, where the traditional stigmata of aging are a manifestation of loss of skin integrity. This results from a decreased effect of photoaging on black skin. In the lower third of the face, a thicker dermis and subcutaneous tissues results in the development of jowling and rounding of the lower face.

As the desire for cosmetic surgery continues to grow among African Americans, it is essential that the facial plastic surgeon develop a thorough understanding of the aging process that is unique to this population. The traditional approaches to aesthetic facial surgery and surgical rejuvenation may not apply to persons of African descent. Ultimately, an understanding of these principles will lead to a precise assessment and surgical plan, resulting in more predictable surgical outcomes and increased patient satisfaction.

References

1. American Society of Plastic Surgeons. Cosmetic demographics. 2006. Available at: http://www.plasticsurgery.org/media/statistics/loader.cfm?url=/commonspot/security/getfile.cfm&PageID=23762. Accessed April 8, 2008.
2. Mattory WE. Ethnic Considerations in Facial Aesthetic Surgery. Philadelphia, PA: Lippincott-Raven; 1998.
3. Harris MO. The aging face in patients of color: minimally invasive surgical facial rejuvenation—a targeted approach. Dermatol Ther 2004;17:206–211
4. Friedman O. Changes associated with the aging face. Facial Plast Surg Clin North Am 2005;13:371–380
5. Taylor SC. Skin of color: biology, structure, function, and implications for dermatologic disease. J Am Acad Dermatol 2002;46:S41–S62
6. Montagna W, Carlisle K. The architecture of black and white facial skin. J Am Acad Dermatol 1991;24:929–937
7. Fisher GJ. The pathophysiology of photoaging of the skin. Cutis 2005;75(Suppl 2):5–9
8. Munavalli GS, Weiss RA, Halder RM. Photoaging and nonablative rejuvenation in ethnic skin. Dermatol Surg 2005;31:1250–1261
9. Gloster HM, Neal K. Skin cancer in skin of color. J Am Acad Dermatol 2006;55:741–760
10. Koch RJ, Hanasono MM. Aesthetic Facial Analysis. In: Papel I, ed. Facial Plastic and Reconstructive Surgery. 2nd ed. New York, NY: Thieme Medical Publishers; 2002:135–144

11. Hantash BM. Traction alopecia. Available at: http://www.emedicine.com/derm/topic895.htm. Accessed April 8, 2008.

12. Springer K, Brown M, Stulberg DL. Common hair loss disorders. Am Fam Physician 2003;68:93–102

13. Goldstein SA, Goldstein SM. Anatomic and aesthetic considerations in midfacial rejuvenation. Facial Plast Surg 2006;22:105–111

14. Barretto RL, Mathog RH. Orbital measurements in black and white populations. Laryngoscope 1999;109:1051–1054

15. Gosain AK, Amarante MT, Hyde JS, Yousif NJ. A dynamic analysis of changes in the nasolabial fold using magnetic resonance imaging: implications for facial rejuvenation and facial animation surgery. Plast Reconstr Surg 1996;98:622–636

16. Romo T, Abraham MT. The ethnic nose. Facial Plast Surg 2003;19:269–277

17. Porter JP, Olson KL. Analysis of the African-American female nose. Plast Reconstr Surg 2003;111:620–626

14

Rejuvenation of the Aging East Asian Face

Jeffrey M. Ahn and Jason P. Sulkowski

It has been a traditional maxim that the peoples of East Asia (hereinafter, Asians) "age better" than Caucasians do.[1] Even so, increasing numbers of Asian patients have been seeking out facial rejuvenation surgeries including facelifts and blepharoplasties. As the nations of East Asia become wealthier and progressively more Westernized, there is less bias against individuals seeking cosmetic procedures to reverse the aging process.[2]

The differences that contribute to the younger appearance of Asian adults are also responsible for causing standard cosmetic procedures that were developed on a primarily Caucasian population to need varying degrees of adjustment. Asians have thicker skin with more elastic fibers and do not develop fine wrinkles such as Caucasians do.[3] This thick skin, however, gives Asians a propensity to develop hypertrophic scars, obliging the surgeon to take care to conceal the incisions. The Asian mesocephalic face is rounder and flatter than the Caucasian face, which tends to be long and narrow. This is due to more prominent zygomatic arches and zygomas. As a result, surgeons must adjust their facelift technique to avoid complications of excessive stretching of skin over these more prominent areas. Bearing in mind features such as these allows one to better accommodate the specific idiosyncrasies of the Asian face.

One should not immediately assume that all Asians have thicker, more pigmented skins. Among the peoples of East Asia, those from Northeast Asia (roughly Korea, Japan, and northern China) tend to have lighter-color skin with less pigmentation than do the peoples of Southeast Asia. Therefore, it would be prudent to subclassify their skin type into finer categories to enhance the rejuvenation treatment result and minimize the possibility of complications. In this chapter, we will focus on the surgical treatments available that are tailored to the aging Asian face. But before this, we would like to briefly discuss the less invasive treatment options for these patients such as Botox (botulinum toxin type A; Allergan, Inc., Irvine, CA) and filler injections, peels, and intense pulsed light (IPL) and laser treatments.

◆ Minimally Invasive Treatments of the Aging Asian Face

Just as in Western countries, Botox injections for facial wrinkles are widely popular among Asians for the treatment of wrinkles. It is the senior author's experience that Asian patients tend to require larger dosages of the toxin than do Caucasian patients to achieve the equivalent results. Also, in thicker-skinned patients, the combination of Botox injection and filler injection is ideal for the treatment of deeper wrinkles with permanent skin changes such as glabellar furrows. Thicker Asian skins tend to accommodate the filler injections well with less possibility of skin irregularities.

On the other hand, one should be extremely careful about applying chemical peels and skin resurfacing lasers on Asian faces because of the possibility of hyperpigmentation and hypertrophic scars. In fact, only light to medium-depth chemical peelings are recommended, and one should refrain from deep peels on these patients. These patients should be fully warned about prolonged erythema (typically 2 to 3 times longer than in Caucasian skin) and possible worsening of pigmentation that can become permanent.

Hyperpigmentation is a popular concern among Asians in general. Therefore, laser and IPL treatment are widely sought-after procedures in East Asian countries. The senior author recommends the use of the second-generation intense pulsed light (I2PL) device with an extra filter as an added safety feature. Again, it would be prudent to start these treatments at the lowest settings and try spot testing whenever possible. This principle also applies to other laser and skin-tightening procedures in Asian patients with thicker skin to avoid the complication of permanent scarring and hyperpigmentation.

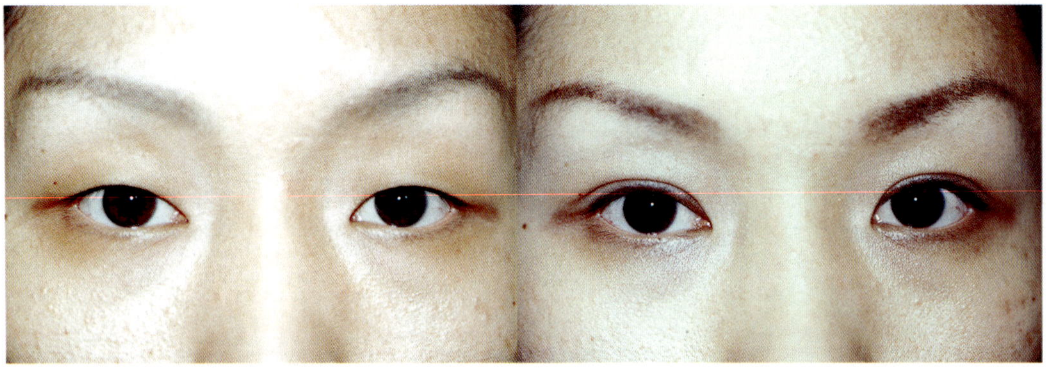

A B

Fig. 14.1 (A) Preoperative view of the Asian eyelids with no supratarsal folds. (B) Postoperative view of the Asian eyelids after the creation of the supratarsal folds.

◆ Upper Blepharoplasty

The upper blepharoplasty is a common procedure sought by Asian patients, many of whom are younger individuals who desire creation of a supratarsal fold to have a more aesthetic appearing eye (**Fig. 14.1**). In an elderly individual, this same procedure is able to correct mild blepharoptosis that makes the eyes look tired. By simply creating a supratarsal fold in an eyelid without it, mild to moderate form of blepharoptosis is corrected by the tucking effect that the double eyelid fixation has on the excess eyelid skin.

When considering an Asian patient who desires an upper blepharoplasty, it is important to consider the specific aesthetics of the Asian eye and to understand what kind of result is being sought. Details such as the size of the supratarsal fold and the medial epicanthal fold can be altered through surgical technique and must be fully discussed with the patient beforehand.[4] Even in those patients whose blepharoptosis necessitates the skin excision, the surgeon should be careful to avoid excessive removal of the skin because this can lead to the Westernization of their eyelids (**Fig. 14.2**). Asians with thicker skins are prone to form hypertrophic scars in medial and lateral canthal regions as well as unsightly large and asymmetric supratarsal folds that are difficult to correct and sometimes irreversible.

◆ Lower Blepharoplasty

As many Asian patients age, their lower eyelids begin to bulge and sag as a result of a herniation of the infraorbital fat pad. Just as in Caucasian patients, a lower blepharoplasty can be performed for Asians to reverse these changes and produce a more youthful appearance. Often this can be accomplished with a transconjunctival fat removal especially in younger patients, which will leave behind no scar and acts to minimize the infraorbital bulge (**Fig. 14.3**).

On the other hand, in older individuals, this type of simple procedure may not be sufficient, and more aggressive treatment will be necessary (**Fig. 14.4**). A subciliary incision can be made to access the fat pad, and skin excision can be performed to address the excess skin and wrinkles. Because Asians have thicker skin with higher likelihood of forming visible scar, the subciliary incision that allows the hiding of

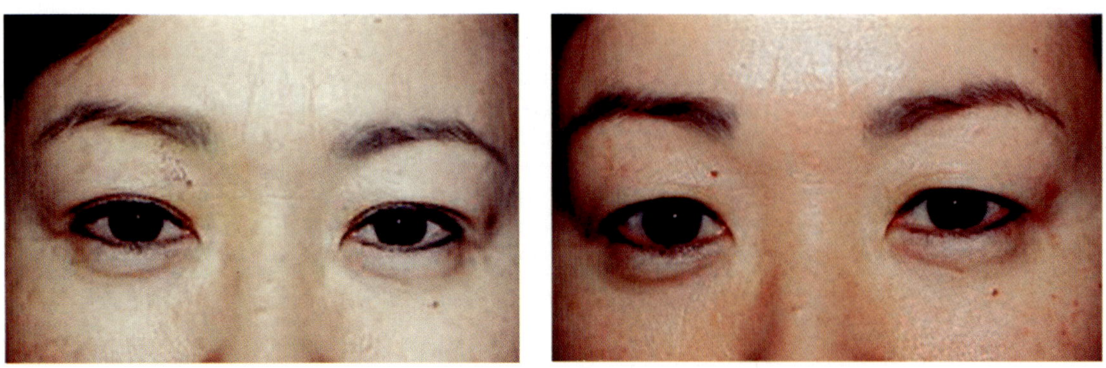

A B

Fig. 14.2 (A) Preoperative view of the aging Asian eyelids. (B) Aging Asian eyelids after upper blepharoplasty with conservative skin excision and creation of the supratarsal folds.

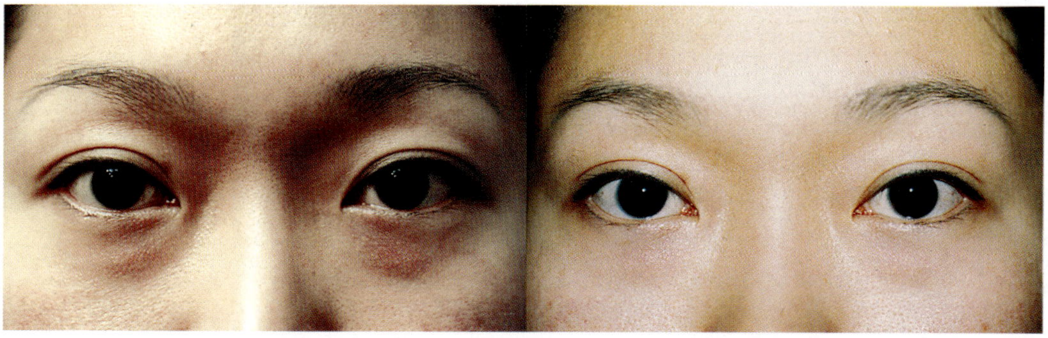

A B

Fig. 14.3 Transconjunctival lower blepharoplasty to address the fat herniation: (**A**) preoperative view; (**B**) postoperative view.

the scar underneath the eyelashes is preferred. In addition, a medial fat repositioning is also used to improve the nasojugal groove.

◆ Endoscopic Forehead and Brow Lift

The endoscopically assisted subperiosteal forehead lift is a procedure that was thought to be inappropriate for Asian patients given their different facial characteristics. Indeed, the typically larger, more sloping forehead shape of Asians makes it technically challenging to dissect and lase the glabellar area via endoscopic incisions. However, surgeons who specialize in the Asian face, including ourselves, have shown that this technique can be successfully applied to the Asian patient seeking to reduce brow ptosis and forehead wrinkles.[5] The use of carbon dioxide laser with flexible tip is especially useful to effectively address the muscles causing deep glabellar wrinkles, which are often located at a farther distance from the endoscopic incisions in these patients with wider foreheads. Puffiness of the upper eyelids and sagging of the lateral eyebrow are frequent complaints among middle-aged Asian women that can be effectively corrected using endoscopic forehead lift technique. The senior author believes it is better to avoid the excision of upper eyelid skin in Asian patients whenever possible, and endoscopic forehead lift allows the surgeon to improve the blepharoptosis without the visible scar or unnatural alteration of the supratarsal folds (**Fig. 14.5**). Extensive subperiosteal undermining down to and sometimes beyond the malar eminence is necessary to improve the sagging of the relatively thick and heavy midface of Asians (**Fig. 14.6**).

◆ Combined Endoscopic Brow Lift and Lower Blepharoplasty

The endoscopic forehead lift and lower blepharoplasty performed in one setting is a very popular combination chosen by the middle-aged Asian patients in the senior author's practice. By repositioning the brow and removing the forehead wrinkles, the upper eyelid ptosis is effectively treated, eliminating the need of the upper eyelid skin excision, which is often the cause of unnatural appearance and alteration of the patient's Asian features. Therefore, the combination of the endoscopic forehead lift and lower blepharoplasty addresses the aging upper face and midface of

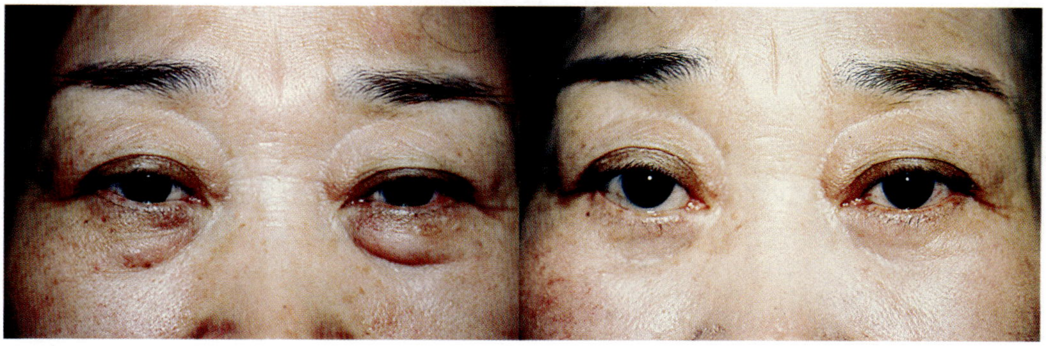

A B

Fig. 14.4 Lower blepharoplasty with skin excision via subciliary incision. Subciliary incision makes the hiding of the scar easier in Asian patients: (**A**) preoperative view; (**B**) postoperative view.

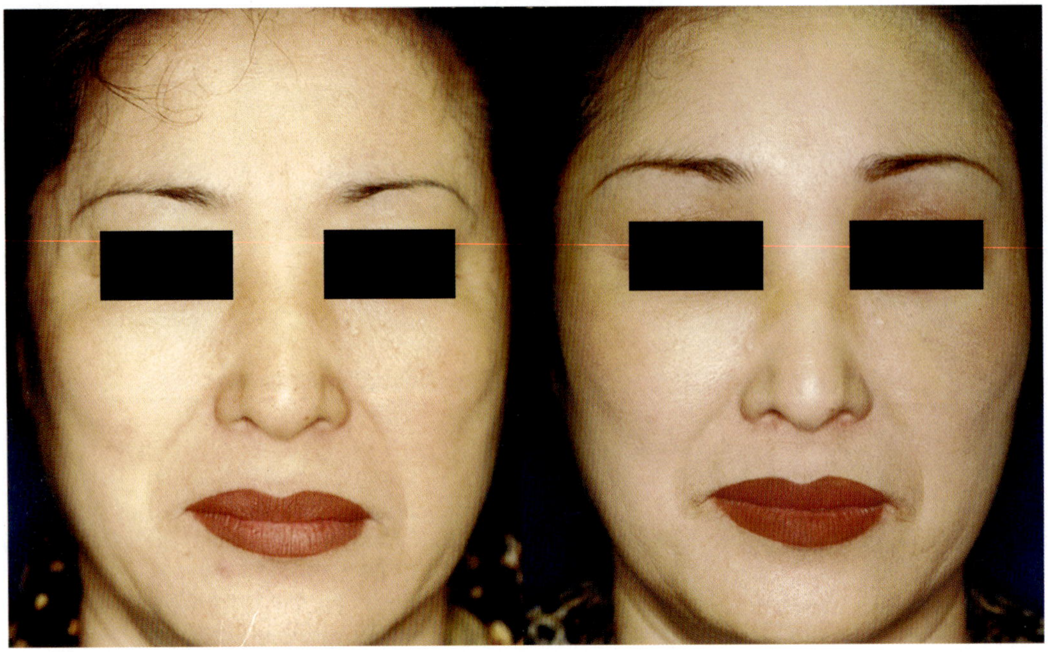

A B

Fig. 14.5 Endoscopic forehead lift in an Asian patient: (**A**) preoperative view; (**B**) postoperative view.

the Asian patients while preserving their natural ethnic appearance (**Fig. 14.7**). Because most Asian women notice the first sign of aging in the upper half of their faces, many middle-aged Asian patients choose this combination of procedures before considering the cheek and neck lift. In addition, the Endotine device (Coapt Systems Inc., Palo Alto, CA) can be concomitantly used during the endoscopic upper facelift in those patients who are more concerned

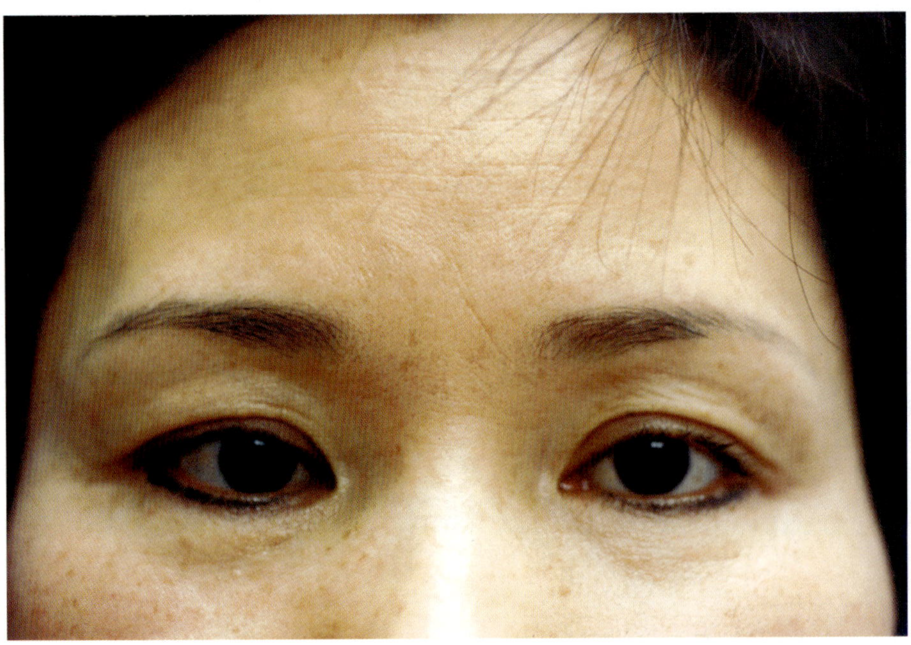

Fig. 14.6 Asian midface with thick skin and subcutaneous soft tissue.

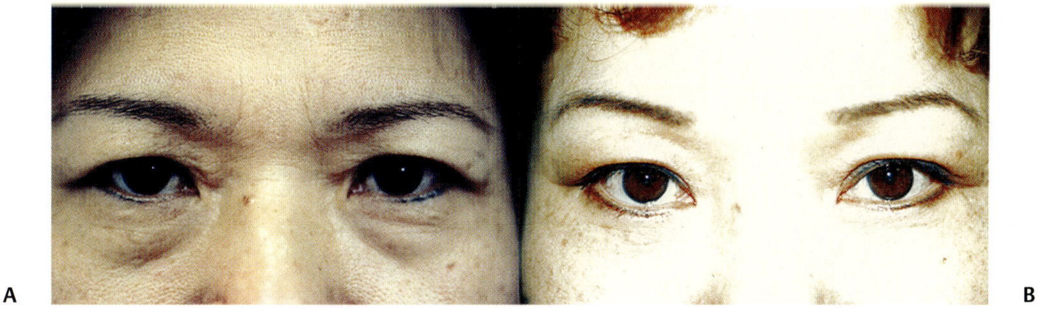

Fig. 14.7 The combination of endoscopic forehead lift and lower blepharoplasty, which allows the rejuvenation of the aging Asian upper face with minimum alteration of the underlying ethnic features: (A) preoperative view; (B) postoperative view.

about the sagging of the midface but reluctant to undergo cheek and neck facelift because of the preauricular scar.

◆ Facelift (Cheek and Neck Lift)

Again, the characteristic thicker Asian skin and superficial musculoaponeurotic system (SMAS) layers often cause the result of the standard facelift technique to be short-lived. The senior author uses extensive deep plane dissection and sturdier fixation of the SMAS flap to the deep temporal fascia and submastoid fascia to circumvent this problem. Weaker fixation frequently cannot be sustained during the immediate postoperative period with extensive edema, which is typically much more impressive in Asian faces.

First, short skin flap is developed anterior to the retrotragal incision, which is preferred in Asian facelifts. Then deep plane or sub-SMAS dissection is carried to the level of melolabial folds. Buccal fat pads are identified and plicated. Then the SMAS flap is pulled posteriorly and superiorly so that it can be sutured to the firm deep temporal fascia just superior to the attachment of the auricle (**Fig. 14.8**). Plication sutures typically employed to fix the SMAS flap in the preauricular region are not sufficient to provide longer-lasting

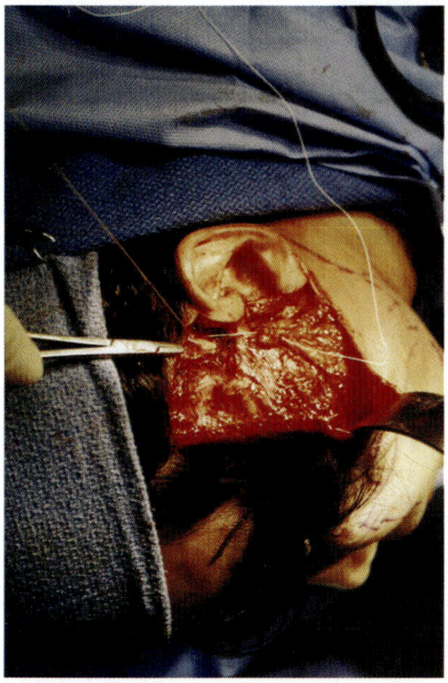

Fig. 14.8 During the Asian facelift, extended SMAS flap is sutured to the deep temporal fascia just superior to the attachment of the auricle. This type of rigid fixation allows the effect of the lift to survive through the immediate postoperative period of edema, which often is much more extensive in Asian patients.

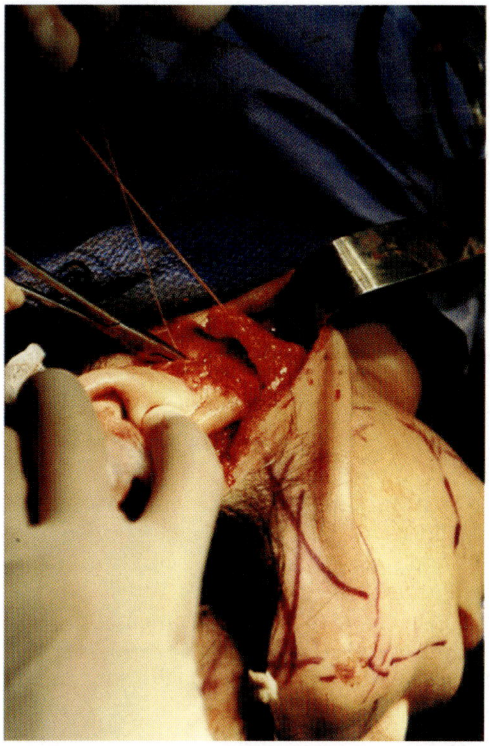

Fig. 14.9 Tailored platysmal flap is being sutured to the rigid submastoid fascia.

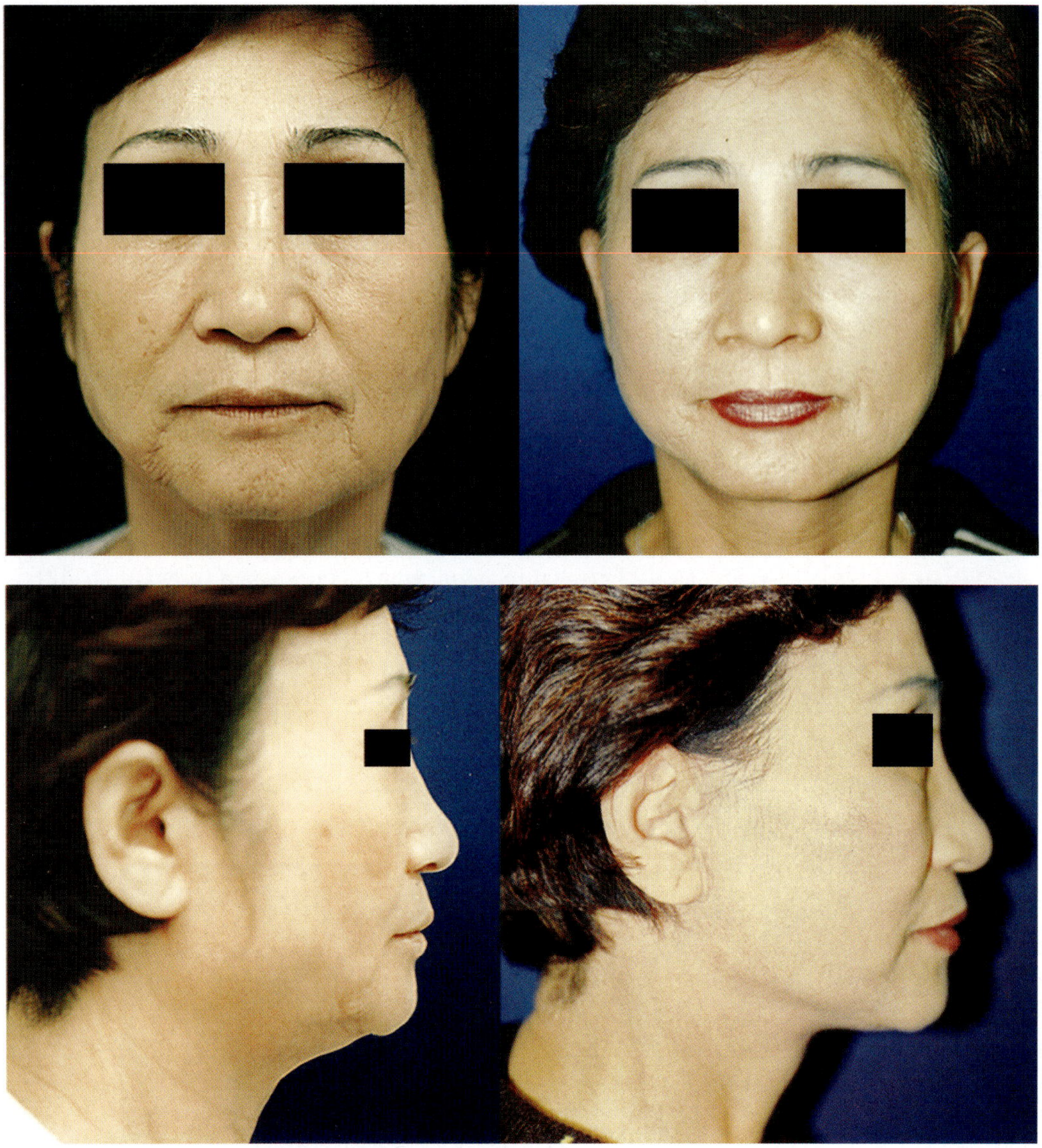

A B C D

Fig. 14.10 Aging Asian face that underwent cheek and neck lift employing the rigid SMAS fixations shown in **Figs. 14.8** and **14.9**: preoperative (**A**) frontal and (**C**) lateral views; postoperative (**B**) frontal and (**D**) lateral views.

result in Asians with thick skin, subcutaneous tissue, and SMAS layer. In addition, the platysmal portion of the SMAS is tailored and pulled posteriorly to be sutured to the immobile submastoid fascia (**Fig. 14.9**). With this maneuver, one can create nicely contoured submental/cervical angles that last over the years. Anterior plication sutures are usually not needed as the dehiscence between the anterior margins of the platysma is relatively rare in Asians. Moreover, incisions used for the anterior platysmal plication often leave visible scars in these patients. Again more aggressive plication techniques are employed, and every possible effort is made to hide the incision scars (**Fig. 14.10**).

◆ Conclusion

There are many surgical techniques available to the facial cosmetic surgeon to help an Asian patient achieve facial rejuvenation. When approaching any patient, the surgeon must take care to consider not only the patient's anatomic but also his or her cultural differences to help understand and achieve the unique goals that the patient desires. This is particularly true in Asians for whom many standard cosmetic procedures are in need of adjustment to accommodate their unique features. Being aware of this will lead to more aesthetic, longer-lasting results and leave the patient more satisfied.

References

1. Shirakabe Y, Suzuki Y, Lam SM. A new paradigm for the aging Asian face. Aesthetic Plast Surg 2003;27:397–402
2. Lam SM. Aesthetic facial surgery for the Asian male. Facial Plast Surg 2005;21:317–323
3. Onizuka T, Hosaka Y, Miyata M, Ichinose M. Our mini-facelift for Orientals. Aesthetic Plast Surg 1995;19:49–58
4. Castro E, Foster JA. Upper lid blepharoplasty. Facial Plast Surg 1999;15:173–181
5. Kim IG, Oh KJ, Baek DH. Personal experiences and algorithm of endoscopically assisted subperiosteal face lift in orientals for 5 years. Plast Reconstr Surg 2001;108:1768–1779

15

Hair Replacement Surgery

Mark M. Hamilton

Tremendous progress has been made in hair restoration over the half-century since its introduction. What a great step forward for men and women with hair loss it was when Norman Orentreich introduced the concept of hair transplantation in 1959.[1] Yet the field of hair restoration has had to overcome the reality of the initially effective yet so very unnatural results. Fortunately, progress has brought this field to an era where dramatic results are possible with the most natural of appearances. This chapter will review some of the essential features that allow results not possible as recently as a decade ago.

◆ A Brief History

The first hair transplant procedures involved use of grafts (or plugs) of 15 to 20 hairs each. These grafts were able to relocate large amounts of hair but were completely unnatural. Even today, patients are concerned about having a "doll's head" appearance. Over the ensuing decades, however, grafts became progressively smaller until minigrafts and micrografts became the state of the art in the 1980s.[2,3] With this decrease in graft size came a more natural result and an increased acceptance of hair transplantation.

Probably the two most significant advances of the past 20 years have been follicular unit grafting as well as incisional slit grafting.[4] These techniques combined have brought hair transplant to the point of achieving the most natural results possible today. Both will be discussed in greater depth later in this chapter.

Other procedures commonly used in hair restoration in the past, but much less so today, include scalp flap procedures as well as scalp reductions. Scalp flap procedures were most often either a Juri flap[5] or a variant of this. These flaps allowed the transfer of a large amount of hair with one flap providing almost immediate results. Their downsides, however, were many. The hairline created was abrupt and unnatural, the scars long and difficult to cover, and the procedure itself technically challenging and of moderate risk. With the improvements in hair grafting techniques, these flaps have become rarely used.

Scalp reductions offered the promise of removing large amounts of hairless scalp, particularly in the crown, without decreasing the amount of available donor hair. The downsides of scalp reduction, however, soon became obvious.[6] These included scarring, creation of unnatural hair growth patterns (slot formation), stretch back, and a decrease in donor density. Again, with improved grafting techniques, their use has been limited.

◆ Patient Evaluation

The initial consultation is the time where patient selection occurs as well as where a treatment plan is made. An important part of this is an in-depth analysis through a focused history and a physical exam.

The vast majority of hair loss in men is due to androgenetic alopecia. This is recognized by the classic pattern and progression as well as a family history. In most women, the cause is not always so clear-cut but is most often of genetic origin as well. In the cases in both men and women where the cause of hair loss is not obvious, a more detailed history, physical, and workup should be considered.

A good starting point is to consider alternative causes of hair loss. These include fever as well as stress, both of which would be associated with an acute onset and fairly rapid progression. Endocrine disorders such as hypothyroidism and hormonal changes (pregnancy/menopause) may also lead to hair loss. Other causes include nutritional deficiencies (especially iron), chemotherapy, as well as recent infection. A review of current medications may reveal one that is associated with hair loss. These include β-blockers, oral contraceptives, hypercholesterolemia medications, as well as Coumadin (crystalline warfarin sodium; Bristol-Myers Squibb, New York, NY).

Scarring is another common cause of hair loss. Most often, this is due to previous cosmetic surgery as seen with facelifts or forehead lifts. Other sources of scarring include lichen planopilaris and discoid lupus.[7]

Traction alopecia is seen with hairpieces or hair weaves. This occurs gradually over time in the areas of greatest tension and is usually obvious to the patient. This is a strong argument for these patients to move forward with hair transplantation to lessen the progression of their hair loss.

Alopecia areata is an unusual autoimmune disorder that results in distinct patches of hair loss that change over time. History as well as scalp biopsy can confirm the diagnosis. Medical treatments of some benefit exist. Fortunately, however, for most the condition is temporary and resolves over time. Another unusual cause of hair loss is trichotillomania. This is an obsessive compulsive disorder where repetitive pulling of hair leads to hair loss.

The workup of hair loss may include some or all of the following tests: complete blood count, electrolytes, antinuclear antibody, VDRL (Venereal Disease Research Laboratory), ferritin and iron levels, thyroid hormone levels and thyroid stimulating hormone, and testosterone and dehydroepiandrosterone levels. A scalp biopsy as stated above may be useful.

◆ Nonsurgical Treatments

Men as well as women have continually been bombarded with alternatives to surgical approaches, most of which have limited value. These include oral medications and topical treatments as well as hairpieces. Of all the medications and supplements available, only two, minoxidil and finasteride, have a proven history. Minoxidil's hair growth benefits were discovered during its use as an antihypertensive. It has now been used as a topical treatment (Rogaine; Upjohn, Kalamazoo, MI) for more than 2 decades. It can be used by both men and women. Minoxidil is available in a 5% concentration over the counter. Minoxidil limits hair loss primarily in the crown with little benefit along the frontal hairline. In addition, its ability to stimulate hair growth is limited. Most find the application time consuming and cumbersome. Given the modest results, it has developed limited popularity.

Of more benefit is finasteride (Propecia; Merck, Whitehouse Station, NJ). Finasteride is taken orally once daily. It acts as a 5-α reductase inhibitor decreasing the concentration of dihydrotestosterone at the hair follicle. Its use is indicated only in men. Studies have shown that 9 out of 10 men will see some results. Two thirds will see visible regrowth. The combination of ease of use with minimal side effects and a fairly effective result has made finasteride the gold standard for medical treatment of hair loss.

Low-level light (laser) therapy is a promising yet poorly understood or documented phenomenon. These technologies do seem to have the ability to stimulate hair growth and sometimes quite dramatically. Most of these realized successes, however, have been reported through personal communication or advertisements. Large multicenter studies will be needed in the future to document expected results and define what role this technology will play in hair rejuvenation.

◆ Patient Selection

An important part of creating a treatment plan is determining expected future hair loss. A detailed family history can be helpful. Because androgenetic alopecia is genetically based, extent and pattern of hair loss in other family members can serve to estimate where the patient may go over time. In addition, a patient's recent history of hair loss can be used to estimate future progression. A rapidly balding patient with extensive hair loss in his father, a grandfather, and a brother will want to take a more conservative approach. A patient with a stabilized hair pattern for 10 years and no family history can take a more aggressive approach.

Age obviously plays a role here as well. Young patients, no matter what the history, need a more cautious approach. Rarely should a patient under 20 years of age undergo a transplant procedure. In older patients, hair loss is often stabilized or if still progressing a final pattern can be more easily predicted.

Physical exam of the patient will reveal several important considerations, including classification of hair loss, extent of donor hair, quality of hair, as well as skin/color similarity. A variety of classification systems have been put forth to quantify hair loss with the most common being the Norwood system.[8] This system rates the patient's extent of hair loss from 1 to 7, with 7 being the most advanced.

Extent of donor hair is the primary determinant of how much transplantation can be done at the present time. This is partly determined by extent of hair loss as in the Norwood classification. It is also determined by the hair density of the donor region. This can be decreased in patients with previous transplantation or in those with diffuse thinning, such as seen in female hair loss.

Hair quality is another important factor.[4] This includes a variety of factors such as hair density, the texture of hair, hair color, and curl. Ideal patients would have coarse curly hair of a lighter color and high density. Fine, sparse hair that is straight and dark would in general be the least ideal.

A similarly related factor is skin color and the contrast it provides to the patient's hair color. In general, less contrast is better. Matching of skin and hair color is ideal. Think dark hair and how visually better this would be on dark skin versus light skin.

◆ Important Numbers

Numbers play an important role in planning for hair transplantation. It is important to keep several in mind. On average, a full head of hair has 100,000 hairs. Each follicular unit on average has around 2.1 hairs, so there are ~50,000 follicular units on a full head of hair. Approximately 25% of these follicular units (12,500) are in the occipital donor area of the scalp. In general, one half or 6250 follicular units can be harvested before there is noticeable thinning or distortion of this area.[9] Also, on average, each square centimeter of donor tissue contains 100 follicular units.

If transplanting a completely hairless area, the total number of grafts can be calculated based on measurements and use of the above numbers. If there is 5 cm × 10 cm, then the total area will be 50 cm^2. Without any balding, this area would contain 5000 follicular units. To achieve coverage in this area where thinning will not be visualized, more than half, or 2500 or more follicular units, must be transplanted.

◆ Donor Harvest

A variety of techniques have been used over the years to obtain donor hair. At the present time, harvesting of grafts through an elongated fusiform excision is the procedure of choice. The area for the hair to be harvested is first marked out with a skin marker. This is typically done in the occipital area at or above the external occipital protuberance. Hair can also be harvested from the temporal area as an extension of an occipital incision or on its own. Length and height are determined based on the number of grafts needed and scalp laxity. In general, 100 (around 200 hairs) follicular units can be harvested from 1 cm^2 of donor scalp.[10] Depending on scalp laxity, donor strips can be anywhere from 8 to 15 mm in height. In my practice, donor strips are created ~1 cm in height to help minimize tension and improve donor scars. If 1500 grafts are needed and the patient has good donor density, a 15- × 1-cm excision would be designed.

Once the donor strip is marked, hairs in this area are shaved to around 2 mm in height and the hair above is taped up. The area is anesthetized by first injecting slowly and in small amounts with 1% lidocaine with 1:100,000 epinephrine through a 30-gauge needle. Once adequately anesthetized, tumescent injections are performed to improve ease of dissection. Tumescence helps to lift the donor strip from the underlying tissue minimizing the chance for vascular or nerve injury. Although not typical, we do prepare and drape the donor area.

The donor strip is harvested with a standard no. 15 blade beveled in the appropriate fashion. The strip is taken in a subcutaneous plane preserving some tissue below the hair follicles. It is immediately placed in iced saline solution. The donor site is first approximated with towel clamps and then closed with interrupted as well as running locking 3-0 Prolene suture (Ethicon, Somerville, NJ).

A relatively new technique of harvesting donor grafts is follicular unit extraction (FUE).[11] FUE is performed by using a 1-mm punch to separate follicular units from the surrounding tissue down to the level of the mid dermis. The follicular unit is then extracted at this point with forceps. The advantages of this technique are the avoidance of strip excision and the potential (although small) for a widened scar, avoidance of sutures, and the ability to harvest grafts of exact hair count as needed.

There are, however, many issues with follicular unit extraction. The process is technically challenging as well as tedious compared with that of strip excision. In addition, many, if not most, patients are poor candidates because of problems at the tissue level with the extraction portion of the procedure. Another major problem with the technique is the large surface area incised during the procedure. This is estimated to be 8 times that with traditional strip excision. This requires patients to have hairs trimmed in a much larger donor area. In addition, it theoretically increases the potential risk to remaining potential donor grafts exponentially. For all of these reasons, the indications for and use of follicular unit extraction remain limited.

◆ Hairline Design

Creating a natural hairline is one of the great challenges of hair transplantation. Placement is critical. Two guidelines are facial proportion and distance from the glabella. Classic teachings on facial proportions dictate that the face can be divided vertically into three equal thirds. These three segments are from the chin to the columella, from the columella to the glabella, and from the glabella to the frontal hairline. This formula allows for a general idea of hairline placement based on an individual's features.

In general, hairlines typically are placed around 8 cm above the glabellar area. This can be altered based on a patient's previous hairline as well as age. With age, hairlines should be placed further from the glabella to give a natural-looking recessed hairline (**Fig. 15.1**). Design of a full, low hairline of a 20-year-old in a 65-year-old will look silly as well as unnatural.

Another feature to creating a natural hairline is not creating a stark line between transplanted and nontransplanted zones. A close inspection of natural hairlines will reveal a transition zone where the hairline is highly irregular and of varying density. It is natural to often find single hairs isolated in front of the hairline.

Creation of this irregular hairline has been described by Stough and Whitworth[12] as well as others. Once a hairline is marked out, we intentionally place recipient sites in front of as well as behind the line. This helps to avoid an obvious, rigid line of demarcation.

◆ Recipient-Site Creation

The other major advance of the past 20 years is the development of incisional slit grafting.[3] Round grafts require the removal of recipient tissue for placement. This results in a vascular insult to the subcutaneous tissue and its associated vascular network.

With incisional slit grafting, recipient sites are created with a small knife. In our practice, a 1.3-mm knife is used along the frontal hairline and a 1.5-mm knife everywhere else. This allows minimal injury to the surrounding tissue and immediate placement of the graft in a snug pocket with surrounding healthy vascular tissue.

Use of incisional slit grafting has been estimated to improve graft take by a factor of 2. The risk of scarring is decreased. In addition, existing hairs are less traumatized minimizing the risk of effluvium of hairs already present in the recipient area.

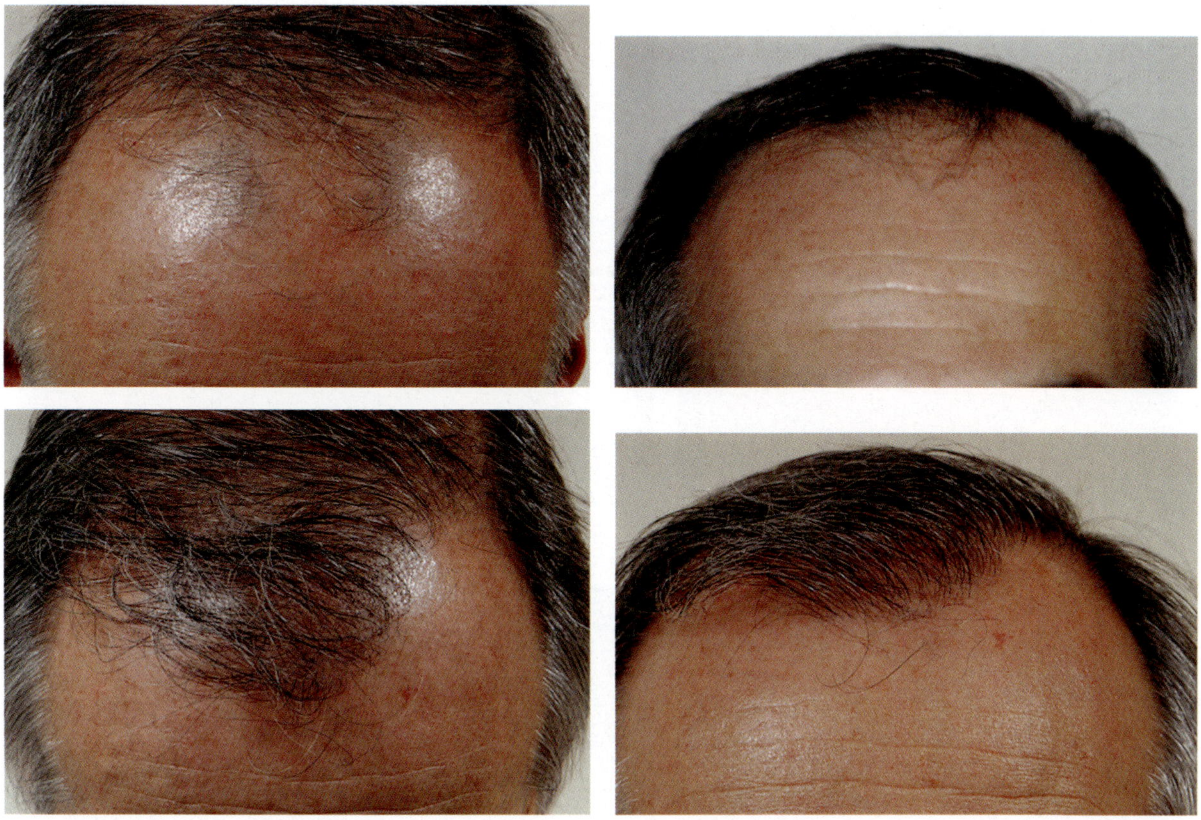

Fig. 15.1 Photographs of an older patient (**A, B**) before and (**C, D**) after hair transplantation. Note creation of narrow, slightly recessed hairline to create a natural result.

Hair direction is critical in creation of the recipient area. Beveling should be done at an angle somewhere between 25 and 45 degrees. Hair growth pattern should be carefully followed. Along the frontal hairline, incisions are beveled anteriorly. This becomes more lateral as one extends posterior. In the crown, creating the natural swirl pattern is critical. Throughout the temporal and occipital areas, the direction is downward and posterior.

◆ Follicular-Unit Hair Grafting

The great extent of the improvement in hair grafting over the past 50 years is due to an improvement in the grafts themselves. Graft size progressively decreased, until in the 1990s micrografts including single-hair grafts became a common practice. The ultimate goal, however, has always been to create a "natural" appearance, and further understanding of what is natural came in an article by Headington.[13] In this article, he described the natural clustering of hair follicles at the skin surface in groups of anywhere from one to four hairs. Further understanding of this anatomy came in an article by Bernstein,[14] where it was recognized that below the surface of the skin these hair shafts would frequently diverge, leading to "splay" of the individual hair bulbs. Follicular-unit grafting was developed to keep this complex anatomic unit intact.

Follicular-unit grafting can best be described from the following personal communication by Limmer[10]: "Follicular unit transplantation is by definition the redistribution of naturally occurring follicular groupings of one to four hairs, rarely more, removed from the donor area by single bladed elliptical excision, careful microscopic dissection beneath the binocular stereoscope, and reimplantation in the bald recipient zone in a needle tunnel or a very small slit incision. Donor tissue is carefully trimmed into such follicular units removing 'bald' donor tissue. Bald tissue is not removed from the recipient zone to minimize damage . . . ."

With follicular-unit grafting, the achievement of natural, nonsurgical-looking results is possible (**Fig. 15.2**).

Magnification and lighting are important elements in dissecting these follicular units. Dissection under the microscope brings both of these together and is the ideal method for graft preparation. This can also be accomplished with light boxes that provide back light and loupes or some other form of magnification.

Another key component is highly trained technicians. To efficiently cut high-quality grafts takes experience and repetition. Many hair transplant candidates are aware of the ability to cut and place thousands of high-quality grafts in a

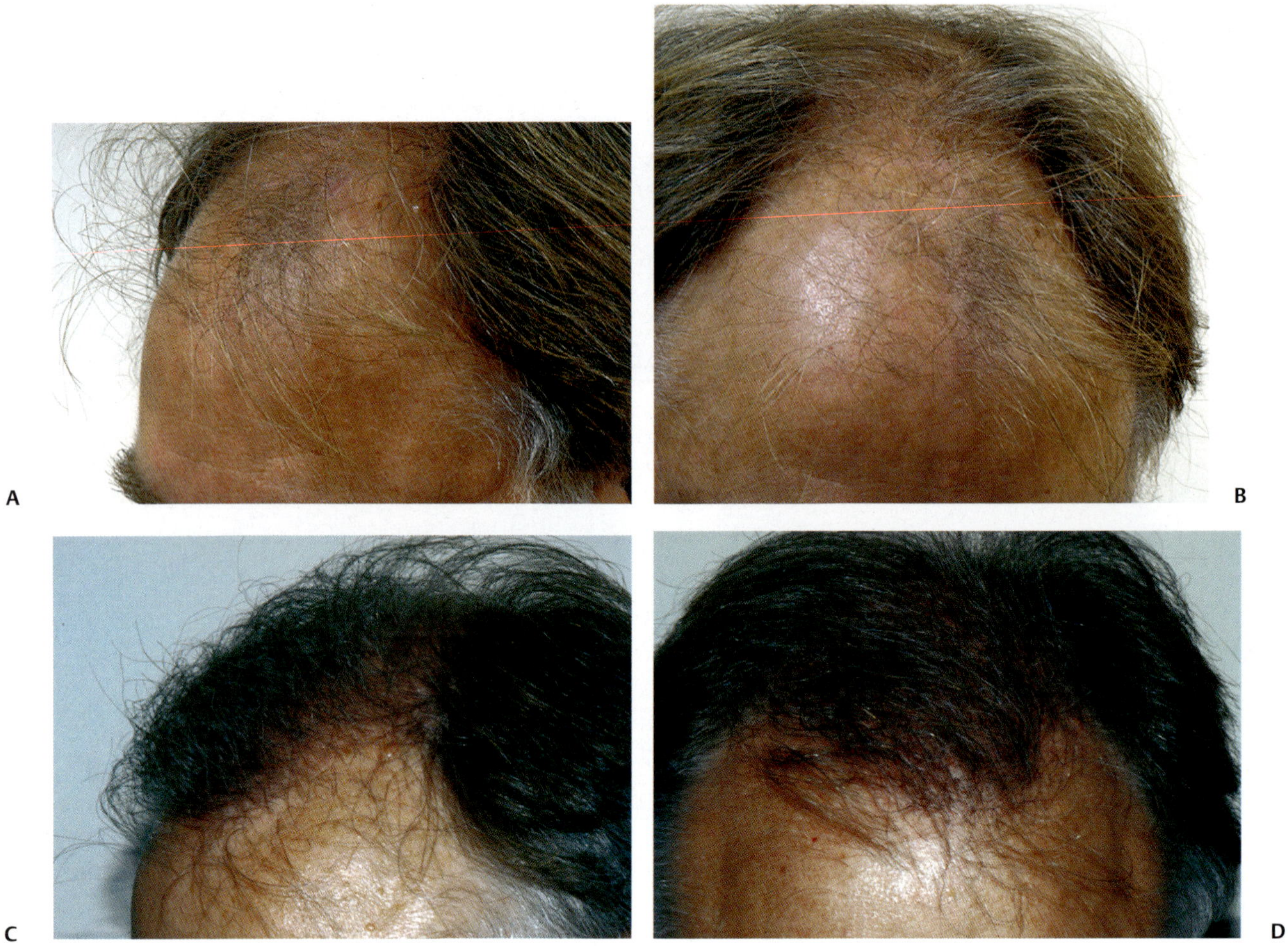

Fig. 15.2 Photographs of a patient (A, B) before and (C, D) after hair transplantation with follicular-unit grafting.

short period of time. It is essential to have two or three experienced technicians to accomplish this.

Grafts in our practice are placed with jeweler's forceps using some magnification. Atraumatic handling is critical to minimizing injury to the hair follicle. The graft can be grasped by the small amount of fat that surrounds the hair shaft. Placement is done in the direction of recipient-site creation, typically using a cotton swab to help the graft into position. Grafts can be placed as recipient sites are made or, as in our practice, as a separate step.

Grafts should be placed with the skin of the graft just above the skin surface. Placement too high will lead to noticeable bumps, or *cobblestoning*. Placement too low will lead to obvious depressions, or *pitting*. Light pressure may be briefly applied if bleeding develops.

◆ Postoperative Care

After completion of the procedure, the patient's hair is sprayed with tap water and combed to reveal any buried hairs. A light pressure wrap is applied over the donor region and around the forehead. A scarf is lightly tied over the recipient area and the patient is discharged home. Patients are seen the next day to remove the dressing, replace any displaced grafts, as well as review wound care.

Care for the patient includes spraying the donor area 3 to 4 times a day with a spray bottle. The hair may be washed with a cup of water at 72 hours. Showering and combing should not be done for a week. Sutures are removed at 10 days. Patients are instructed not to do any strenuous activity for 2 weeks and no heavy lifting for 3 weeks.

Patients are continually reminded about the telogen phase that follows hair transplantation. An appointment is typically made at the 3-month point primarily for giving reassurance. A final result can be expected in 7 to 8 months and a second session is typically not done until this point.

Some surgeons have reported success with minimizing hair shock by having patients use minoxidil regularly after surgery. Another product with reported benefits after surgery is GraftCyte (Procyte Corp., Redmond, WA).[7] This too has been reported to minimize hair shock as well as crusting and redness immediately after surgery.

◆ Hair Transplantation in Women

Hair transplantation among women has lagged behind that among men, although the need is just as high. It has been estimated that 10% of women will develop female pattern hair loss.[7] Interest among women does now seem to be growing, and the author has seen this in his practice. The majority of hair loss in women is due to female pattern hair loss. The classic pattern involves thinning throughout, but primarily over the vertex, crown, and upper sides of the head. Hormonal changes often play a role, with acceleration often seen during pregnancy and menopause. Typically, the frontal hairline is spared.

As in men, hair is harvested from the occipital area. In women, a thinning donor area does seem to be more of an issue. It is important to establish realistic goals in consultation. With limited grafts, determining what areas women are most concerned about or are most difficult to cover is imperative. This allows focusing of limited resources on those areas.

Grafts of larger size may be used when transplanting in areas well camouflaged by existing but thinning hair. This allows placement with minimal injury to the recipient area with maximal improvement in density.

Eyebrow, Eyelash, and Body Hair Transplantation

The ability to transplant other areas of hair loss has improved greatly as the size of hair transplants has grown smaller. Single-hair grafts are especially beneficial when transplanting these off-scalp areas. Two areas that have received increased attention for transplanting in recent years include the eyebrow and eyelashes.

Eyebrows have a functional importance as well as an aesthetic role. Their presence facilitates blockage of bright light as well as serving to keep forehead perspiration away from the eyes. From an aesthetic standpoint, they are an important part of expression of a variety of emotions. In addition, eyebrows are continually analyzed as well as modified for purposes of beauty.

Many women develop thinning or loss of the eyebrows over time. A wide variety of medical conditions including hypothyroidism as well as congenital conditions can lead to hair loss in this area. Probably the most common cause for hair loss in this area is trauma. This includes aggressive techniques of hair removal and burns as well as accidental traumatic injury.

Use of transplantation of the eyebrows was described as early as was transplantation on the scalp.[15] A critical part of a natural-looking eyebrow is the use of single-hair grafts. The ideal position of an aesthetic eyebrow has been well described.[16] Discussing eyebrow design before the procedure is critical. This can be done in front of the mirror marking a recommended pattern and eliciting patient comment.

Donor hair grafts for nonscalp work are typically performed just as with scalp transplantation. Eyebrow and eyelash transplantation, however, is one area where follicular-unit extraction may be of particular benefit. For complete re-creation of both eyebrows, between 200 and 250 grafts will need to be harvested and placed.[17] A 19-gauge needle can be used for insertion sites. Direction and angle are critical. Medially, brow hairs tend to all direct in a cephalic direction. As the brow arches laterally, the direction shifts to a more lateral direction. At the inferior edge, hairs project slightly cephalad; superior edge projection tends to be somewhat caudal. At all points, the needle should be inserted at an acute angle to the skin surface mimicking the natural hair growth pattern (**Fig. 15.3**).

Eyelashes play an equally critical role from an aesthetic as well as functional standpoint. Their re-creation is even more technically challenging. Transplantation is this area for years has been for mostly reconstructive purposes. With recognition of improved techniques, eyelash transplantation for cosmetic purposes has increased dramatically in recent years.

The most accepted technique involves implanting hairs in the eyelid with a sewing-type technique.[18] Hair is harvested

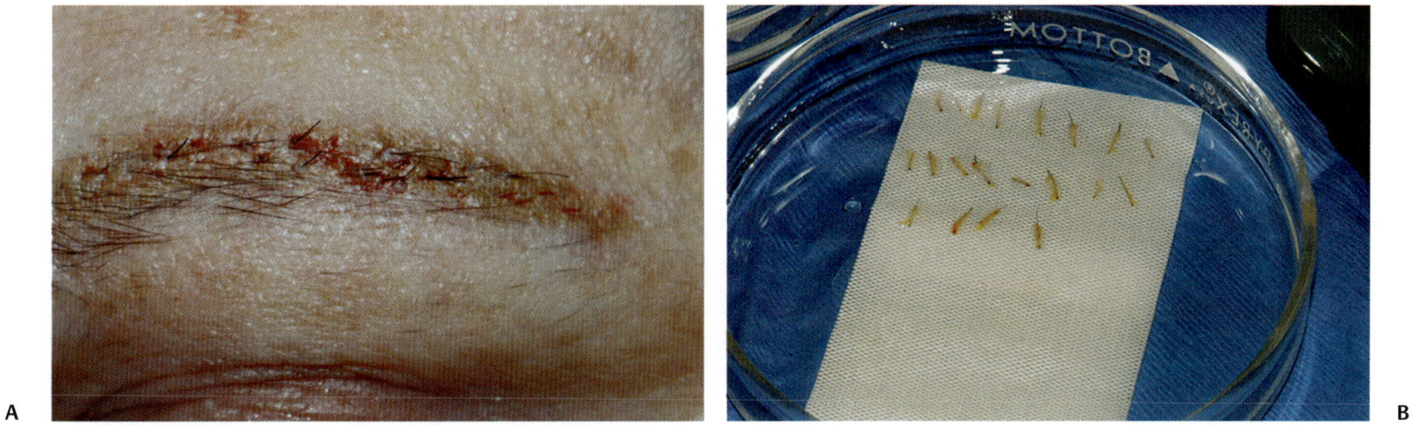

Fig. 15.3 (**A**) Thinning eyebrow immediately after placement of hair grafts. (**B**) Single-hair grafts created for use during hair transplantation to the eyebrow.

as in standard hair transplantation except the hairs are left long (10 cm). Typically anywhere from 20 to 40 hairs are transplanted per eyelid when doing so for cosmetic purposes. Once harvested, hairs are threaded through the eye of a French surgical needle. The needle is then inserted into the upper eyelid starting 6 to 10 mm above the lid margin. The needle is threaded down to the lash line and advanced out between existing lashes. With careful attention to direction, the follicle is pulled into the newly created tunnel. The hair is then cut short to release the needle and prevent dislocation of the existing follicle. The process is then repeated.

After the procedure, care is used to prevent dislocation. Glasses or goggles are worn the first week afterward. Makeup should not be worn for 1 week. Continuous care of transplanted hair is required. It must be trimmed and curled every 4 to 6 weeks.

Other potential areas of off-scalp transplantation include the chest, the pubic region, and facial hair such as sideburns, moustache, and beard. Expect increased interest among patients as awareness of these techniques grows.

◆ Revision Hair Transplantation

Hair transplantation is a procedure that should be associated with very high satisfaction. Complications are unusual, and with appropriate counseling and good technique, results should be predictable. There are, however, many patients who present for revision work. Two of the most common reasons seem to be transplants done with large grafts years ago and poor donor scarring.

One of the most disappointing patients to see in public for the hair transplant surgeon is the patient who had his procedure years ago and has the classic "corn row" appearance. The bad name these results gave hair transplantation has taken years to remove. On the other side, these can be some of the most rewarding patients to care for. These patients have typically suffered years of ridicule. They often suffer low self-esteem. Their appearance often affects both their personal and professional life.

The first to describe correction of large-graft transplantation was Lucas.[19] Since then, many have put forth similar techniques with their own modification. The two main features of corrective surgery include partial or complete removal of the large grafts and camouflage with follicular-unit grafting.

Grafts can be partially or completely removed. Our practice is to use a 3-mm punch to remove slightly more than two thirds of the graft. A 4-0 Prolene stitch is then used in a mattress fashion to close the defect. The portion of the harvested graft is then recycled as several smaller grafts for use during the procedure. Usually partial removal of the first two rows of grafts combined with camouflage provides good correction of the plug appearance.

Camouflage is performed by surrounding existing plugs with dense packing of follicular unit grafts. In addition, if possible, extension of the frontal hairline 1 to 2 cm anterior to the line of plugs will further hide the larger grafts (**Fig. 15.4**).

In certain patients, request for removal of all the grafts may be made. Though certainly possible, they must be aware of the markedly decreased rate of take from grafts that are harvested and retransplanted. Some patients may not have adequate donor hair for camouflage. In these patients, removal of more than just a few rows of grafts will be required.

Fortunately, most donor regions can be closed in a linear fashion with single-layer suture closure, and a more than acceptable scar will result. In a few patients, however, a wide or unacceptable scar may result. In addition, poor technique, such as harvesting too wide a strip or multiple excisions from the same area, will result in expectedly poor outcome. Correction of these scars can be done using several techniques.

Repair of a scar with closure done in the same fashion as a trichophytic incision used for forehead lifting can be beneficial. This is done in such a way that the superficial dermis and epidermis of one wound edge overlaps the deep dermis and follicle-bearing region of the other wound edge. This allows hair growth through the wound edges camouflaging any widening that may occur.

A w-plasty excision and closure of a widened scar will help to change the direction of tension as well as disperse areas of widening that may occur. This technique is very effective if scalp tension is not unusually high.

When a patient presents with a markedly widened scar and unusually high scalp tension, tissue expansion may be required. Tissue expansion is a well-described technique that allows increased tissue for closure minimizing tension. As with all scar repairs, aftercare is important. Restricting activity for the first several weeks afterward is critical to minimizing tension.

◆ Complications

Fortunately, hair transplantation is a procedure in which complications are rare, and serious events almost never occur. As with most surgical procedures, bleeding is always a concern. Making sure patients are off any blood-thinning medications 2 weeks prior to a procedure helps to prevent bleeding problems. Usually, any bleeding in the donor area during the procedure can easily be controlled with bipolar cautery. Either temporary light pressure or reinjection of an epinephrine solution can control bleeding in the recipient area during the procedure. A pressure bandage is applied to the donor area for 24 hours after the procedure. If bleeding does occur, either in the donor area or the recipient area, pressure should be applied first. Most postprocedure bleeding should be controllable with pressure, and a return to surgery should be rare.

As with any surgery, infection is also a concern but extremely rare due to the vascularity of the scalp. All of our patients are placed on an antibiotic with adequate staphylococcal coverage starting the day before surgery and for

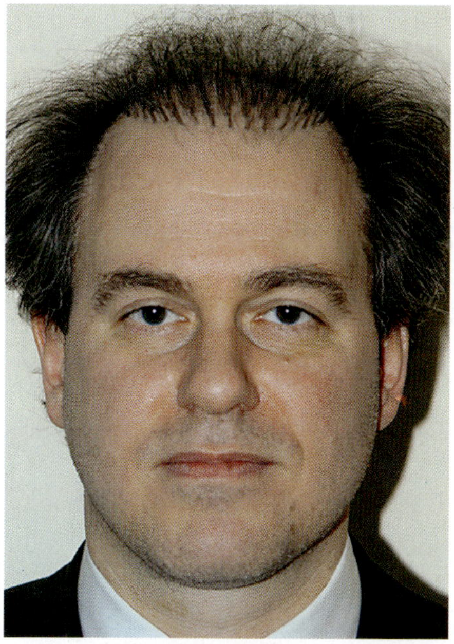

A

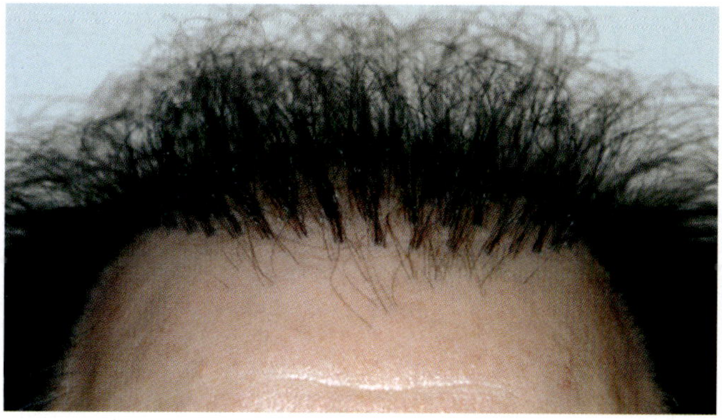

B

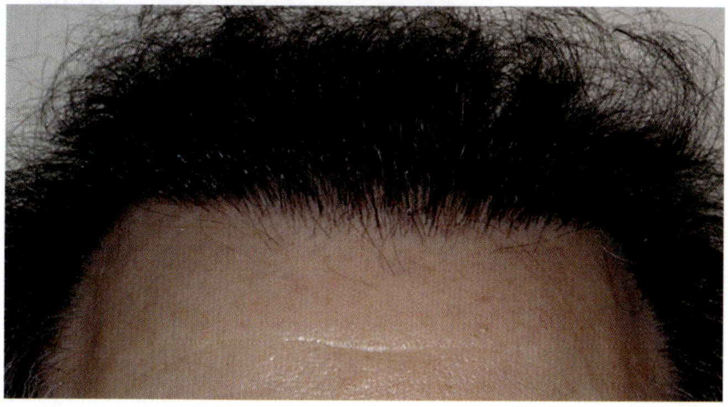

C

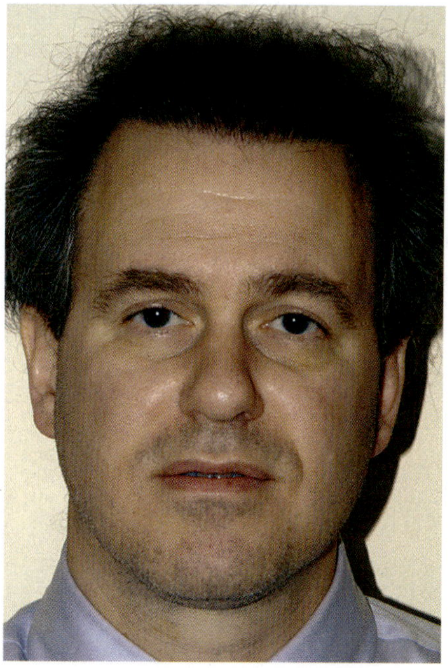

D

Fig. 15.4 (A, B) Before and (**C, D**) after images of a patient who underwent partial removal and replacement of large grafts anteriorly as well as follicular-unit grafting. Procedure performed for correction of "pluggy" appearance from large-graft transplantation done elsewhere.

3 days afterward. The most common source of infections is ingrown hairs as well as small cysts that form after surgery. Typically, drainage and oral antibiotics are more than adequate to treat these. Swelling and edema after hair transplantation can be fairly dramatic due to all of the fluid injected in the scalp during the procedure. A short burst of steroids can help to minimize this.

Scarring, particularly in the donor area, can be a significant issue. Any history of keloid formation should be sought. Keloid formers should obviously be approached cautiously. The potential for donor scar widening and hair loss, however, can occur in any patient. Keys to minimizing this include attention to detail in closing, leaving sutures in for a period of at least 10 days, and emphasizing avoidance of strenuous activity for a period of at least 2 weeks after surgery.

In the recipient area, problems with scar formation or cobblestoning or pitting (development of surface irregularity) can be an issue. Careful graft placement at the appropriate height will help to minimize surface irregularity. Use of the least traumatic method for recipient sites will also help to minimize scarring. In our practice, a 1.3- or 1.5-mm knife is used, which minimizes vascular injury and preserves healthy recipient tissue.

Poor graft take is an issue all hair transplant surgeons will face at some time. Obviously, using the best techniques possible will go a long way toward minimizing this occurrence. When this does develop, review of techniques and methods may reveal possible errors and the opportunity for correction. On the rare occasion that this has occurred in our practice, a complimentary treatment to compensate for the poor graft take is helpful in minimizing the disappointment of both the patient as well as the surgeon.

◆ Conclusion

Tremendous advances have been made in the past 20 years in both the medical as well as surgical treatment of hair loss. Biotechnology offers the hope of even more dramatic developments such as synthetic hair and hair cloning. With public awareness of these advances, we can expect increased interest in and more patients presenting for hair restoration.

References

1. Orentreich N. Autografts in alopecia and other selected dermatologic conditions. Ann N Y Acad Sci 1959;83:463–469
2. Marritt E. Single-hair transplantation for hairline refinement: a practical solution. J Dermatol Surg Oncol 1984;10:962–966
3. Stough DB IV, Nelson BR, Stough DB 3rd. Incisional slit grafting. J Dermatol Surg Oncol 1991;17:53–60
4. Dow S, Whitworth JM. Hair replacement techniques. In: Papel I, ed. Facial Plastic and Reconstructive Surgery. 2nd ed. New York, NY: Thieme Medical Publishers; 2002:299–308
5. Juri J. Use of parieto-occipital flaps in the surgical treatment of baldness. Plast Reconstr Surg 1975;55:456–460
6. Norwood OT, Shiell RC, Morrison ID. The complications of scalp reduction. J Dermatol Surg Oncol 1983;9:831–839
7. Epstein JS. The treatment of female pattern hair loss and other applications of surgical hair restoration in women. Facial Plast Surg Clin North Am 2004;12:241–247
8. Norwood OT, Shiell RC. Hair Transplant Surgery. 2nd ed. Springfield, IL: Charles C. Thomas; 1984
9. Venkataram M. Changing trends in hair restoration surgery. Indian J Dermatol Venereol Leprol 2006;72:103–111
10. Limmer BL. The density issue in hair transplantation. Dermatol Surg 1997;23:747–750
11. Rassman WR, Bernstein RM, McClellan R, Jones R, Worton E, Uyttendaele H. Follicular unit extraction: minimally invasive surgery for hair transplantation. Dermatol Surg 2002;28:720–728
12. Stough DB, Whitworth JM. Constructing the zig-zag hairline: architectural considerations. Poster presented at: International Society of Hair Restoration Surgery; San Francisco, CA; October 1999
13. Headington JT. Transverse microscopic anatomy of the human scalp: a basis for a morphometric approach to disorders of the hair follicle. Arch Dermatol 1984;120:449–456
14. Bernstein RM. A neighbor's view of the "follicular family unit." Hair Transplant Forum Int 1998;8:23–25
15. Fujita K. Reconstruction of the eyebrow. La Lepro 1953;22:364
16. Rafaty FM, Brennan G. Current concepts of browpexy. Arch Otolaryngol 1983;109:152–154
17. Gandelman M, Epstein J. Hair transplantation of the eyebrow, eyelashes and other parts of the body. Facial Plast Surg Clin North Am 2004;12: 253–261
18. Gandelman M. Eyelash reconstruction and aesthetic augmentation. In: Barrera A, ed. Hair Transplantation. St. Louis, MO: Quality Medical Publishing; 2002:168
19. Lucas MW. Partial retransplantation. A new approach in hair transplantation. J Dermatol Surg Oncol 1994;20:511–514

16

Rejuvenation of the Aging Nose

Ted A. Cook and Brian W. Downs

The aging nose presents a unique set of obstacles to rhinoplasty surgeons. In addition to the typical forces of healing and scar contracture acting on the youthful nose, the aging nose features the altered anatomy and physiology of aging added to an already-complicated, three-dimensional structure. Approaching the aging nose requires an appreciation of the nuances of the preoperative, intraoperative, and postoperative phases of the patient interaction. Correction of this deformity has both cosmetic and functional implications and can be quite rewarding to the conscientious surgeon.

◆ Nasal Anatomy and Function

Nasal anatomy is commonly divided into three layers, each of which is often considered separately for surgical purposes but must ultimately unite as a harmonious whole. The *inner lining* refers to vestibular skin and nasal mucosa. The middle layer of the nose is composed of the *nasal skeleton*: the complex cartilaginous and bony framework that supports the nose, preventing collapse. The outer layer is composed of epidermis, dermis, and subcutaneous tissue of varying depths depending on the location craniocaudally on the nose. The aging nose features alterations in all three of these layers. This has direct surgical and functional implications that must be considered during preoperative planning and intraoperative execution. In keeping with our belief that nasal anatomy and function are closely related, these factors will be discussed simultaneously.

Understanding the internal nasal valve is critical to understanding function and dysfunction of the aging nose. First described by Mink,[1] the internal valve is defined by the caudal septum, adjacent upper lateral cartilage (ULC), inferior turbinate, and floor of the nose. Aside from aesthetic concerns voiced during the patient encounter, significant time and effort are expended to accurately assess the internal nasal valve preoperatively. Likewise, many of the treatment options discussed later focus on this same structure.

The outer layer of skin and subcutaneous tissue over the nose, like these tissues elsewhere on the body, undergoes changes during the aging process. The skin becomes thinner with a flattening of the dermal-epidermal junction and a reduction in the collagen content of the dermis. This thinning is thought to be related somewhat to hormonal influences, becoming exaggerated in the postmenopausal female. Evidence suggests that this is reversed with hormone replacement therapy.[2] The direct surgical implication is that dorsal and tip irregularities are more prominent in the presence of this thinner envelope. This is most pronounced over the dorsum where the skin is already thinnest. Direct and careful palpation of both the dorsum and tip during the preoperative encounter can be helpful in determining skin thickness.

Though the nasal bones themselves remain fairly stable, the cartilaginous skeleton of the nose undergoes significant change with aging. The ULCs become softer and weaker, leading to a nonsupported internal nasal valve and functional nasal obstruction. We refer to this phenomenon as *resorbed or palpably-absent ULCs*. This is exacerbated by the unraveling of the *scroll region*—the junction of the ULCs and lower lateral cartilages (LLCs). In youth, the ULCs and LLCs have a "yin-and-yang" relationship, one locked into the other with intervening fibrous connections (**Fig. 16.1**). With age, the scroll assumes a flattened, almost flaccid configuration, contributing to a lengthening of the lower third of the nose and tip ptosis. These changes are manifest over the dorsum as a pseudohump and an exaggerated supratip depression (**Fig. 16.2**). Atrophy of the premaxillary fat pad aggravates this deformity.[3] Concomitant with these changes, the LLCs themselves soften and the nasal alae lose their resilience.

Moreover, aging changes are present in the region of the columella and caudal septum. The attachments of the septum to the medial crurae are weakened, leading to a lengthening of the membranous septum. Fibrous attachments between the domes and medial crurae relax, which can lead to a "winging" of the medial crural footpods and worsening obstruction (**Fig. 16.3**).

These anatomic changes together serve to change the configuration of the nares, directing airflow more

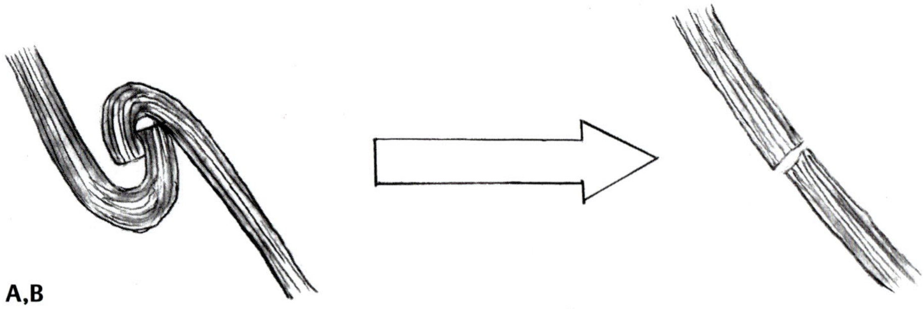

A,B

Fig. 16.1 (**A**) Schematic of the intact scroll region in the youthful nose. (**B**) Unraveling of the scroll region in the aging nose.

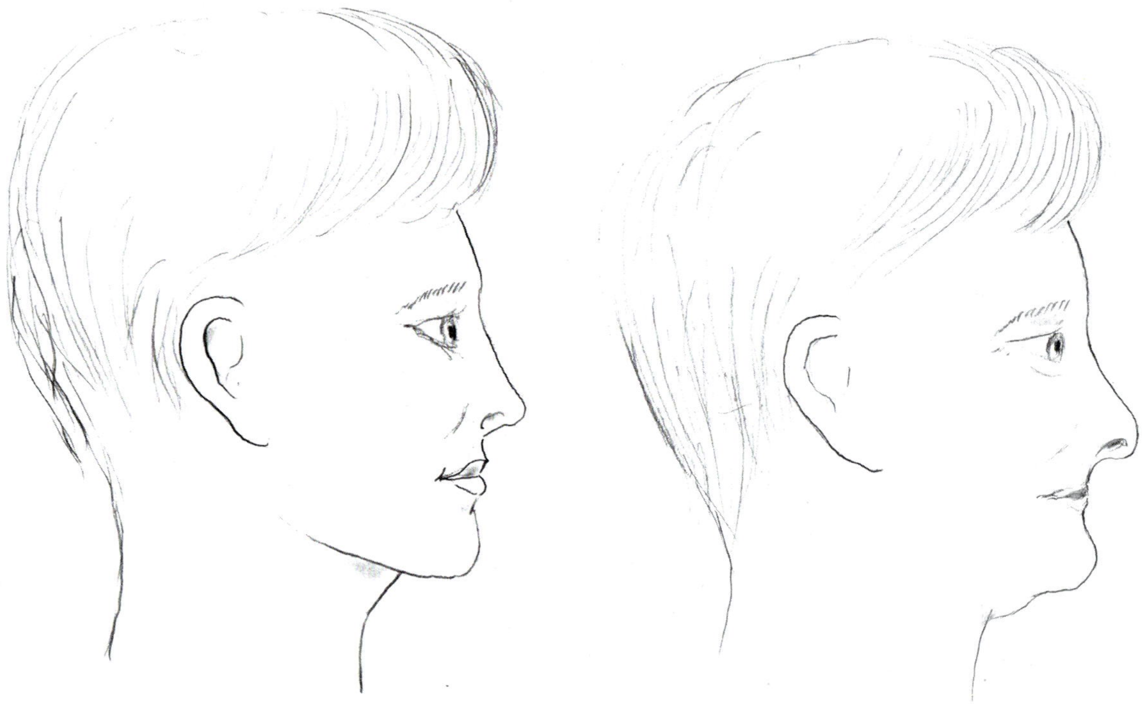

A B

Fig. 16.2 (**A**) The youthful profile. (**B**) The aging profile demonstrating exaggerated dorsal pseudohump and tip ptosis.

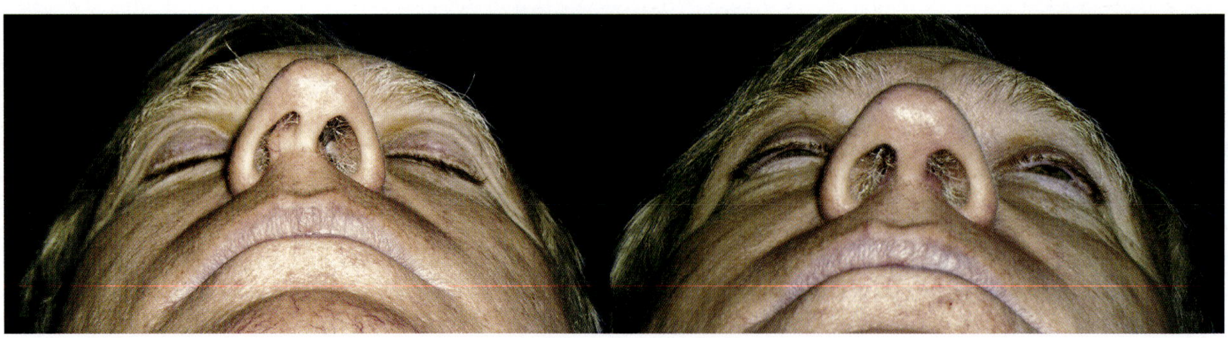

A B

Fig. 16.3 (**A**) Winging of the medial crural footpods in the aging nose. (**B**) Correction of this deformity by suture securing the medial crural footpods to a stable caudal septal extension graft.

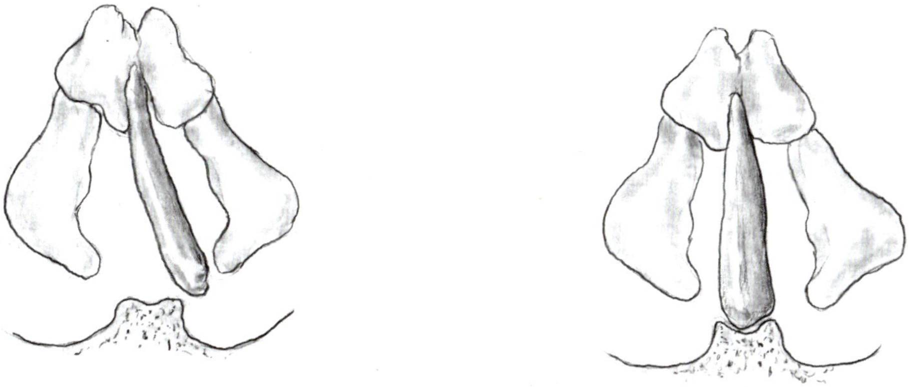
A
B

Fig. 16.4 (**A**) Schematic of left-sided septal spur and cartilaginous redundancy along the maxillary crest potentially exacerbated by ptosis of the nasal tip. (**B**) Septal deflection corrected with caudal end secured in the midline.

superiorly in the nasal vault and producing more turbulent airflow. Particulate matter is then filtered less efficiently by the nose. As the body's hydration status declines, nasal mucosa becomes dry and atrophic with uneven islands of mucus. This filtration inefficiency and static areas of mucus can lead to the sensation of cough and postnasal drip that plagues many patients in the sixth decade and beyond.[4]

In our experience, a septal deflection often accompanies these changes in the aging nose. Anecdotally speaking, this is more often on the left side (**Fig. 16.4**). We hypothesize that this anatomic defect is secondary to generalized descent of the nasal tip such that over time, the inferior aspect of the quadrangular cartilage is "made redundant" by the primary problem, nasal tip ptosis. As the septum slides off the maxillary crest, a spur is formed, further contributing to the nasal obstruction. Why this occurs more often on the left side is unknown.

The muscles of facial expression located in the midface region, like muscles elsewhere in the body, undergo changes with age. Specifically, the dilator naris muscle innervated by cranial nerve VII is partially responsible for nasal valve competence. Like muscles elsewhere in the body, it would be expected to atrophy with age, becoming less effective. Perhaps more importantly, the dilator naris responds to nasal airway resistance. In the presence of less nasal airflow (less resistance), the muscle can become less active until complete cessation of function is reached.[5] This can theoretically lead to a completely adynamic nasal valve. For example, aging individuals who are chronic mouth breathers with nasal obstruction may have causative anatomic factors as outlined above and neurophysiologic ones as well.

Analysis of the aging nose from an aesthetic standpoint must take these changes into account. Preoperative planning and postoperative satisfaction depends on recognition of the characteristics of the aging nose. Specifically, the ptotic tip also leads to an exaggerated supratip depression. Combined with tip ptosis and relatively stable nasal bones, this leads to formation of a dorsal pseudohump. Failure to recognize this altered anatomy may lead one to reduce the dorsum in this instance instead of supporting the middle third and tip of the nose.

◆ Preoperative Evaluation

As with all patients, the aging rhinoplasty patient should undergo a thorough preoperative history and physical examination. The history is of increasing importance, as age is accompanied by increasing medical problems and medication usage. Caution is warranted when patients are taking nonsteroidal anti-inflammatory drugs, Plavix (clopidogrel bisulfate; Bristol-Myers Squibb, New York, NY), and warfarin, as well as any herbal supplements that cause bleeding. This becomes a point of emphasis when one considers that we use no nasal packing postoperatively. For herbal supplements, one good rule of thumb is that agents with names that begin with the letter "G" can potentially predispose patients to relative anticoagulation or postoperative bleeding: ginger, gingko, ginseng, and garlic.[6] Vitamin E poses a similar risk.

Other specific questions in the history inquire about duration and course of nasal obstruction/deformity, any previous trauma, presence of inhalant allergies, prior surgery, and use of over-the-counter remedies such as Breathe-Right strips (CNS, Berkley Heights, NJ). The recently developed and validated Nasal Obstruction Symptom Evaluation (NOSE) scale provides a quick and easy glimpse at preoperative symptom severity and postoperative success.[7,8]

The preoperative physical examination is critical to developing a successful operative plan for the aging nose. We advocate following a standard approach with each patient progressing in order from inspection to palpation to internal examination. As stated above, palpation of the nose is of paramount importance. This allows the tactile sense to further define visual impressions and to aid in analyzing convexities, concavities, and irregularities. Skin thickness is also best appreciated by palpation. Disorders such as rhinophyma, the advanced form of acne rosacea, should be ruled out during physical examination. Finally, size and strength of the ULCs and the scroll region should be assessed with palpation, with special attention paid to nasal valve competency. Manual elevation of the nasal tip accompanied by a subjective improvement in nasal airway should alert the examiner to the presence of nasal tip ptosis causing functional impairment.

The internal nasal examination is an essential component of the evaluation of the aging nose. Standard anterior rhinoscopy is performed with a speculum to document any obvious lesions, masses, or septal spurs. However, it is the examination of the base of the nose without a speculum that is often most helpful. This angle highlights both static and dynamic collapse at the internal nasal valve. Furthermore, inserting a wax curette and manually lateralizing the ULC is helpful in predicting success with nasal valve surgery. Patients presenting with signs or symptoms worrisome for rhinosinusitis are offered in-office diagnostic sinonasal endoscopy. Indeed, some rhinoplasty surgeons routinely perform this for all septorhinoplasty consultations.[9] Though we stop short of this, patients considered for surgery of the aging nose are referred to our rhinology colleagues for rhinosinusitis evaluation when warranted. Combining functional endoscopic sinus surgery with functional rhinoplasty has been shown to be successful in published studies for patients well into their eighth decade of life.[10,11] Though diagnostic testing such as acoustic rhinometry and rhinomanometry is frequently employed to aid in diagnosis and treatment planning for nasal surgery, we do not routinely perform these tests.

As with any procedure with rejuvenation potential, patient motivations should be carefully elicited during the preoperative process. A desire for functional improvement in the nasal airway is often sought in conjunction with aesthetic concerns. It has been suggested that merely correcting the aging effects on the nose can restore approximately 5 years to the aging face.[12] Caution should be exercised when recommending surgery to the patient who is acutely adjusting to a life change or requesting surgery at another's behest. In our experience, psychologically stable patients with reasonable expectations have the highest postoperative satisfaction.

◆ Surgical Intervention

Though numerous nonsurgical interventions for functional and aging nasal disorders have been advocated (such as biofeedback),[13] our patients undergo primarily surgical intervention. Careful consideration is given to surgical approach and mode of anesthesia when addressing the aging nose. We always consider the endonasal approach with either an intercartilaginous or a cartilage-splitting incision for all rhinoplasties with the external approach reserved for patients needing further tip refinement. In our hands, the endonasal approach is also generally faster—perhaps a secondary consideration but relevant for some patients seeking correction of the aging nose in whom significant medical comorbidities exist. As a general rule, with all patients over the age of 60 years, we consider the nasal bones to be somewhat more fragile, the periosteum to be thinner and less capable of healing well, and the subcutaneous soft tissues to be more atrophic than in the younger nose. Therefore, we try to be as conservative as possible in our surgical approach to the rhinoplasty and in performing each portion of the procedure itself. The combination of intravenous sedation and local anesthesia is also appealing for all rhinoplasty because this avoids the cardiovascular stress and lability of induction and emergence seen with general anesthesia. This is probably even more important when operating on the aging nose patient population. Anecdotally, emergence from general anesthesia is generally when most of our bothersome postoperative bleeding occurs and, though seldom severe, avoiding emergence altogether with the use of intravenous sedation is helpful. Of course, a necessary part of the equation regardless of mode of anesthesia is the presence of a skilled anesthetist.

The majority of our interventions for the aging nose addresses functional nasal obstruction. The etiology is most often either internal nasal valve collapse, tip ptosis, or a combination of the two. Multiple internal nasal valve operations have been described including spreader grafts,[14] onlay spreader grafts,[15] "autospreader" grafts,[16] and flaring sutures.[17] Injectable fillers have even been used.[18] A comprehensive review of these techniques is beyond the scope of this chapter. However, our preferred nasal valve correction is the *butterfly graft.*[19] Adapted from a description by Claus Walter,[20] this technique employs conchal cartilage to support the nasal sidewalls, correcting internal valve collapse by acting as "an upper lateral cartilage replacement graft"—effectively replacing structural support lost in the scroll region (**Fig. 16.5**). This graft can be placed endonasally or externally and is readily accepted by patients, with the donor site at the ear rarely an issue. A highly effective intervention, the butterfly graft was shown to have 97% success at achieving total resolution of nasal obstruction in functional secondary rhinoplasty.[19] This concept has been modified for treating the aging nose with functional obstruction by using alloplasts placed via an external dorsal incision.[21] Though we have not used it, this technique theoretically could accomplish the same goal.

Tip ptosis is managed by a variety of methods depending on the surgical approach taken. Placement of a columellar strut into a precise pocket over the nasal spine followed by suturing the medial crurae to it is one reliable method. We prefer septal cartilage for the strut when present. However, we agree with Romo et al that porous polyethylene (Medpor; Porex Surgical, Inc., Newnan, GA) is also an excellent choice[22] and, in our hands, can be placed externally or with a limited endonasal incision. If a cartilage-splitting approach is planned, dependable tip rotation can be achieved by emphasizing the cephalic trim of the LLCs laterally. If significant septal work is to be done and a straight L-shaped piece is available, we do not hesitate to perform septal transplant with medial crural stabilization to improve tip ptosis. Other reliable methods of tip ptosis correction include tongue-in-groove[23] if a straight caudal septum exists. Though described specifically for the ptotic aging nose, we do not

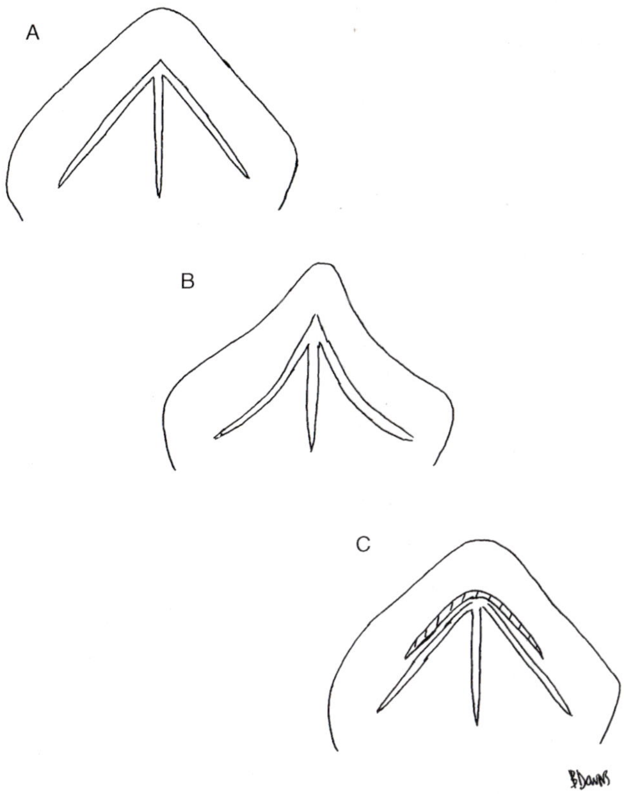

Fig. 16.5 (**A**) Schematic of the well-supported nose (nasal base view, cross section through ULCs and septum). (**B**) Narrowing of the internal nasal valve due to midvault weakness in the aging nose (nasal base view, cross section through ULCs and septum). (**C**) Correction of ULC weakness in the aging nose with butterfly graft. Butterfly graft is shaded (nasal base view, cross section through ULCs and septum).

routinely perform direct skin excision at the radix, or the "nose lift" operation.[24]

A smaller proportion of aging patients suffer from external nasal valve collapse, either in isolation or in combination with the above two phenomena. These patients often present with dynamic collapse of "floppy" fibrofatty tissue of the distal nasal alae. Placement of conchal cartilage alar batten grafts is indicated in these cases, either by the external rhinoplasty, endonasal, or alotomy approach. If butterfly grafting is performed for internal valve collapse, this usually obviates the need for alar battens, even if there is a component of external valve collapse as well. Again, if no suitable ear cartilage is available, we use prepackaged Medpor alar battens placed via an alotomy approach.

The remainder of the aging septorhinoplasty operation is performed as per routine. True dorsal humps are taken down if indicated, although we are conservative for all bony work in these patients. Some have even advocated altering osteotomy paths as patients age.[25]

◆ Postoperative Care

Details of postoperative care vary little in the aging rhinoplasty patient. A nasal dressing consisting of paper tape and thermoplastic splint is placed for 5 to 7 days. No packing is used. All patients receive postoperative antibiotics and steroids, the latter having been shown to decrease postoperative edema after rhinoplasty.[26] Of course, prior to prescribing steroids, medical comorbidities such as diabetes mellitus are considered, and steroids are withheld in appropriate cases. Virtually all cases are performed in the outpatient setting (**Fig. 16.6**).

A 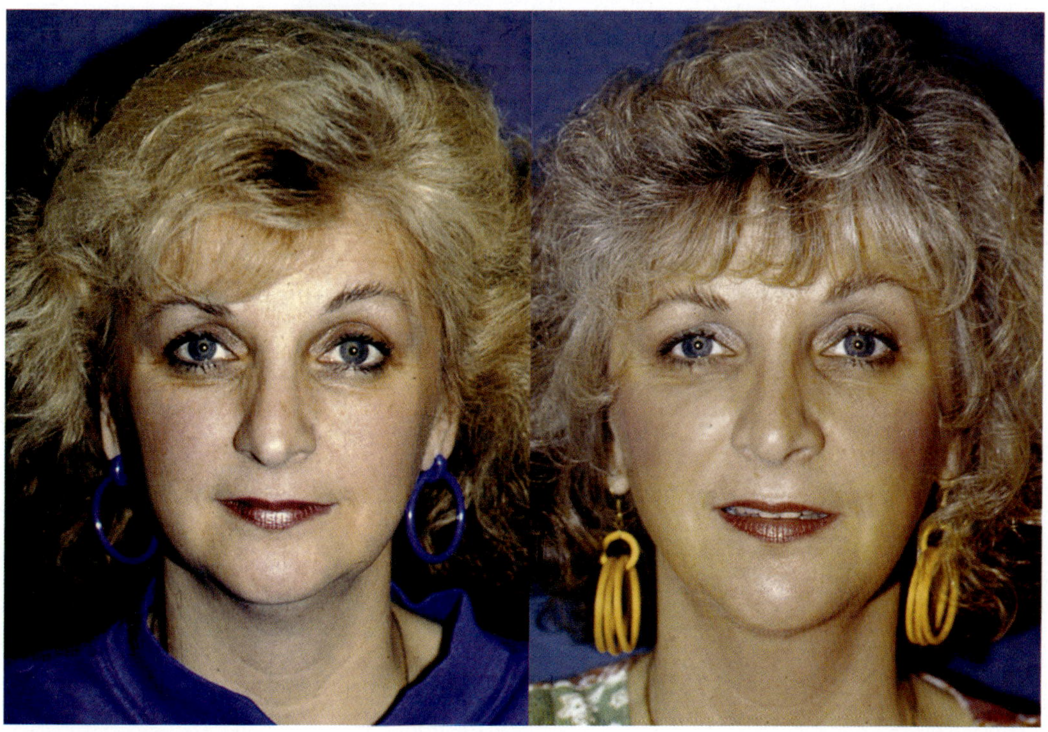 B

Fig. 16.6 (**A**) Preoperative frontal view demonstrating pseudohump formation and tip ptosis in the aging nose. (**B**) Postoperative view.

(Continued on page 174)

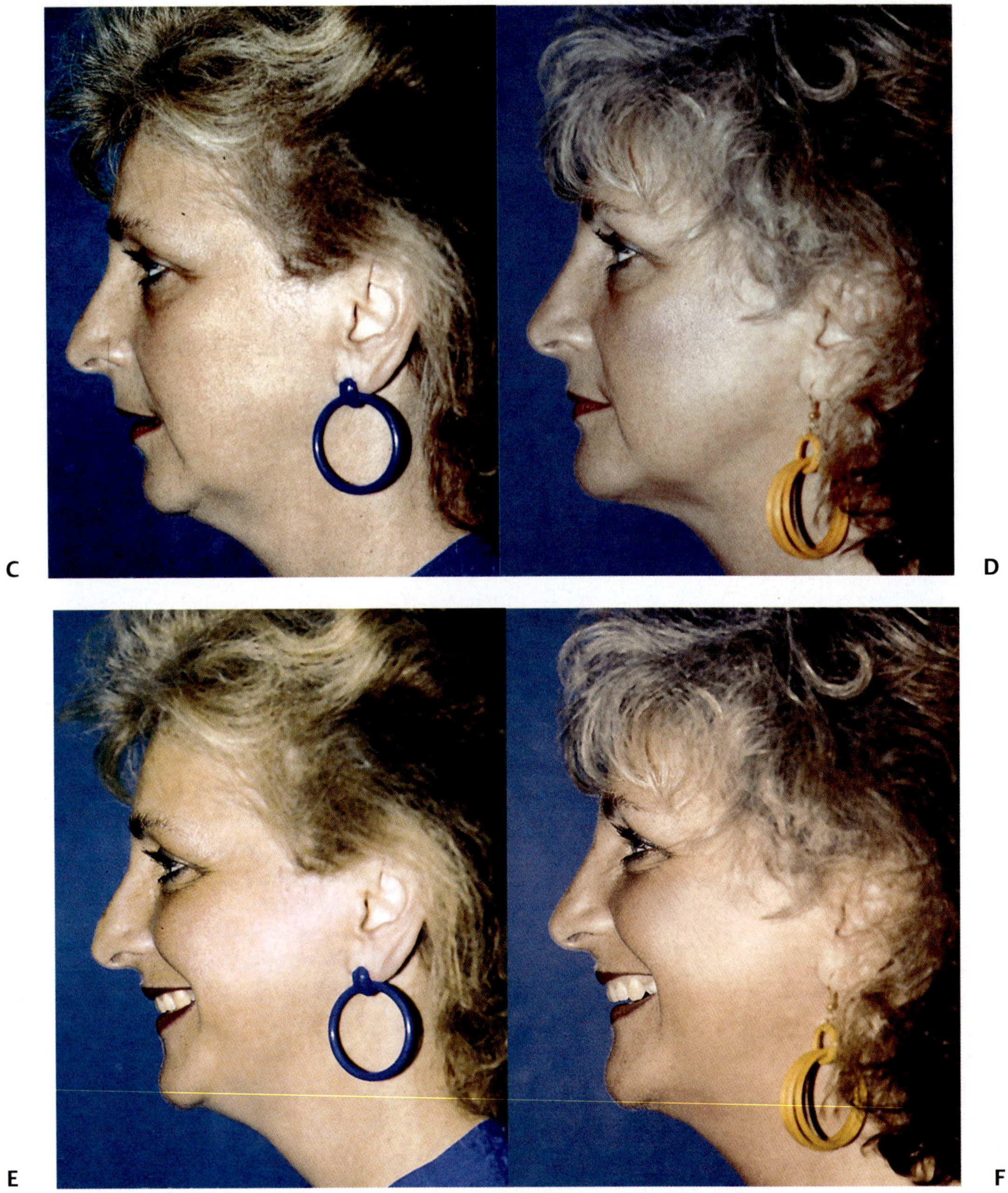

Fig. 16.6 (*Continued*) (**C**) Preoperative left lateral view. (**D**) Postoperative left lateral view. (**E**) Preoperative lateral smiling view. (**F**) Postoperative lateral smiling view.

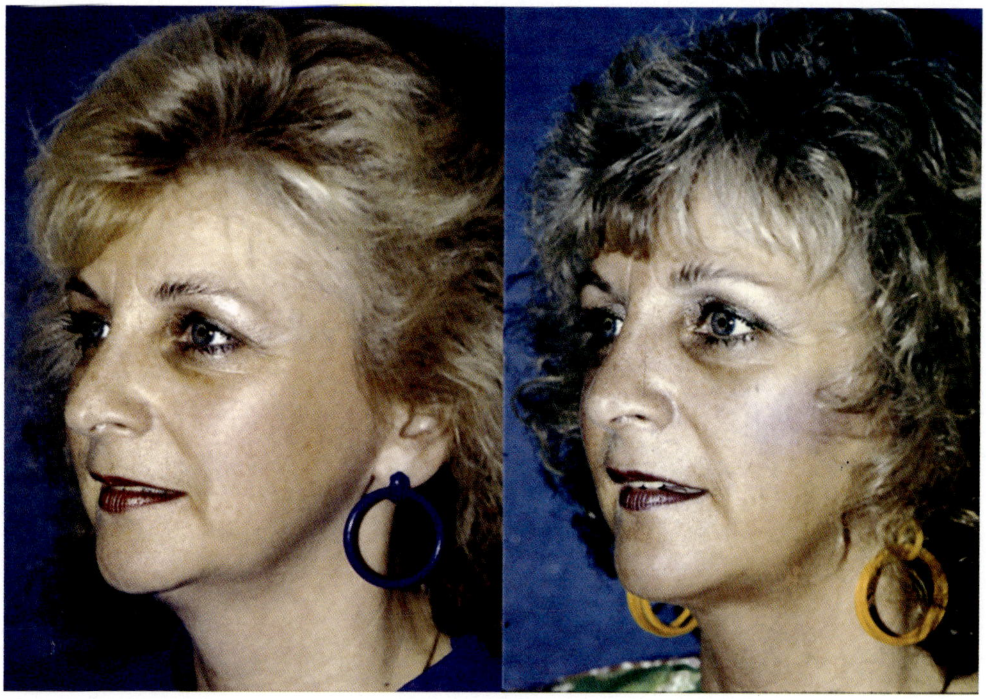

G H

Fig. 16.6 (*Continued*) (**G**) Preoperative left oblique view. (**H**) Postoperative left oblique view.

◆ Conclusion

Rhinoplasty on the aging nose is both challenging and fulfilling. We find this population to be among the most grateful of all patients in facial plastic surgery. Careful planning and execution can lead to a high level of postoperative satisfaction for both patient and surgeon.

References

1. Mink PJ. Le nez comme voie respiratorie. Presse Otolaryngol (Belg) 1903:481–496
2. Sumino H, Ichikawa S, Abe M, et al. Effects of aging, menopause, and hormone replacement therapy on forearm skin elasticity in women. J Am Geriatr Soc 2004;52:945–949
3. Anderson JR, Ries WR. Rhinoplasty: emphasizing the external approach. New York, NY: Thieme Medical Publishers; 1986
4. Ries WR, Rathfoot CJ. The aging nose in rhinoplasty for facial rejuvenation. Facial Plast Surg 1996;12:197–203
5. Mann DG, Sasaki CT, Suzuki M, Fukuda H, Hernandez JR. Dilator naris muscle. Ann Otol Rhinol Laryngol 1977;86:362–370
6. Heller J, Gabbay JS, Ghadjar K, et al. Top-10 list of herbal and supplemental medicines used by cosmetic patients: what the plastic surgeon needs to know. Plast Reconstr Surg 2006;117:436–445
7. Stewart MG, Witsell DL, Smith TL, et al. Development and validation of the nasal obstruction symptom evaluation (NOSE) scale. Otolaryngol Head Neck Surg 2004;130:157–163
8. Most SP. Analysis of outcomes after functional rhinoplasty using a disease-specific quality-of-life-instrument. Arch Facial Plast Surg 2006;8:306–309
9. Lanfranchi PV, Steiger J, Sparano A, et al. Diagnostic and surgical endoscopy in functional septorhinoplasty. Facial Plast Surg 2004;20:207–215
10. Lee JH, Sherris DA, Moore EJ. Combined open septorhinoplasty and functional endoscopic sinus surgery. Otolaryngol Head Neck Surg 2005;133:436–440
11. Marcus B, Patel Z, Busquets J, Hwang PH, Cook TA. The utility of concurrent rhinoplasty and sinus surgery. Arch Facial Plast Surg 2006;8:260–262
12. Guyuron B. Analysis and treatment of the aging face. Dermatol Clin 1997;15:659–664
13. Vaiman M, Shlamkovich N, Kessler A, Eviatar E, Segal S. Biofeedback training of nasal muscles using internal and external surface electromyography of the nose. Am J Otolaryngol 2005;26:302–307
14. Sheen JH. Spreader graft: a method of reconstructing the roof of the middle nasal vault following rhinoplasty. Plast Reconstr Surg 1984;73:230–237
15. Murakami C. Nasal valve collapse. Ear Nose Throat J 2004;83:163–164
16. Quatela V. Discussion. Presented at: Portland Rhinoplasty Course, 2006
17. Park SS. The flaring suture to augment the repair of the dysfunctional nasal valve. Plast Reconstr Surg 1998;101:1120–1122
18. Nyte CP. Spreader graft injection with calcium hydroxylapatite: a nonsurgical technique for internal nasal valve collapse. Laryngoscope 2006;116:1291–1292

19. Clark JM, Cook TA. The 'butterfly' graft in functional secondary rhinoplasty. Laryngoscope 2002;112:1917–1925

20. Walter C. The use of composite grafts in the head and neck region. Otolaryngol Head Neck Surg 1977;4:7–10

21. Hurbis CG. An adjustable, butterfly-design, titanium-expanded polytetrafluoroethylene implant for nasal valve dysfunction: a pilot study. Arch Facial Plast Surg 2006;8:98–104

22. Romo T, Soliemanzadeh P, Litner JA, Sclafani AP. Rhinoplasty in the aging nose. Facial Plast Surg 2003;19:309–315

23. Kridel RWH, Scott B, Foda H. The tongue-in-groove technique in septorhinoplasty. Arch Facial Plast Surg 1999;1:246–256

24. Johnson CM, Anderson JR. Nose-lift operation: an adjunct to aging-face surgery. Arch Otolaryngol 1978;104:1–3

25. Rohrich RJ, Hollier LH, Janis JE, Kim J. Rhinoplasty with advancing age. Plast Reconstr Surg 2004;114:1936–1944

26. Hoffmann DF, Cook TA, Quatela VC, et al. Steroids and rhinoplasty. A double-blind study. Arch Otolaryngol Head Neck Surg 1991;117: 990–993

17

Developing and Maintaining a Successful Facial Cosmetic Surgery Practice

Jon E. Mendelsohn

Today's facial cosmetic surgery practice is more complex, competitive, and confusing than ever before. The economic changes in health care have mandated a shift in conventional practices, transferring reconstructive and insurance-based surgery to cosmetic surgery. With significant increases in nonsurgical and minimally invasive surgical procedures, the competition between specialties is greater than in the past.[1] Facial plastic surgeons are just one of the main specialty groups in this environment. Today, however, we also see other fields not traditionally thought of as providing cosmetic procedures entering this competitive environment. Even non–medical doctors, such as oral surgeons and dentists, are now offering many so-called nonsurgical cosmetic procedures such as Botox (botulinum toxin type A; Allergan Inc., Irvine, CA), dermal fillers, skin peels, laser treatments, and even surgical procedures such as facelifts, brow lifts, and rhinoplasties. Although these trends seem to be on the rise, taking the right proactive steps to achieving a successful practice in facial plastic surgery will help guide you toward the top of the competition and a fulfilling professional career.

The development of a successful facial cosmetic surgery practice involves knowledge of the market, planning, commitment to allocating resources, appropriate leadership and management, marketing, and precise execution, as well as a well-thought-out plan with achievable and predetermined goals. In this chapter, I will present information gathered from my own personal experience over the past decade, in which I established a solo facial cosmetic surgery practice in Cincinnati, Ohio, performing cosmetic procedures. Although I have made many mistakes and learned many hard lessons over the past years, I can now impart that the development and maintenance of a successful cosmetic facial surgery practice requires a well-thought-out strategy and the ability to execute the plan without hesitation.

I would like to mention at the outset that the definition of a successful practice is ultimately subjective. All of us would like to make a decent living and probably, by our nature, lead the competition, but I would also caution that success is also found in the amount of time we spend with family, our relationships, and ourselves. Although this chapter will not help you balance those things, you must nevertheless be aware of the consequences you may face in a tunnel-visioned pursuit of the successful facial cosmetic practice.

◆ The Business Plan for the Facial Cosmetic Surgery Practice

Business Management

If there is one critical component to developing and maintaining a successful facial cosmetic practice, it lies within the process of creating a business plan. A thoughtful plan will bring clarity and objectivity into the evaluation of goals, successes, and failures. The business planning process will also bring about an increased efficiency in regard to the use of a practice's human and capital resources.[2] This process of strategic planning will bring organization, focus, and discipline to those involved in making the practice successful. A well-thought-out and deliberate plan will also increase the likelihood of meeting or exceeding practice goals.

Preparing the Plan

Developing a long-term strategic business plan requires a vision for future options. When thoughtful evaluation of such options occurs, the practice builds a road map that it may begin to follow. This long-term vision will be achieved when shorter-term objectives are met—generally the result of a well-prepared marketing plan. It is the marketing plan along with other components of a strategic business plan that needs to be wisely developed so that goals and expectations can be measured and quantified. Simply stated, a strategic marketing plan should bring you one step closer to fulfilling tomorrow's vision and meeting long-term goals.

The strategic business plan should address at least a few basic questions:

- What do we want the practice to be like in 12, 24, and 36 months?
- What products or services do we want to continue to offer, introduce, or change?
- What needs to be done *now* to meet the demands of the future practice (i.e., remodeling or acquiring facility, obtaining certifications, staff development, hiring key personnel, etc.)?
- How many providers will we have? What will be the specialization of each provider?
- What trends are occurring that may affect the practice in the future?

Answering the above questions will assist in the process of developing an awareness of the long-range implications of short-term events or emerging trends. This is the essence of thinking strategically.

Unfortunately, many practices only think "in the moment" and chase other practices that appear to be ahead of the pack in terms of marketing, facility development, or service implementation. What often occurs with this lack of perspective is that the short-term actions do not fit within the context of the long-term plan. In fact, a practice may not have developed a long-term plan in the first place. Required for the practice to have the best opportunity for achieving its long-term goals is the ability to think strategically and to recognize, understand, and appreciate the strategic business planning process.

Successful practices develop the ability to continually evaluate the marketplace and their own internal systems, as well as to modify their plans to progress toward their vision. Yearly strategic planning meetings may work for some practices; however, to increase the likelihood of success, it may be beneficial to meet more frequently to respond quickly to the changes in the market. Often, despite the best intentions, a business will seem to be tracking well when a down period occurs. During these times, an emotional decision is often made to pull marketing and impulsively change course. Marketing dollars may be impulsively added to an area without a plan to sustain that direction—resulting in impulse purchasing.

Whereas this has happened to all of us, this emotional mistake can be prevented when a plan is strategically prepared and the business goals are being tracked. Although many practices play "follow the leader" with the perceived benefit of reducing marketing costs, in the long run, the practice that does this has not developed the discipline or understanding that it takes to be successful. To begin the process of successful strategic planning, a series of preparatory or planning tasks are suggested.

Developing a Vision Statement

The vision statement is an overall picture of what the business will look like in the future. It addresses who you are and what you are about. It also outlines in general terms how the business will accomplish its goals. What is it that will make you the best? How will you meet patients' expectations? Simply stated, the vision is the skin in which your business will operate in the future (**Table 17.1**).

Developing a Mission Statement

Defining the mission of your practice involves several preparatory steps that should be executed over a period of time, rather than rushed through as though they were a school assignment. **Table 17.2** shows some of the steps that are basic to any business model and can be found in any business planning textbook or Web site. Completion of these tasks should result in an action plan that will serve as a road map for the practice. The mission statement answers the question, "Who are we and what do we want to become?"

Developing a strengths, weaknesses, opportunities, and threats (SWOT) analysis is the first step in defining your current position and will help establish an effective strategy that builds upon your strengths, minimizes your weaknesses (which are internal), takes advantage of your opportunities, and defends against threats (which are usually external). Developing a market and practice assessment will guide you in a specific strategic direction (**Table 17.3**).

The vision statement can be easily prepared by defining the reasons for being in practice and what your personal and professional goals are (**Table 17.4**). A mission statement provides more detail about how the vision of the practice is fulfilled.

Table 17.1 Example of a Vision Statement

Vision Statement
We will strive to consistently meet or exceed the service and care expectations of our patients. We will maintain a comfortable, warm, and pleasing environment for our patients. We will strive to be available and accessible and to ensure we provide an appropriate amount of time for each patient. We will strive to offer state-of-the-art facial plastic surgery services through our practice and our referral network of providers. We will ensure the most compassionate and convenient care setting for our patients. We will do so by investing in staff education and new treatment modalities. We will provide them the tools necessary to most effectively and efficiently perform their jobs while reinforcing the basic tenet of providing excellent customer service. We will reward our employees with above-average compensation packages. We will plan and invest wisely in the future of our practice. We will diversify our service lines and invest in new technology in a conservative and well-thought-out manner. We will put in place financial controls and benchmark our operating results internally and with our peer group while striving to provide an above-average return to the shareholders.

Table 17.2 Basic Steps for Creating a Business Plan

- Prepare a SWOT (strengths, weaknesses, opportunities, and threats) analysis.
- Assess your current environment.
- Complete a competitive analysis for your market.
- Assess the financial health of your practice.
- Translate your mission statement into specific long-term goals and short-term performance objectives.
- Identify critical success factors and high payoff activities (HPAs)
- Develop your strategy.

Developing Your Strategy

With the vision and mission statement and the associated analyses completed, you are ready to translate all of this information into a strategic plan, with specific and relevant goals and objectives. This plan, however, should remain a work in progress, to be revisited and revised as new information becomes available from ongoing analysis of the market and practice. Questions that should be considered regularly are:

1. Is the current strategy appropriate for the changes that have occurred?
2. What changes need to be considered to diminish internal weaknesses and external threats?
3. What can be done to take advantage of new opportunities to advance the competitive position of the practice?
4. What are the best ways to maximize the strengths of the practice?

Table 17.3 Developing Assessments

External Assessment

1. What are the demographic characteristics of the market?
2. What is your market share for your key service lines?
3. Who are your competitors?
4. What is their market share?
5. What market strategies do they employ?
6. What do you perceive to be their strengths and weaknesses?

Practice Assessment

1. What are our strengths and weaknesses? (see example In Table 17.4)
2. What do we perceive to be potential opportunities and threats for the practice?
3. What is the state of our current financial health?
4. Are we practicing in an efficient and effective manner?
5. How do employees feel about their work environment?
6. Do our facilities meet our current and future needs?
7. How do patients feel about their experience with the practice?

The strategy is to be tweaked, but not completely redesigned, to achieve greater success in the business in which you are competing. Should you recognize problems for which there are no easy changes, a consultant may be useful to help guide the next relevant steps.

Executing the Plan

Whereas much time, energy, and effort is spent generating a written plan, its success or failure lies squarely in its implementation and execution. Spoken from personal experience,

Table 17.4 Example of a Mission Statement

Our Mission

1. Our mission is to provide compassionate and personalized care to our patients, to create an environment that motivates and satisfies our employees and stimulates and rewards our physicians, and to ensure financial stability for all stakeholders.
2. Associates will be compensated based on performance and alignment with the vision statement.
3. We will develop and maintain a world-class performance and evaluation system in which associates participate in both the risks and rewards of the business.
4. We will clearly communicate our vision and mission statements with all associates on a regular basis.
5. Our revenues will meet or exceed the 75th percentile of all comparable practices in the United States.
6. We will grow at a rate of 7% per year.
7. We will exceed revenues of $2.5 million per year.
8. By the 5th year of business, we will exceed $3 million per year of revenue.
9. By the 7th year, we will offer additional services to increase the revenues to $4 million per year.
10. We will seek only profitable growth.
11. We will publish on average one notable educational work every 2 years targeting the lay public.
12. Our practice will be a fun place to work for both owners and associates.
13. We will solicit employee feedback and input on all business matters.
14. We will create a comfortable yet professional working environment where associates feel at ease and productive.
15. We will hire only the most qualified and most capable in the cosmetic surgery field, and they will receive outstanding training and work experience, as well as long-term growth opportunities.
16. Within 5 years, we will be the most recognized cosmetic surgery practice in the region.
17. We will develop and maintain a highly visible community presence. Our marketing and promotional materials will be distinctive and will be highly visible in all of our prospects' places of business.
18. We will contribute community services and focus on philanthropic activities to better the community at large.
19. The owners and all associates will participate in unpaid community service as a way of giving back to society beyond the scope of the business.

Source: Maller BS. Implementing Your Strategic Plan. Incline Village, NV: BSM Consulting Group, 2002. Reprinted with permission.

Table 17.5 Factors Contributing to Successful or Unsuccessful Implementation of the Written Plan

- Physician leadership and commitment to the plan
- The assignment of the right people, with the right skill sets, to the right positions on the team
- The process of holding team members accountable
- Established buy-in from all team members
- Clearly defined goals and objectives
- Realistic timelines for implementing tasks
- A well-designed financial plan that supports the long-term goals
- Periodic evaluation, measurement, and quantifying of practice goals

it is relatively easy to establish a reputable practice and achieve moderate success. However, it is extremely difficult to truly separate your practice from others and to define it as exceptional and unique to maintain a competitive advantage.[3] Several factors that contribute to the successful or unsuccessful implementation of your written plan are shown in **Table 17.5**.

◆ Positioning Your Practice for Sustained Success

How do you position your practice for continued success? Presuming that the first steps have been taken, you must integrate the strategic plan with the operational functions of your practice. This means establishing the right team, creating a solid marketing plan, having fiscal policies for financing the practice, and developing a management team capable of moving the process forward.

Employees must possess the necessary skill sets to achieve practice objectives dictated by the strategic plan. Although employees may have helped establish the current status of the practice, its future growth is dependent on the ability of staff members to change and grow if necessary. If the necessary skill sets do not exist and training is too costly or difficult, the practice must hire the right individual(s) through recruitment. An effort should be made to pair the skill sets of the individual with that of the needs determined by the plan.

The marketing plan is also a necessary component of the strategy to implement practice goals. This document will serve as the road map for how the practice will follow its business plan for the year. The plan needs to carefully evaluate a variety of options based on the current and anticipated future market environment. It should also be a reflection of the overall practice strategy.

Establishing and maintaining a budget is of critical importance. The budget provides the financial means to implement the agreed-upon strategy. Stated simply, it forces you to "put your money where your mouth is." When you begin to assign dollars to the plan, you begin to focus on your specific needs. The budget will also ensure that resources are efficiently used and that sufficient funds are allocated to the most critical components of the strategy.

Budgeting

A budget is a critical component of the overall strategic plan. It is the tool that can help the most in evaluating the financial impact of the initiatives of the plan. Once the financial analysis has been completed, decisions can be made in a timely and deliberate manner, rather than rashly, based on gut feelings. Practices that recognize, develop, and apply rigorous financial analysis consistently achieve greater success. It is not uncommon for practices to consider a potential opportunity, only to have analysis indicate that the risk contemplated is too great in relation to the potential benefit.

The best method of evaluating a budget is to take a look at historical data that incorporate a 9- to 12-month period of time. It is important to look at the core business, as well as any new initiatives that were undertaken over that period of time, to help obtain an accurate assessment for the year ahead. The numbers of facelifts or peels performed are likely standard items that would be evaluated in a facial plastic surgeon's budget. However, the introduction of a laser technology such as Fraxel (Reliant Technologies, Mountain View, CA) or other new advances should be evaluated closely so that "good" money is not put forth after "bad." An accountant or other financial advisor may be beneficial in establishing consistencies for future planning. Internal reporting may also be helpful and can be easily set up in-house through standard computer software.

The budget should also include the anticipated future costs associated with planned expansion, equipment needs, marketing, providers, and so forth. As resources and capital are limited, this process helps to guide the practice toward its goal, without "breaking the bank" and reallocating resources in an attempt to maintain cash flow. By preparing a budget that reflects the initiative of the plan, an accurate assessment for future revenue and expenses will aid in the overall implementation of the plan.

Completing Your Action Plan

There are several important features of completing the plan. First of all, there must be clearly defined goals, each with specific directives. The directives need to be written in a clear, actionable language. Each also requires that there is a responsible person assigned to it with a deadline for execution. If these guidelines are followed, employee ownership of the items will result in completion and accountability of each task, which will dovetail into a reward system for all involved parties.

Overall responsibility for the plan needs to be assigned to a single person, typically the director of operations. Whereas this may be assigned to a physician with leadership ability, most busy physicians will have difficulty executing these responsibilities with the little time they have. It is important that the director holds the respect of the other associates and possesses the organization and communication skills to follow through with projects and pay attention to detail. If the practice manager assumes this responsibility, he or she must provide progress reports to the physician owner on a regular basis. These reports should include action plans with notations on the progress made on each initiative.

Physician Leadership

The role of the physician in the process is twofold. Generally, it is the physician's responsibility to educate the team to increase the likelihood of buy-in. The associates need to understand the value of their efforts and the goals of the practice and must also understand how they will benefit from its implementation.

When a physician leads these efforts, he or she usually fails to direct the change required for sustainable goal achievement. Although physicians may want to delegate the responsibility of communicating plan details to the administrators or managers, it is recommended they resist this temptation. Whereas these individuals are critical in the implementation of the plan, it is the physician who bears the responsibility to communicate the message to the rest of the team. However, generally, the physician has neither enough time nor the right information to effectively communicate and implement the plan. Asking for help or advice is a far better answer than embarking on a venture based on a gut feeling or inadequate information. Solicit the opinion of colleagues or trusted advisors before rolling out any major initiatives.

Committing to the Process

Although turning your practice's written strategic plan into reality comes with challenges, success is possible. Remember that a practice should approach strategic planning as an integrated process that features a firm commitment to implementation. A well-documented action plan supported by a strong physician leadership team is essential to success. However, successful implementation is also contingent on limiting financial risks and ensuring the plan is having a positive impact on the financial health of your practice.

Financial Evaluation

The next area meriting consideration is associated with evaluating your progress. The use of certain financial tools will aid in limiting risk and ensuring that your strategic plan is having a positive financial impact. When planning, it is useful to undertake a break-even analysis. A break-even analysis will clarify whether planned objectives are possible. They are often used to evaluate opportunities for purchasing new equipment, bringing on other providers, expansion, or other capital-intensive proposals.[4]

This analysis will allow you to make wiser decisions as to how much new business is required to meet your break-even point. For example, let us say you are considering a new laser that costs $100,000.00. If the fee charged per patient for that new laser is $5000.00, then it might appear that you need to perform 20 such treatments to recover your investment. While this is probably adequate, it would be wiser to look at other costs involved with implementing the device. These include such things as provider salary, time, allocation of space, marketing costs, other in-office staffing costs, disposable costs, and so forth. When this is done properly, it helps focus on what the true goals and costs are so that a better and more educated decision can be made. Simply stated then, a break-even analysis suggests what level of business activity is necessary to cover expected costs.

Cost Categories

Cost categories generally include fixed and variable expenses. Fixed expenses usually do not vary with the volume of patients treated. Examples of fixed overhead include facility rental, most staffing costs, and insurance. Although there is a limit to how much volume can be handled with a certain level of fixed overhead, maximizing this potential is the main goal. If the volume goes up or down significantly, it may be necessary to either increase or reduce overhead.

On the other hand, variable overhead expenses are proportional to the level of business activity. An example is the cost of goods associated with the sale of skin care products, or a proportion of operating room personnel salaries, and so forth. Variable expenses will fluctuate with the number of patients treated or with the amount of revenue generated by the practice. In one sense, increasing the variable expense should be associated with increased revenue, as it often becomes a production number based on how active the practice is.

The Basics of Financing

When deciding to open a new facial cosmetic surgery practice, the method of accounting practices needs to be selected. This accounting method is a set of rules used to determine when and how income and expenses are to be reported. The main goal is to establish a method of accurately reporting income and expenses. There are several accounting methods that you may chose from.[5] Even though most practices primarily provide services, selling pharmaceutical or other products may be considered inventory under IRS guidelines and may lead to a change in accounting method. The choices of accounting method are relatively simple as shown in **Table 17.6**.

Cash Method

The cash method of accounting requires the inclusion of income that is actually or constructively received during the year and deduction of expenditures in the tax year in which they are actually paid. Gross income includes the fair market value of property or services received during the year. If income is computed by changes in inventory, as may occur with retail sales, the accrual method of accounting must be used.

Table 17.6 Accounting Methods

A taxpayer can choose one of the following accounting methods: Cash method Accrual method Combination Choosing the right method for a practice is likely to be based on the way financial recordkeeping is maintained. Simple systems involving cash-based transactions will likely lead to the cash method of accounting, whereas more sophisticated recordkeeping may lead to the accrual method. Some situations may require a certain method for tax reporting. Such decisions should be made in consultation with your practice accountant.

Accrual Method

The accrual method requires income and expenses to be included in the taxable year when the service is rendered or the expense is acquired, regardless of the time payment is received or made. Income is recognized only when all the events have occurred that fix the right to receive the income and the amount can be determined with reasonable accuracy. Expense is incurred in the taxable year in which all the events have occurred that established the fact of the liability, the amount of the liability can be determined with reasonable accuracy, and economic performance has occurred with respect to the liability.

Combination Method

Generally, it is possible to use any combination of cash, accrual, and special method of accounting if the combination clearly shows income and is used consistently.

Equipment Financing Options

Whether you are starting a new practice or transitioning an existing one, you will have a need to acquire new equipment. In the facial cosmetic surgery practice, this may occur even more frequently, as the demands to offer cutting-edge technology easily require the expenditure of hundreds of thousands of dollars. New equipment may also be needed to replace inoperable or outdated items. In either event, decisions must be made regarding the manner in which the equipment is to be acquired. Each of the options offers advantages and disadvantages depending upon the goals of the practice.[6]

Cash Payment

Cash payment involves writing a check from the practice bank account for the purchase price of the equipment. The transaction is simple: the vendor is paid, and the practice then owns the equipment. This option represents the most common method used by practices, especially for low-cost items. The value of the equipment is fully deductible as a depreciation expense over subsequent years. In recent years, even higher-cost items, up to $100,000.00, could be eligible for an accelerated depreciation. Because no interest or finance charges are involved, cash payment is usually the least costly option. The disadvantage to this method is that it requires the practice to have sufficient cash to make the purchase and to meet other payment obligations. The biggest problem arising from cash payment occurs when the practice has insufficient funds to pay year-end profits for salaries, profit sharing, taxes, and other year-end financial obligations. This problem is often the result of cash outflows being greater than the depreciation expense charged for the year. When this occurs, other options such as bank financing or leasing may be preferable.

Bank Financing

Bank financing involves taking a conventional bank loan from a lender. Most banks actually pursue physician practices and consider them to be good credit risks. This transaction involves vendor payment from loan proceeds, with the repayment term and interest rate subject to loan provisions. The practice owns the equipment, even though the bank may retain a lien on the equipment until the loan is paid in full. With bank financing, the cost of the equipment purchase is fully deductible as depreciation and interest expense. Ideally, the loan term will correspond with the depreciation term, avoiding the unbalanced cash flow problems associated with cash payment. The interest rate for many of these loans usually fluctuates, as it is often tied to the prime rate.

Bank financing assumes that the practice has sufficient means to ensure repayment, and the institution will confirm this from tax returns and financial statements. Often, banks require personal guarantees from the physician for repayment of the loan and to ensure the best possible terms.

Leasing

Leasing is similar to bank financing as the equipment is available to the practice in exchange for a monthly payment. In effect, the practice pays to use the equipment rather than paying to own the equipment. Leases typically allow the practice to acquire ownership at conclusion of the lease, commonly for $1.00 or for 10% of the then-current fair market value.

There are two types of leases that may be obtained. With capital leases, the acquired asset is booked on the balance sheet, which yields depreciation and an interest expense on the income statement. With an operating lease, the payments are deductible as a business expense. With each type of lease, cash flow is balanced as cash outflows and deductibility are matched. The payment amounts are determined by application of a lease factor, depending on equipment value and the lease term. Unlike bank loans, the lease factor and resultant payments are usually fixed at constant values during the term of the lease. Rates will vary among leasing companies, and competitive bids should be obtained from at least three leasing companies.

Similar to banks, prospective lessors will request practice financial documents for review.

The total costs involved in leasing tend to be greater than those involved in bank financing, especially if state sales tax applies to the entire lease payment. However, when leasing is tied to equipment supply/maintenance discounts or other manufacturer offers, overall costs can be quite competitive.

The decision to finance new equipment then is based on several factors. If you are uncertain as to the best method of acquiring new equipment, consulting a financial advisor may be useful.

Acquisition of new equipment is usually undertaken through cash purchase, bank financing, or leasing. Each option offers various benefits and disadvantages, depending on the circumstances and objectives of the practice.

The Financing Decision

The best decision for the practice depends on several factors:

- Cash position: Does the practice have sufficient cash available for the intended financing method and its future cash obligations?
- Overall costs: How does the sum of total payments for the intended financing method compare with other methods?
- Tax treatment: Will the intended financing method produce tax benefits or tax problems?
- Future plans: Will the intended financing method allow for needed future acquisitions without depleting the cash or credit capacity of the practice?

These questions should be evaluated with the help of the practice accountant or other qualified financial advisor.

◆ Establishing the Proper Office Layout

One of the first decisions in setting out to establish a successful facial plastic surgery practice is establishing the proper office layout. For the purposes of this discussion, it will be assumed that the goal is to establish a space with the appropriate requirements to obtain accreditation through a respected organization. As the practice itself may be established in either a free-standing building or office complex, the choice may be more related to the overall financial and personal views of the physician. Although ownership of the real estate offers long-term financial advantages, the specific geographic location may be an important reason to lease space. Space requirements can also vary depending upon the type of practice and the number of providers anticipated. The space itself should be well planned and designed to maintain a professional, comfortable, nonthreatening, private, and customer-centric look and feel. This should also reflect the overall feel of the practice reflected in the vision statement. It is this culture that will lead to successfully establishing and achieving your vision.

The general design of the space should also provide privacy for the cosmetic patient. The flow should be structured so that new patients follow a path from waiting area to consultation room through computer imaging, nursing, and so forth, in which they will have very little exposure to other patients, such as those undergoing skin care or postsurgical care. One of the difficulties with adding cosmetic services to an existing noncosmetic practice is the challenge of meeting the cosmetic patient's need for privacy. While it can be and is performed successfully by physicians, establishing certain "cosmetic" days can be challenging, as one cannot always predict when the rhinoplasty or facelift patient will arrive unexpectedly. For this reason, when cosmetic services are of priority for the practice, establishing a separate area or, even better, a different office location that sees only cosmetic patients should be considered, even if only for 1 day a week. This creates the impression for cosmetic patients that they are in the right place, being treated by the facial cosmetic surgery specialist.

If an operating suite is planned, the design should incorporate more than one operating room. This is important in terms of maximizing the efficiency of the surgical suite, even if it is a single-provider practice. Whereas the cost of the second operating room may seem like an unnecessary expense, the greater cost is in the time lost prepping the single operating room. If there is a retail component to the practice (i.e., skin care products, vitamins, makeup, etc.), it should ideally be displayed on the right side of the office as the patient enters the practice. Human psychology of space suggests that we typically will turn and browse items placed in this orientation. The next time you are in a department store, pay attention to where the sale items are placed. Promotions, new procedures, or information that you would like to share with your patients should also be displayed in this location.

A similar psychology exists as it pertains to colors and office decor. Color, without our realizing it, can have a profound effect on how we feel both mentally and physically. The power of color, as was suggested by the ancient Egyptians and pre-Columbian Americans, has been used to help with healing throughout the centuries.

A few of the emotional associations that humans tend to have with certain colors are mentioned below. These are important to keep in mind to create the mood you are seeking. Green is a color associated with calming and healing, and blue has been shown to reduce blood pressure, slow the heart rate, and lower body temperature. Blue is also a color that reflects reliability and trustworthiness. In contrast, red has been shown to raise blood pressure and can be associated with blood and danger; thus, red is probably not the best choice of color for a surgery center. Yellow is also a color that has been associated with deceit and also associated with hazards. **Table 17.7** evaluates colors, but the purpose here is to be aware of the subliminal messages you may be sending to your patients just by the colors that appear in the office.

Table 17.7 Color Associations

Blue
Represents peace, tranquility, calm, stability, harmony, unity, trust, truth, confidence, conservatism, security, cleanliness, order, loyalty, sky, water, cold, technology, and depression Can slow the pulse rate, lower body temperature, and reduce appetite Is considered a business color because it reflects reliability Is often considered to be the safest global color
Black
Represents power, sexuality, sophistication, formality, elegance, wealth, mystery, fear, evil, anonymity, unhappiness, depth, style, evil, sadness, remorse, anger, underground, technology, mourning, and death
Green
One of most-often-cited favorite colors Represents nature, environment, health, good luck, renewal, youth, vigor, spring, generosity, fertility, jealousy, inexperience, envy, and misfortune Cool quality soothes, calms, and has great healing powers Is often worn in operating rooms by surgeons
Orange
Is considered a warm color like red, but to a lesser extent; orange expresses energy Has luminous qualities and has been used for attention-getting purposes, such as on caution signs
Purple
Represents royalty, spirituality, nobility, ceremony, mystery, transformation, wisdom, enlightenment, cruelty, arrogance, and mourning Is considered an exotic color
Red
Is the color that we pay the most attention to. It is the warmest and most energetic color in the spectrum. Is associated with love, valentines, danger, desire, speed, strength, violence, anger, emergency exit signs, stop signs, and blood Can evoke a fight-or-flight response, raise blood pressure, and make the heart beat faster
White
Is what we see when all colors come together in perfect balance Represents reverence, purity, simplicity, cleanliness, peace, humility, precision, innocence, youth, birth, winter, snow, good, sterility, and marriage
Yellow
Represents joy, happiness, optimism, idealism, imagination, hope, sunshine, summer, gold, philosophy, dishonesty, cowardice, betrayal, jealousy, covetousness, deceit, illness, hazard, spirituality, and inspiration

There are certain colors that may be trendy or signs of the times. And depending on the market in which you are located, these may be desirable colors to choose for certain aspects of your design.

Setting Up an Office-Based Surgery Suite

The basic design of the office suite is critical to patient flow and efficiency, yet the design of the surgical suite requires greater attention to detail. As there are several licensing agencies, the requirements for establishing an office-based surgery center will vary. In the past, undergoing the accreditation process was optional. Today however, many boards mandate that their surgeons comply with policies that state that surgical services must be provided in an establishment that meets certain accreditation guidelines.[7] As this is a patient care and liability issue, if you are establishing a space in which you intend to provide surgical services, it would be a mistake not to have it accredited.

◆ Certifying Agencies

The three main certifying agencies include Medicare, the American Association for Accreditation of Ambulatory Surgery Facilities, Inc. (AAAASF), and the Accreditation Association for Ambulatory Health Care (AAAHC). Although there seem to be some major differences in what each agency requires, Medicare seems to have the most specific rules requirements, particularly on issues such as room types, locations, sizes, and ventilating and air-filtration issues. Medicare bases its rules on the National Fire Protection Association Codes. Medicare certification is not required, but it does have some advantages. Selecting this certification method allows you many advantages if you decide that insurance reimbursement is part of the overall business model. Another advantage is that Medicare certification is free, whereas other agencies charge a fee and also have fees on a regular basis. It can be difficult, however, to get Medicare to come out and inspect your facility. It also can be a little more costly as the minimum requirement for an operating room is 360 square feet, which may be wasted space for a practice focused solely on facial cosmetic procedures.

The problem of Medicare taking an excessive amount of time to finally certify a site has been partially solved by what is known as "deemed equivalency." Rather than take a year to schedule a certification, Medicare allows the other agencies to check on the Medicare rules and grant the practice a "deemed equivalency."

Finally, Medicare requires that certain procedures be followed as outlined in the Medicare *Policy and Procedure Manual*. This includes procedures for administrative policies, quality assurance, facility staff requirements, ancillary services, anesthesia requirements, facility rules and regulations, and documentation including medical records, infection control, and patient care procedures. Documents required by Medicare include written agreements with ancillary staff and consulting services, medical staff bylaws, board of directors' bylaws, and corporate bylaws. The Medicare guidelines also state that the ambulatory surgical center (ASC) must be a separate facility with no overlapping of staff or patient care and must also comply with state licensure requirements. The facility must also have a governing body that assumes full legal responsibility for determining, implementing, and monitoring policies for ensuring that health care is provided in a safe and effective manner.

In summary, certification by an accrediting agency is a must in today's environment. With running a purely cosmetic practice, I personally did not obtain Medicare status, nor did I apply for "deemed equivalency." However, I would recommend doing so if your center will offer other services, as it offers greater flexibility and opportunity for future growth. In certain states, the facility reimbursement for certain procedures far outweighs the cost associated with this type of certification process. If, however, you believe that you will remain a purely cosmetic practice, then the extra expense is probably not worth the effort, and you will be well served to perform these procedures in a center accredited by the AAAASF or the AAAHC.

◆ Developing a Strategic Marketing Plan

In today's competitive and ever-changing marketplace, the success of the facial cosmetic surgery practice relies heavily on the development of a strategic marketing plan. The strategic marketing plan needs to go beyond advertising, public relations, or sales.[8] These disciplines are important in the overall marketing plan but, in and of themselves, do not constitute marketing.

The marketing of professional surgical services requires a patient-centric environment, rather than a procedure or staff-centric environment. The cosmetic procedure's marketing program needs to follow specific operational systems and mimic the practice's management values. Some of the important aspects of this are (1) identifying what current patients, potential prospects, and referral sources desire and require; and (2) developing the proper services, systems, and patient care regimens to satisfy these things.

Like many of the strategic plans that are developed to achieve long-term goals, the marketing plan also represents a dynamic document that can and should be tweaked as necessary. Although periodic modifications of such a plan are essential, it is important that the plan be developed in such a manner that allows specific, measurable goals to be evaluated. To be most effective, however, marketing activities should be ongoing and consistent.

Strategic Marketing Goals

The purpose of a strategic marketing plan is to establish a planned direction for the growth of the practice by generating increased cosmetic procedures and revenues to meet its goals on a long-term basis.

A strategic marketing plan should strive to meet the following goals:

1. Positioning of the practice's cosmetic marketing program in a clear and competitive manner
2. Development of advertising and public relations programs to communicate the points of differentiation of the practice
3. Establishment of a comprehensive referral network from other professionals, aestheticians, salons, patients, and so forth
4. Successfully obtaining staff buy-in to increase the likelihood of the plan's success
5. Development of appropriate internal systems to manage inquiries created by the marketing program
6. Education and training of staff and the creation of appropriate collateral materials such as brochures, videos, Web site, newsletters, direct-mail pieces, and so forth
7. Preparation of a formal budget for marketing programs, media advertising expenditures, and promotional materials

Hitting Your Target Audience

The goal with any targeted marketing plan is to reach a selective audience that fits the demographic of your patients. Obviously, if you can access data that screen for your target market, the overall plan becomes more efficient and less costly. Understanding psychographic profiles as well as the geographic, age, income, and population density are some of the important key elements to assist with this process. Local organizations can also be helpful such as the Chamber of Commerce, mail-list houses, marketing agencies, as well as your own database. In addition, the more information you can collect and use about your own patients, the more you can acquire similar prospects.

Basic Tenets of Marketing

Although there is much data from several different fields as to how much money should be spent on annualized marketing, it is important to keep several things in mind. The first is that money that is spent should develop and maintain the brand of the practice. The materials should consistently reinforce your brand from medium to medium. This should not be a "shot in the dark" approach, rather a thoughtful approach defined by identifying the niche market that you are after.

It has been said that marketing dollars should reflect a certain percentage of next year's anticipated revenue. This means that if you intend to generate $1 million next year, you should consider spending a percentage this year on marketing. Numbers range from 3 to 20%, in this example $30,000.00 to $200,000.00 allocated for marketing. I personally believe that an aggressive budget for marketing is just below 10%. Whatever your goals and comfort level, the budget, once set forth, should be maintained as to avoid impulse changes that do not support the overall vision and strategic plan.

The plan should be developed to encompass a specific time frame; often this is 1 year. A very useful technique in helping to establish guidelines and goals is to develop a plan that uses low, expected, and high projections. For example, let us say that we are currently performing 100 facelifts per year, and our goal is to increase that by 20% in the following 12 months. Our expected goal then is 120 facelifts. We would then set a low goal of around 110 facelifts (or a 10% increase) and a high goal of 140 facelifts (or an increased of 40%). Although this is established for the next 12-month period, it may also be used to develop the marketing plan over the next 12, 24, and 36 months, respectively. In essence, a 3-year marketing plan is established. The value of setting these goals in a measurable manner cannot be understated. It offers the practice the ability to tweak the plan as market conditions change and allows you to stay calm and to avoid impulse decisions that will negatively impact your practice.

Developing a Creative Brief

Developing a creative brief can make a big difference, when done properly. The creative brief has been described as the most important document for an agency working to help promote business products or services.

A creative brief is a document that is typically written by the creative director in a marketing agency. It is where all the information, including background, product features, objectives, and target audience, is obtained from your practice and distilled down and passed along to the "creatives" in the agency. The document must give the creative team enough clear information to enable them to fully understand the practice's requirements and to produce a creative execution that will fulfill them (**Tables 17.8, 17.9, and 17.10**).

Table 17.8 Creative Brief: First Example

Hair Replacement: Male Perception
Project Description: Develop print advertising campaign to alter consumer perception of the social stigma associated with hair transplants and increase sales of transplant procedures
Target Audience: Males experiencing hair loss
Consumer Insights: Even though consumers are knowledgeable of procedure advancements, hair transplants are not socially accepted as an alternative to preventative medications and topical applications:
Outcome is perceived as unnatural
Painful procedure
Expensive
Copy Strategy: Because of medical advancements, hair transplant procedures are a welcome alternative to hair loss.
Brand Equities
Immediate results
Permanent results
Virtually pain-free
Highly trained staff
Confidentiality
Natural-looking results
Caring, informative doctors
Brand Character: The perfect procedure for an active, healthy lifestyle
Communication Mandatories
Logo
Web site URL
Phone number
Tagline

Table 17.9 Creative Brief: Second Example

Hair Replacement: Female Perception
Project Description: Develop print advertising campaign to increase consumer awareness and sales of hair transplants
Target Audience
Primary: Males experiencing hair loss
Secondary: Females in the key position to influence men
Consumer Insight
Women are just as concerned about their loved one's hair loss.
Men seek women's approval.
Feeling good about oneself leads to a healthy relationship.
Copy Strategy: Women, as the biggest influencers of men, can provide the motivation and empowerment for men to have hair replacement.
Brand Equities: The perfect procedure for an active, healthy, and youthful appearance
Immediate results
Permanent results
Natural-looking results
Confidentiality
Virtually pain-free
Highly trained staff
Caring, informative doctors
Brand Character: The perfect procedure to look your best. Hair replacement provides a more youthful and appealing appearance while giving a boost of confidence and relieving the paranoia of hair loss.
Mandatory Communication
Logo
Web site URL
Phone number
Tagline

Table 17.10 Example Creative Development Plan: Proposed Budget and Time Frame

Week 1 (Project One)	**Budget ($)**
Research design elements for hair, advanced lift, and overall business	300
Week 2	
Present 4 mood boards for approval	
Mood boards describe the overall feel of design communication.	
Two boards for the hair transplant area and two boards for facelift and overall business	
Weeks 2 and 3 (Project Two)	
Research trends, competition, and insights from employees, patients, and potential customers	1,875
Week 4	
Present three creative briefs	450
Each creative brief will give direction for the development and execution of creative work in the areas of hair transplant, facelift, and overall business.	
Week 6 (Project Three)	
Present advertising concepts and placement plan	1,725
We will present nine different creative boards (three for each creative brief). Each board will consist of a headline, tagline, and thumbnail sketch depicting the potential visual. These boards are considered roughs to be used for direction approval.	
Billing and payment is based on project	**Total $4,350**

A good brief will result in efficient, good-quality creative output that meets your needs. A poor brief often results in wasted time and unworkable or inappropriate solutions that result in an undesirable outcome.

What Should a Creative Brief Contain?

The style of the briefing form will change from agency to agency, but in general, the essential elements of the document remain the same. The creative brief should make clear the following:

- What are the objectives of the promotion?
- What do we want it to do?
- How do we want the target audience to react?
- Who is the target audience?
- Not just demographics, but lifestyle, attitudes, and so forth
- What will we be saying?
- Tone of voice? Brand personality?
- What type of media is to be used?
- Guidelines for execution: anything that must be included or avoided
- Budget
- Timing

What a Creative Brief Will Reveal

Once the creative brief has been developed, specific problems and challenges can be evaluated and solutions sought to overcome them. Additionally, this process will help establish both primary and secondary benefits to the consumer, which will be beneficial both for them and for achieving your own business goals.

The development of the design mandatory is also something that will come from this process. This document specifies design elements, such as the colors, sizes, fonts, and logos, that will be consistent throughout the all branded materials.

Medium and Placement

With all of the planning, budgeting, and creative process developed, the next step is getting your message out to the audience who will be influenced most into taking action. Selecting the medium and the actual placement of an advertisement are crucial to success. The goal here is to minimize expense and maximize visibility. This may be done by positioning the advertisements in a far forward, right-facing position in a magazine, or even on the inside of the cover or on the back cover itself. It is the creative process that will drive both the best placement of the advertisement as well as the best message for the medium in which it is placed.

Strategic planning and formal budgeting of media advertising segments are essential parts of marketing a successful cosmetic practice. Once this process has been achieved, targeting the proper mix of consumers within a market area can maximize return on investment, allowing even further opportunities for increased revenues and growth of the current business.

◆ Office Management

Every year we attend conferences to share new techniques and review old ones. We often see presentation topics such as "What I have learned over the past 25 years in practice." And every time one of these presenters stands up, a common theme seems to exist, and that is the challenges faced with the facial cosmetic surgery team. It seems that if you can create a vision, develop strategic plans, budget properly, and generate happy patients, you will be a success, and this is true to some degree; however, the potential to fail increases greatly without the proper cosmetic surgery team.

There are several important steps to building a dynamic and successful cosmetic surgery team. It is critical to retain top performers and establish a positive and winning environment. Not surprisingly, most practices realize from their own experience that the lack of teamwork leads to patient care issues, inefficiencies, low morale, greater stress, wasted time addressing staff controversies, and ultimately higher staff turnover and reduced satisfaction and success.[9]

One of the main goals to establishing a productive team is to hire and retain top performers. Management needs to

Table 17.11 Questions Necessarily Addressed by Physicians and Management Team

1. Do we encourage high performers to excel in our practice?
2. Do we consistently ask our staff what is going well and where can we improve?
3. Have we created an environment that attracts quality people?

Table 17.12 Commonly Reported Reasons Why Individuals Leave Companies

The most commonly reported reasons why individuals leave companies are:

1. Lack of recognition and appreciation
2. Feeling stressed and overworked
3. Not feeling a part of a team and not getting along with fellow employees
4. Lack of leadership/management
5. Work is not meaningful
6. Feeling as though they are not contributing
7. Lacking clear job descriptions
8. No career path or training
9. Low salaries and/or benefits
10. Lack of vision or understanding of their role

assess the needs of the organization and closely evaluate its progress. Certain difficult questions need to be addressed honestly by the physicians and management team (**Table 17.11**). The answers to these questions will also help make it clearer why staff members leave the practice (**Table 17.12**).

It is therefore of critical importance for the practice to rank itself in these areas and commit to these fundamentals if it is to retain the right personnel and build a high-performance team. Unfortunately, physicians are not generally the right managers for their own practice. Although establishing the vision and developing trust with the team is critical for the team to be successful, the physician attempting to run his own practice generally does not do well. This is not to say that many physicians are incapable of managing day-to-day operations; however, if you have established a successful practice, the time available to devote to managing the practice does not exist. Therefore, the practice manager or the director of operations is vital to long-term success.

After hiring the right people and getting them in the right positions,[10] the next ingredient to successful team development is a winning environment.

Retaining good people and creating a high-performance team can only happen with strong leadership. This can be created when goals are established and clearly communicated to the team. Every individual is to be aware of his or her role in this process, and the contributions and efforts of the team are recognized so that everyone shares in the successes of the practice.

Detailed job descriptions are a good way to communicate team member roles. A team member must know her job specifics and expectations. She must clearly understand how her position fits into the vision of the practice. She also must be held accountable for performing those duties appropriately through annual, semiannual, or quarterly reviews. A review serves as a report card that measures what team members are doing well and where they need to improve. Building a team starts with goals, roles, and reviews; however, a team will only succeed if management recognizes team members, shows appreciation for their efforts, and shares successes with them. Recognition and showing appreciation does not have to be complicated. Simply saying hello or good morning to a team member, thanking him after a difficult session, or complimenting him on handling a difficult patient can have a tremendous impact on morale. Make it a habit to "catch" team members doing things right—and acknowledge them for it. Praise works wonders on staff morale. A firm commitment to attracting and retaining top personnel, developing goals, defining roles, and recognizing accomplishments of team members will eliminate many battle lines and lay a firm foundation on which to build an enduring, winning team.

Approaching the Difficult Employee

If you manage people, eventually you will come across a difficult person. These people will hurt the team spirit and the productivity of your practice. If you are able to better understand why these individuals act the way they do, you will be better able to observe, predict, and guide them in a more productive manner.

Several important things need to be maintained for the team to be successful. The first is that you must maintain a positive attitude and be direct, descriptive, and nonjudgmental. It is important to focus on the detrimental *behavior* rather than the offending person. It is also important to not be judgmental, as we may not know all of what is occurring in the individual's life that may be contributing to the behavior.

Next, we need to be prepared with the facts, not gossip or rumors. If the unacceptable behavior came to you secondhand, your approach to the individual must be different than if you witnessed it personally or if you experienced the implication directly. Secondhand information must be validated or admitted to by the source before we move on to deal with it. This always helps us attack the problem, not the individual. By using a 360-degree evaluation, the situation and the facts can be more accurately obtained and the situation managed more efficiently. This analysis involves obtaining information from all parties and assimilating the facts to better understand the nature of the issue. However, it also is important to hold the offending parties accountable as per the policy and also to be sure that all parties understand how the situation was addressed.[10]

When addressing a difficult employee, it is important to (a) maintain eye contact; (b) watch the tone of your voice; and (c) time the discussion appropriately. Only after these three aspects of your communication are optimized can you then focus on the message you need to deliver to the difficult employee (**Table 17.13**)

Table 17.13 Dealing with Difficult Employees

Here is a list to help remember when dealing with difficult employees: 1. Remain positive. 2. Be direct, descriptive, and nonjudgmental. 3. Be prepared with facts, not gossip or rumors. 4. Address the problem; do not attack the person. 5. Maintain eye contact (also be aware of your body language). 6. Watch your tone of voice and timing. 7. Focus on the message, restating it as appropriate and necessary. Here are some additional guidelines: 1. Realize that the behavior is often predictable. Look for patterns. 2. Expect that behavior will impact others. 3. Know when to withdraw and turn to experts such as medical and psychological professionals (even if you do some personal counseling). 4. Try to discover the root causes of the problem so they can be addressed most appropriately, either by you or other professionals. 5. *Do not* try to provoke anyone into quitting or getting fired. Most employees are worth saving with some coaching and a solid approach to getting them to change or to accept help. 6. Always deal with the issue of an employee's performance rather than criticizing him or her personally.

Remember, timing is just as important here as in all other aspects of life. When something unacceptable happens, supervisors need to take enough time to ensure they do not blurt out things they will regret or have to withdraw later; however, they also need to make sure they do not let things drag on unaddressed for too long.

In addition to realizing the importance of our reactions and attitudes, we must also sometimes arrive at the conclusion—or at least proceed on the premise—that the difficult person will probably not change. We can ultimately only be responsible for our behavior and for how the behaviors of others are allowed to affect us. This is crucial as the task that we have in dealing with difficult people is more about us than it is about them. We are the ones charged with the responsibility of putting an end to the behavior that upsets the team or reduces productivity. The difficult employee usually recognizes his own behavior and is waiting for someone to take action.

Types of Difficult Employees

Table 17.14 is a handy reference tool for dealing with the various types of difficult employees[10] and includes numerous scenarios involving typical difficult employee types. Perhaps you do not recognize any of them among your staff.

Table 17.14 Action Plans for Various Types of Problem Employees

Symptoms	Suggested Action Plan
The Complainer • Voices lots of complaints but few, if any, suggestions • Even imagines problems • Appears blameless and innocent • Feels he must get personal opinions across • Gets worse if ignored • Includes disillusioned youth and perfectionists	1. Try to find the cause. 2. Listen; do not agree or disagree. 3. Avoid accusations. 4. Ask specific questions. 5. Stick to the facts. 6. If his complaints are job-related, determine whether he is unable or unwilling to perform the required duties. 7. Take appropriate action.
The Subversive Sniper • Often wants to move up • Seeks to undermine her supervisor (you) and make you look foolish • Is extremely passive-aggressive • Puts on a friendly face but snipes behind your back	1. Make it clear that you are aware of her ways. 2. Give specific, job-related orders. 3. Set necessary limits regarding behaviors that will not be tolerated.
The Busybody • Is a professional meddler • Believes he knows everything (and is usually wrong) • Likes to drop in anytime to gossip and relate his latest discovery	1. Visit him privately. 2. Help this person see how whispered charges hurt the whole unit. 3. Do *not* act like a prosecutor with a hostile witness. 4. Keep him busy, leaving little time to gossip. 5. Focus on the problem, its impact on his work and that of others, and take necessary corrective action.
The Maybe Person • Talks a good game • Usually does not produce • Procrastinates, hoping a better choice will present itself	1. Pinpoint work objectives; commit her to a project in advance; and cover who does what for whom and by when. 2. Make your expectations clear. 3. Seek any other causes. The source is not always shiftlessness; sometimes employees might be acting out of fear, inability, confusion, or boredom. 4. Determine what is applicable and take appropriate action.
The No Person • Is sometimes a perfectionist • Avoids mistakes at any cost • Loses hope and shares feelings with all when things go wrong • Extinguishes hope in others, smothering all creative sparks	1. Employ compassion and patience, not contempt. 2. Use him as a resource for others. 3. Use this person as your personal character-builder. 4. Run new ideas past him for critique before moving ahead.

(Continued on page 190)

Table 17.14 (*Contined*) Action Plans for Various Types of Problem Employees

Symptoms	Suggested Action Plan
The Explosive Employee • Blows up if threatened • Needs to prove herself • Has concrete answers for everything • Opposes any variations in process • Becomes irritated and impatient if plans are resisted • Deals with all others in the above manner	1. Do not expect change. 2. Let her run down, then regain her control after she explodes. 3. Show you take her opinions and others' seriously, and that there is a need to respect all equally.
The Belligerent Aggressor • Bullies his way to achieve what he wants • Embarrasses co-workers, thinking he will gain support of others • Throws temper tantrums • Tries to make supervisor (you) feel you are doing poorly when you are actually doing well	1. Use self-control and be consistent. 2. Do *not* let him pressure you into doing what you do not want to do. 3. Confront but do *not* oppose his accusations of you. 4. Anticipate challenges. 5. Practice what to say. 6. Respond with caution. 7. Set a time to deal with the situation.
The Harasser • Personally attacks co-workers • Avoids the real issue • Tries to set others up as opponents to impress her superior (you) • Cannot be objective	1. Establish and maintain a meeting plan to discuss the concerns. 2. Do *not* allow the discussion to drift. 3. Keep discussions to the point. 4. Refocus conversations as necessary.
The Green-Eyed Monster • Distinguishing mark is jealousy • Believes he should have something not earned • Reacts with spiteful behavior when others get raises or promotions	1. Keep conversations friendly and professional. 2. Avoid being dragged into an argument. 3. Always remind this person that everyone is evaluated or assessed according to his or her own efforts.

If you do, however, this will provide you with a fresh way of looking at your options.

◆ Conclusion

Although establishing and maintaining a successful facial cosmetic surgery practice can be quite challenging, employing some of the above guidelines will certainly increase your odds of success. I have learned, as we all have, by making many mistakes, yet I have always focused on the opportunities for improvement. The greatest challenges are not starting this process, but rather, to continually improve and grow the practice, to be flexible and adaptable to the market, and to be fiscally responsible with planning and budgeting. Without building a solid foundation and without a strategic plan for the future, you may find that costly mistakes prevent you from achieving your vision. But with the proper focus, commitment, and strategic planning, the likelihood of establishing a successful practice is greatly improved.

References

1. Fagien S. The aesthetic surgery business: a competitive sport? Cosmetic Surgery Times 2002;15 Nov
2. Maller BS. Developing Your Strategic Plan. Incline Village, NV: BSM Consulting Group
3. Maller BS. Implementing Your Strategic Plan. Incline Village, NV: BSM Consulting Group
4. Maller BS. Strategic Planning—Financial Considerations. Incline Village, NV: BSM Consulting Group
5. Thorne RL Jr. Choosing the Right Accounting Method for Your Practice. Incline Village, NV: BSM Consulting Group
6. Koval RC. Equipment financing options: different approaches provide differing costs and benefits. Allergan's Dermatology Practice Advisor 2000;Summer. Incline Village, NV: BSM Consulting Group
7. Hannapel CE. Setting up an office-based surgery suite. Cosmetic Surgery Times. 2002;15 Nov
8. Moore JW. Developing a Targeted Media Planning Strategy. Minnesota Refractive Surgery Center
9. Schildmeyer T. Two Critical Components to Building a Dynamic Team. Allergan Practice Consulting Group
10. Godevenos K. Staff Management: Dealing With Difficult Employees. Accord Consulting

18

Scheduling and Following Through with a Cosmetic Surgical Procedure

Jonathan M. Sykes

> "Good judgment comes from experience; experience comes from bad judgment."

The goal of the facial plastic surgeon is to satisfy the cosmetic surgery patient. To achieve this goal, the surgeon must exhibit good judgment in many aspects of medical and surgical practice. Good judgment on the part of the facial plastic surgeon requires focused observation and keen awareness.

A successful outcome in plastic surgery begins with the patient's first contact with the office, continues through the consultation and surgical procedure, and proceeds throughout all postoperative follow-up visits. Most postgraduate plastic surgery education emphasizes surgical technique and how-to-do surgical procedures; however, a successful plastic surgery practice is based on the surgeon's ability not only to complete the operation but also to select patients and attend to their needs and wants. This chapter provides an in-depth look at the process of interacting with the cosmetic surgery patient: the initial consultation, patient photography and imaging, scheduling of surgery, fee agreement, and informed consent. Additionally, postoperative issues such as the follow-up visits, aesthetician services, such as manual lymphatic drainage (MLD) and cosmetics, and dealing with patient dissatisfaction are addressed. It is clear that satisfaction after plastic surgery procedures requires meticulous attention to each of these details. They are as important as the surgical procedure itself.

◆ The Initial Patient Contact

The evaluation process of the cosmetic surgery patient should begin with the initial patient contact. The first contact with the prospective patient is usually a telephone call. The behavior exhibited during the initial phone call is often important and can set the tone for the physician-patient relationship that follows. Every piece of information obtained during the initial (and all subsequent) phone conversations should be used in evaluating whether the patient is an appropriate candidate for surgery. If any abnormal or inappropriate comments are made during any phone conversations with staff, these should be carefully documented in the chart.

The observations of nursing and office staff should be used in evaluating the cosmetic surgery patient. Office staff members often witness patient behavior that is different than the behavior used in front of the physician. The patient who is overly demanding or requires special treatment often will exhibit these traits to office staff. Although patients are often on their best behavior with the surgeon, they may treat the staff with a lack of respect. For these reasons, the opinions and observations of office staff are invaluable, often providing information that is not obtainable by the surgeon.

◆ The Consultation

The initial consultation between the facial plastic surgeon and patient is a complex interaction that involves two-way diagnosis and decision making. The surgeon is evaluating the medical history of the patient and the physical suitability of the patient. The surgeon is also beginning a process of deciding whether or not the patient is a good psychological candidate for surgery. The patient simultaneously is evaluating the surgeon and deciding whether to be operated on by the surgeon.

Most patients seeking a plastic surgery consultation have already thought about the decision-making process regarding surgery. As opposed to noncosmetic surgery patients who often hope that surgeons will recommend that the patient not have surgery, plastic surgery patients desire change and usually request surgery. For this reason, careful communication during the consultation is essential in establishing a healthy and open surgeon-patient relationship. It is important that the surgeon identify characteristics that may predispose the patient toward postoperative dissatisfaction with the surgical result.

The personality characteristics of both the patient and the surgeon are noticeable during the initial consultation. The overt goals of the patient are to evaluate the competence and expertise of the surgeon; that is, "Will the surgeon be able to improve the function and appearance of my face?" The less-stated goals of whether or not the surgeon can care for, and comfort, the patient during the healing process are at least as important as surgical competence is to the patient. Thus, the decision to choose a given surgeon is a complex one based on reputation, perceived competence, empathy, and comfort during the consultation.

The surgeon also has an important evaluation of the patient's psychological profile during the consultation.[1] This begins with the surgeon trying to understand the patient's position and perspective and, importantly, his or her motivation for having surgery.[2] If the surgeon feels that the patient has a poor self-image and is generally an unhappy person, the patient's motivation for surgery may be to create personal happiness. If the surgical results are disappointing to these patients, the resulting dissatisfaction is accentuated. Furthermore, patients with poor self-image are more likely to have surgery not meet their expectations. The failure to meet a patient's expectations usually results from the patient initially having an unhealthy motivation for surgery. All of these factors mandate that the surgeon be aware of the patient's psychological profile and to communicate any potential issues with the patient preoperatively.

◆ Selecting Patients

The first step to obtaining a successful outcome in facial plastic surgery is to carefully select the patient. This requires the surgeon to delve beyond the surface and to determine the patient's inner strength and ability to deal with the postoperative healing process.[3] Surgeons are taught how and when to operate, but the skill of when not to operate requires experience and good judgment. At the end of a surgeon's career, he or she will rarely be disappointed at not having operated on a particular patient; however, operating on the wrong patient (with a poor psychological profile) often creates anger and frustration on the part of both the patient and the surgeon. To exclude or discourage certain facial plastic surgery patients from having surgery, the surgeon must be aware of patient profiles that are problematic. **Table 18.1** lists patients who may be predisposed to unhappiness or dissatisfaction.

Table 18.1 Patients Who May Be Predisposed to Dissatisfaction with Plastic Surgery

Overly demanding
Unrealistic expectations
Poor self-image
Perfectionist
Body dysmorphic disorder
Patient critical of past surgery or medical care
Patients with prior depression or psychiatric disorders

◆ Photography and Video Imaging

The use of photography and imaging by the facial plastic surgeon is both helpful and essential. The patient often requests photographic documentation of the surgeon's competence (i.e., other preoperative and postoperative results) and imaging of their potential postoperative appearance. The surgeon needs photographic documentation as an ongoing learning tool and as a permanent medical record.

Preoperative and postoperative photography allows the surgeon to use surgical planning and to retrospectively look at outcomes of a particular technique. Photographs need to be consistent in lighting, positioning, and background. Archiving of photographs requires easy image retrieval and a system that allows cross-referencing by the surgeon. Accessibility to photographs needs to maintain patient confidentiality and comply with HIPPA regulations.

The five standard views obtained for facial rejuvenation surgery are frontal, lateral (two; left and right), and oblique (two; left and right) (**Fig. 18.1**). These photographs should be taken approximately 3 ft (1 m) away from the patient and should be 3:2 (vertical:horizontal). If periorbital surgery is to be performed, close-up photographs of the periorbital region should be obtained from approximately 2 ft away. These periorbital photographs should also be taken in the above-mentioned five positions. Additionally, a periorbital frontal photograph should be obtained with the patient in upward gaze (**Fig. 18.2**).

Patients often request computer imaging of their potential surgical result. Computer analysis should be performed after the actual consultation and as an adjunct to the consultation. Prediction of results should be done conservatively, and printed documentation of the computer imaging should not be given to the patient. It is very important to avoid "overselling" the outcome of any proposed procedure.

◆ Scheduling of Surgery

An efficient process of surgical scheduling, discussion and collection of fees, and communication of perioperative instructions is essential. Each facial plastic surgery office should have its own method to make the perioperative process flow smoothly. Successful surgical scheduling usually begins with an organized and personable surgery coordinator.

The surgery coordinator in the facial plastic surgeon's office must have good communication skills and a thorough knowledge of the surgeon's goals and abilities. Patients seeking plastic surgery usually have many questions, and friendly and professional attention to these perioperative concerns will often allay fears. The surgery coordinator must also discuss surgical fees and patient payment methods and schedules. Lastly, the coordinator should discuss and schedule postoperative appointments and perioperative instructions. These instructions must be carefully communicated, including medications and supplements to avoid preoperatively and activities to avoid postoperatively.

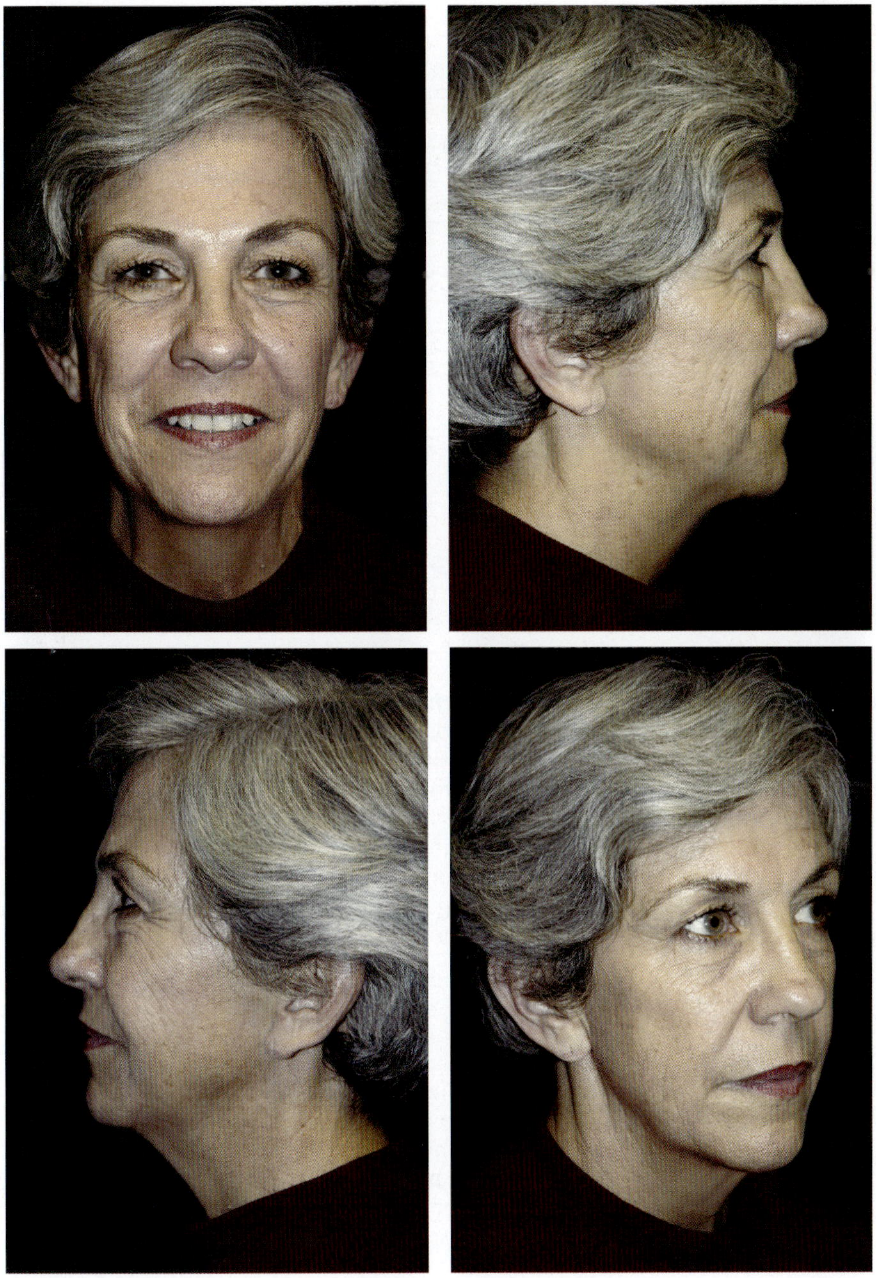

Fig. 18.1 (**A**) Preoperative frontal view. (**B**) Preoperative right lateral view. (**C**) Preoperative left lateral view. (**D**) Preoperative right oblique view.

When deciding on scheduling surgery, some patients have insecurities about their decision. The patient should not feel coerced into scheduling surgery. At the same time, the coordinator should let the patient know that the surgeon's operative time is valuable; vascillation regarding surgery should occur before scheduling surgery, with every attempt to avoid last-minute changes in surgical scheduling. For this reason, it is important that the surgeon have a fee schedule in place that discourages scheduling changes. For example, most offices require a 10 to 25% nonrefundable deposit at the time of scheduling. The surgeon may refund these monies at his or her own discretion (e.g., personal or family illness). The balance of the payment is then required 2 to 4 weeks before the actual surgery. The goal of the nonrefundable deposit is not to be punitive to the patient; rather, this deposit makes the patient (and staff) value the surgeon's time and discourages last-minute changes in surgical scheduling.

◆ Fee Agreement

In that the cosmetic surgery patient is usually paying for his or her surgery, rather than using third-party payers, professional handling of surgical fees is crucial. A fee agreement

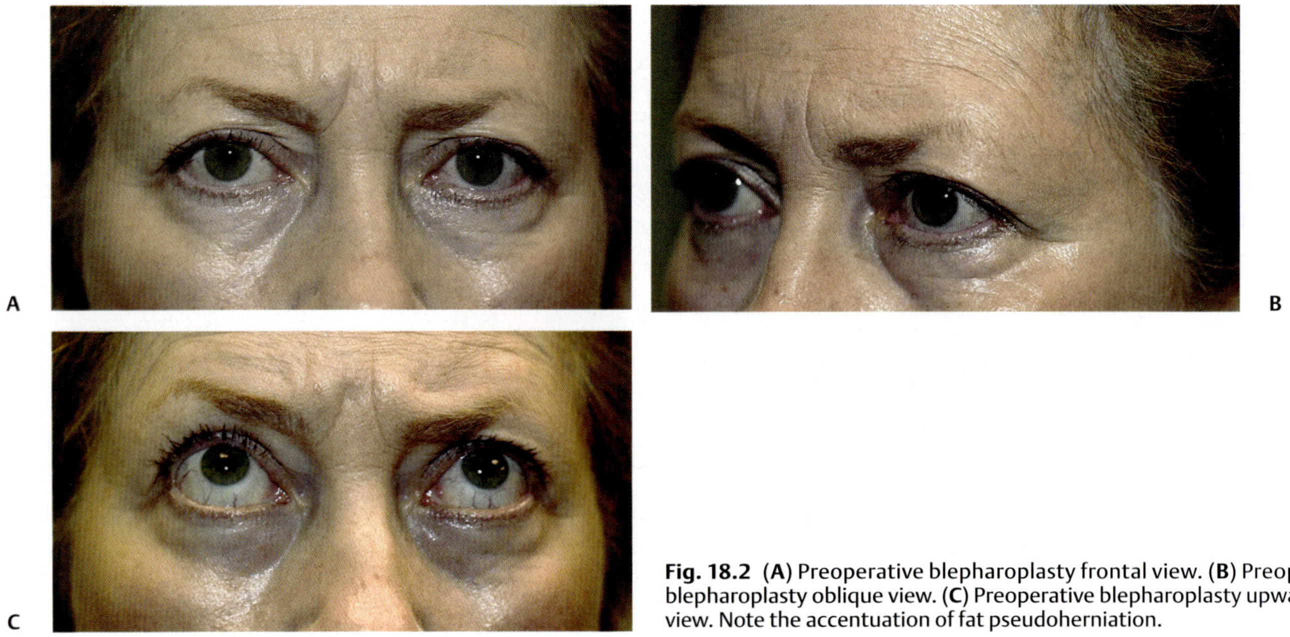

Fig. 18.2 (A) Preoperative blepharoplasty frontal view. (B) Preoperative blepharoplasty oblique view. (C) Preoperative blepharoplasty upward gaze view. Note the accentuation of fat pseudoherniation.

itemizing all surgical fees (surgeon, facility, anesthesiology, implant or laser fees, etc.) should be presented to the patient at the time of the initial consultation. A copy of this should be given to the patient, and a copy is kept in the patient's chart. This serves as a record of the discussed fees and should be easily referenced when the patient schedules surgery. This will avoid inaccurate "guessing" at the amount of previously discussed fees. If the patient decides to change (add or delete) a given procedure(s), a new fee agreement should be written, dated, and maintained in the patient's chart. As stated above, all cosmetic surgical fees should be paid well in advance of the surgery date. This will decrease the incidence of surgical rescheduling. If the patient fails to pay the balance of the surgical fees at the prescribed time, postponement or cancellation of the surgery with loss of deposit will occur.

◆ The Preoperative Visit

During the preoperative visit, two-way communication is extremely important. The surgeon should re-discuss each procedure: the goals, incisions, limitations, risks, and healing expectations. Avoidance of certain preoperative medications and postoperative physical activities is again discussed. The patient should ask questions relating to surgical goals, expectations, and perioperative concerns. At the conclusion of this visit, it is hoped that the patient will feel comfortable with the decision regarding surgery, and most fears should be allayed. Lastly, the timing and intent of postoperative appointments are discussed.

Patients are often anxious in the days leading up to their surgery. Written information including perioperative instructions should be given to the patient, as these will serve as a reminder to the patient who is unable to focus well and remember these perioperative instructions. All postoperative prescriptions are given to the patient at the preoperative visit. These include pain medications, antibiotics (if used), antiemetics, and anxiolytics. If skin resurfacing is to be performed, antiviral medication is also prescribed at this time. Anxiolytic medication (e.g., Valium [diazepam; Roche Laboratories, Basel, Switzerland] or lorazepam) is a useful adjunct in the perioperative period and often diminishes the need for narcotic pain medication.

◆ The Day of Surgery

Preoperative anxiety is often maximal the night before, and the day of, surgery. A social visit with the patient (and his or her family member, if present) just prior to surgery can be calming and reassuring to the patient. Last-minute patient questions can be answered at this time. The family member should be contacted at the conclusion of surgery and told prior to surgery the approximate time of return. Postoperative instructions are again discussed with the patient and family member (or friend).

Prior to surgery, it is important that the patient (and caretaker) be assured that the surgeon can be reached in case of emergency. It is advisable to give the patient the surgeon's page and/or cellular phone numbers to instill confidence and trust. The patient should be phoned on the evening of surgery to answer questions or concerns.

◆ Postoperative Visits

The schedule of postoperative visits should be individualized according to the surgery performed and the patient's specific needs. In most cases, the patient is seen the day after facial aesthetic surgery. This visit may be to remove nasal packing or surgical drains or to evaluate the patient for hematoma, seroma, infection, or wound issues. Eyelid sutures are removed in the 3- to 5-day postoperative range, and facelift/brow lift sutures are removed at days 5 to 7.

It is important that the surgeon realize that the patient is insecure and vulnerable in the immediate postoperative period. Although the patient's healing may be normal and "expected" by the surgeon, the perioperative condition of the patient is entirely new and unexpected to him or her. For this reason, empathy and compassion on the part of the surgeon are essential to successful postoperative communication.

The ability to empathize with patients is very important in all fields of medicine and particularly crucial in plastic surgery. Empathy allows the surgeon to accept the patient's perspective and to understand his or her motivation for surgery. To empathize with the patient, the surgeon must be a caring listener. The patient should experience being heard and accepted. The surgeon can use *reflective listening* to allow the patient to experience being heard. Reflective listening involves repeating what the speaker says to guarantee that the speaker's words and meaning are understood. The surgeon should use short summaries to reflect what he or she hears. The surgeon can use stems such as, "So, you are saying that . . . ," or "You are wondering if . . . ," or "I hear you saying . . . ." The technique of reflective listening should be used in all patient interactions beginning with the consultation and continuing through all postoperative care.

Education of patients is fundamental to all successful patient communications. The patient should feel as though there is shared knowledge in diagnosis and in treatment options. The surgeon should ask the patient about his or her understanding of the condition, why it is occurring, and what is his or her knowledge of possible treatments. This will allow the patient to better accept the surgeon's viewpoint and better assess the treatment options presented. This is particularly important with cosmetic surgery patients, who may be inundated with multiple surgical options from the media and the Internet. If the patients feel as though they have made an educated decision preoperatively regarding their surgical choice, they are less likely to be angry or frustrated postoperatively. It is important for the physician to ensure that the patient understands the diagnosis and treatment options. This understanding is essential to successful patient education.

The last successful physician-patient communication is enlistment. Enlistment is defined as an invitation from the clinician to the patient to collaborate in the decision-making regarding the goals and plan for treatment. The surgeon should offer options, explore the pros and cons of each option, and, with the patient, agree on the best option. The patient should be allowed to weigh all treatment options. This is extremely important in elective cosmetic surgery, which is not a need but a want by the patient. If the patient understands that the surgery is something that he or she desires but does not need, there is less chance for postoperative dissatisfaction. By engaging the patient in the process and enlisting him or her in the decision making, the surgeon converts the patient into a partner.

◆ Perioperative Services

During the first several weeks after aesthetic surgery, many patients are insecure about their appearance and their postoperative surgical result. It is important that the surgeon and staff reassure the patient and administer services to facilitate healing and maximize self-esteem. A complimentary MLD administered by a trained aesthetician often lessens postoperative discomfort and aids in relieving swelling. This is usually performed at approximately 5 to 7 days. A makeup consultation also helps patients camouflage postoperative ecchymosis and bolsters patient confidence. Of course, these services are not replacements for good medical care but should be thought of as adjunctive measures that facilitate the patient's return to his or her daily routine.

Postoperative photography is usually obtained at 3 months, 6 months, and at 1 year. Access to the patient's preoperative photographs is often helpful, as patients often forget many aspects of their preoperative appearance.

◆ Managing the Dissatisfied Patient

Dissatisfaction after cosmetic surgery results in distress for both the patient and the surgeon.[4] Even though a relatively small percentage of cosmetic surgery patients are truly dissatisfied with their result, these few patients usually occupy a large amount of the surgeon's time and energy. Learning to deal with patient dissatisfaction after cosmetic surgery requires significant psychological skills by the surgeon.

The key to dealing with postoperative patient dissatisfaction is communication.[5] As stated in the previous section, successful communication requires empathy and compassionate listening. This will allow the surgeon to identify the specific reason(s) for the dissatisfaction. It is important for the surgeon to avoid the impulse to immediately suggest a solution for the problem; rather, the surgeon should listen carefully and express compassion with the patient. The surgeon should approach the patient with postoperative issues in the same manner that is used during the initial consultation; that is, the surgeon should use a systematic communication style that employs all four E's of communication: engage, empathize, educate, and enlist (**Table 18.2**). This will allow the surgeon to display empathy and compassion to the patient and will usually prevent anger and frustration by the patient.

The cause of patient dissatisfaction after aesthetic surgery is usually the result of unmet expectations. Patients often expect that cosmetic surgery will improve their

Table 18.2 The Four E's of Effective Communication

Engage
Empathize
Educate
Enlist

self-image and self-confidence.[6] In most patients, this is the case. In some patients with significant preoperative issues with their self-image, the surgery actually causes an erosion of self-esteem.[7] Naturally, the patient then transfers his or her feelings of loss of confidence and self-image onto the surgical result. The patient will become extremely sensitive to the reactions and comments of family and friends. Such patients will often become overly concerned with normal postoperative swelling and bruising and will become impatient over normal healing times. It is very important that the surgeon recognize the patient's insecurity over the postoperative healing and surgical results. It is more important to show the patient compassion and empathy than it is to try and assure him or her that the healing is "normal."

As discussed in the Patient Selection section, the best method to obtain a successful outcome in plastic surgery is to carefully select patients. If a patient has significant postoperative dissatisfaction and communication between the patient and the surgeon erodes, the surgeon should use other means to communicate with the patient. This includes using friends and family of the patient to assist communication. Often, a friend or family member may add reason and may help the patient articulate his or her concerns and dissatisfaction. The surgeon should also use a caring staff member to attend all postoperative visits. The presence of other people (staff member, family member) during the visit will foster communication and help avoid anger and frustration. It is very important to carefully document all visits and to have staff members separately document their impressions of the visit.

In rare cases, communication erodes resulting in increased patient frustration and increased surgeon distress. The patient will occasionally ask for financial refund. The surgeon should then consult risk management and his or her insurance carrier. In these instances, a refund or partial refund of the surgeon's fee may be given. This should be given to the patient only after a full liability release is signed by the patient. Refund of fees should terminate the relationship between the surgeon and the patient.

◆ Conclusion

The success of any facial plastic surgery practice requires both the surgeon and staff to pay attention to many details. The surgeon must diagnose the medical/aesthetic condition precisely, choose and execute the surgery carefully, and give caring and empathetic postoperative care. The staff must act in a professional manner to educate the patient, coordinate surgery and office appointments, and collect fees. Use of adjunctive services makes the patient feel important and helps transition from surgery to normal daily activities.

Evaluation and caring for the patient begins with the initial patient contact and proceeds through all postoperative visits. Attention to these perioperative details is often as important as the surgery itself. Careful communication between the patient and the surgeon/staff helps educate the patient and establish realistic patient expectations. Satisfaction of the facial plastic surgery patient requires the surgeon to not only perform surgery well but also completely care for the perioperative needs of the patient.

References

1. Webb WL Jr, Slaughter R, Meyer E, et al. Mechanisms of psychosocial adjustment in patients seeking "face lift" operation. Psychosom Med 1965;27:183–192
2. Edgerton MT, Knorr NJ. Motivational patterns of patients seeking cosmetic (esthetic) surgery. Plast Reconstr Surg 1971;48:551–557
3. Pruzinsky T, Edgerton MT. Body-image change and cosmetic plastic surgery. In: Cash TF, Pruzinsky T, eds. Body Images: Development, Deviance, and Change. New York, NY: Guilford Press; 1990:217–236
4. Goldwyn RM. The dissatisfied patient. In: Goldwyn RM, Cohen MN, eds. The Unfavorable Result in Plastic Surgery: Avoidance and Treatment. 3rd ed. Philadelphia, PA: Lippincott Williams & Wilkins; 2001:8–13
5. Rohrich RJ. The who, what, when and why of cosmetic surgery: do our patients need a preoperative psychiatric evaluation? Plast Reconstr Surg 2000;106:1605–1607
6. Knorr NJ, Edgerton MT, Hoopes JE. The "insatiable" cosmetic surgery patient. Plast Reconstr Surg 1967;40:285–289
7. Cash TF. The psychology of physical appearance: aesthetics, attributes, and images. In: Cash TF, Pruzinsky T, eds. Body Images: Development, Deviance, and Change. New York, NY: Guilford Press; 1990:51–79

19

The Future of Facial Plastic Surgery

Peter A. Adamson and Theodore Chen

Science has the ability to surprise, because it marshals the power of both measurement and art. Neither of these pursuits alone could claim to be science, only the two together. Reconstructive surgery is indeed a science, because it strives for precision in measurement while acknowledging a reality that goes beyond measurement—the unique character of the individual. We can expect it to surprise even its practitioners in years to come.[1]

◆ Past, Present, and Future

> "I never think of the future—it comes soon enough."
>
> —Albert Einstein (1879–1955)

Reflecting on Einstein's words, at the very least it is bold and presumptive to comment upon the future of facial plastic surgery. One can infer a degree of hubris emanating from any such scribe, if not downright foolishness. But our human imagination is indeed a wondrous trait, and upon request flights of fanciful thought are soon filling the mind to meet the challenge. To share the burden of this pursuit, the authors engaged many recognized leaders and innovators in facial plastic surgery to contribute their musings—it should come as no surprise that there were areas of confluent and diverse opinions. It is well recognized that even the greatest inventors rarely foresee the ultimate impact of their invention or innovation. Edison allegedly believed that the main application of electricity would be the light bulb, which would allow people to read after dark. The brightest of minds, apparently, cannot foresee the future. So where does that leave us mere mortals?

It therefore should come as no surprise that a review of articles in *Facial Plastic Surgery* and *Plastic and Reconstructive Surgery* from 1984 to 1988 revealed studies on liposuction, tissue expansion, dermabrasion, fat cell grafting, and polyamide mesh, among others. However, there were no articles on deep plane face lifting, endoscopic lifting, facial transplants, laser skin resurfacing, pulsed light therapies, radiofrequency treatment, or hyaluronic acid fillers—only a few of the advances seen in the past generation. Who could have foreseen these specific developments, and who can truly foresee what the next generation of advances will bring? But let us ponder, if only perhaps to stimulate an idea that will be transformed by one of us into a serendipitous advance for our specialty.

◆ Flashes in the Pan or Foundations for Our Future

> "The future, according to some scientists, will be exactly like the past, only far more expensive."
>
> —John Sladek

The author of this comment may have been referring to endoscopic, laser, or radiofrequency therapies, which have, respectively, attempted to displace scalpels, sutures, and topical skin treatments from our armamentarium but at a much greater expense. There is no doubt these modalities have their essential applications. Notwithstanding their positive impact on the field of facial plastic surgery, they too have followed the curve of innovation (**Fig. 19.1**). Many of us remember buccal liposuction; malar, mandibular, and tear trough implants; platysmal excisional techniques; the "push down" rhinoplasty; and a variety of other procedures that once were in vogue but now have much more limited application. This trend will certainly continue, and many of the techniques, tools, and products that we espouse today will be replaced tomorrow.

The unanswerable question is, "Which ones will be flashes in the pan, and which ones will become new foundations for our future?" Each of us will play our individual role in the acceptance, rejection, and application of new technologies and ideas. There is no doubt that some of our current thinking will prove to be false and discarded. Other parts of our future are already here—we just do not recognize it because it has not been discovered yet.

◆ Which Direction To Go?

> "How can you research the future? It hasn't happened yet."
>
> —Ambrose Bierce, *The Devil's Dictionary*

Today we have two core philosophies jostling for supremacy in facial plastic surgery: minimally invasive versus open procedures. This began with the controversial external or open rhinoplasty procedure in the 1970s. Studies show the

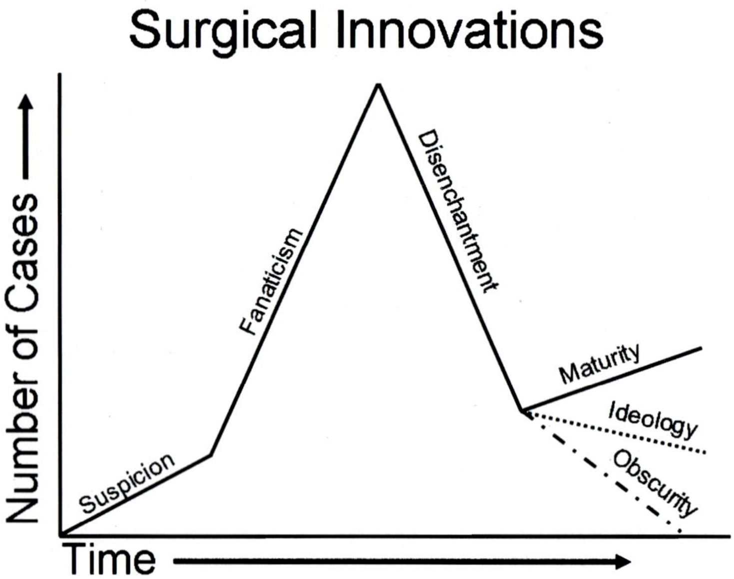

Fig. 19.1 Surgical innovation curve. (From Rogers EM. Diffusion of Innovations. New York, NY: Free Press; 1962. Adapted with permission.)

open approach has been accepted by the majority of facial plastic surgeons and has enjoyed increasing application over the past years.[2] Its use may now be plateauing, however, and who knows what will be the impact of the novel endoscopic septoplasties now being performed. While we have been opening up the nose, we have been expounding upon the virtues of "closing" our surgical approaches to the forehead, midface, and even the lower face. This modern, minimalistic, innovative, technically savvy trend has held sway for the past 15 years, but it is not without its agnostics who feel that open procedures give a longer-lasting, more secure and natural result that cannot always be achieved by endoscopic approaches. Notwithstanding the sophisticated surgical tools and materials we have at our disposal, it should be stressed there is no substitute for excellent surgical technique, whatever the approach. Although very unlikely in the near future, one might conjure that surgery itself may be minimized with the application of genetic and soft tissue engineering that will create the potential to rejuvenate skin, muscle, and fat biologically without any mechanical intervention.

◆ Our Search for Beauty

"I have seen the future, and it is still in the future."

—James Gleick, 2002

Although we know little of the direction that science will lead us, we might presume to possess a little more foresight in how we will perceive beauty, and how this will impact our goal of improving the human visage both reconstructively and cosmetically.

For centuries, we have used the canons of Leonardo da Vinci and others in ascribing mathematical proportions to describe the beautiful face. The Golden Decagon describes the phi ratio of 1:1.618, which represents perfect harmony and which can even be applied to the regional aesthetic units of the face. A more recent concept, koinophilia, which means "love of the average," emanates from Darwinian theory that states that evolutionary pressures operate against the extremes of the population. We are therefore more attracted to others of the opposite sex with "average features." This average is determined uniquely for each person by the constant collection of facial impressions each sees in his or her own environment. The composite human face so encrypted in our mind becomes the most attractive to that specific individual.

As our world becomes a global village with greater travel, migration of people, and interracial reproduction, the paradigm for the average, attractive face is changing. This will undoubtedly continue for the generations to come resulting in increasing attraction by all of us to nonhomogeneous racial features as there is more blending of distinct racial stereotypes. There will be a globalization of beauty. At the same time, there will be an increased acceptance of ethnicity as we live side by side with different races and individuals who still express homogeneous racial features in their appearance. Political, religious, and ethnic realities will likely counter this trend.

It is also recognized that beauty, in contradistinction to attractiveness, is determined by facial features that not only reflect averageness and symmetry but also importantly reflect estrogen in females and testosterone in males. This implies larger eyes, smaller nose, fuller lips, and narrower chin for females, and smaller eyes, larger nose, longer thinner upper lip, and wider jaw for males. Needless to say, much of our work is directed toward procedures that enhance these features: forehead lifting, eyelid lifts, rhinoplasty, lip enhancement, and facelifting, to name but a few. These procedures not only make a woman look more youthful but also more feminine. However, caution must be observed. If any feature is overdone so as to look unnatural, the genuineness of character is lost and the overall effect of the procedure negated. Knowing this, we can expect an ever-increasing effort to achieve natural appearances and a move away from treatments that create trendy looks that are overdone and unnatural. We will

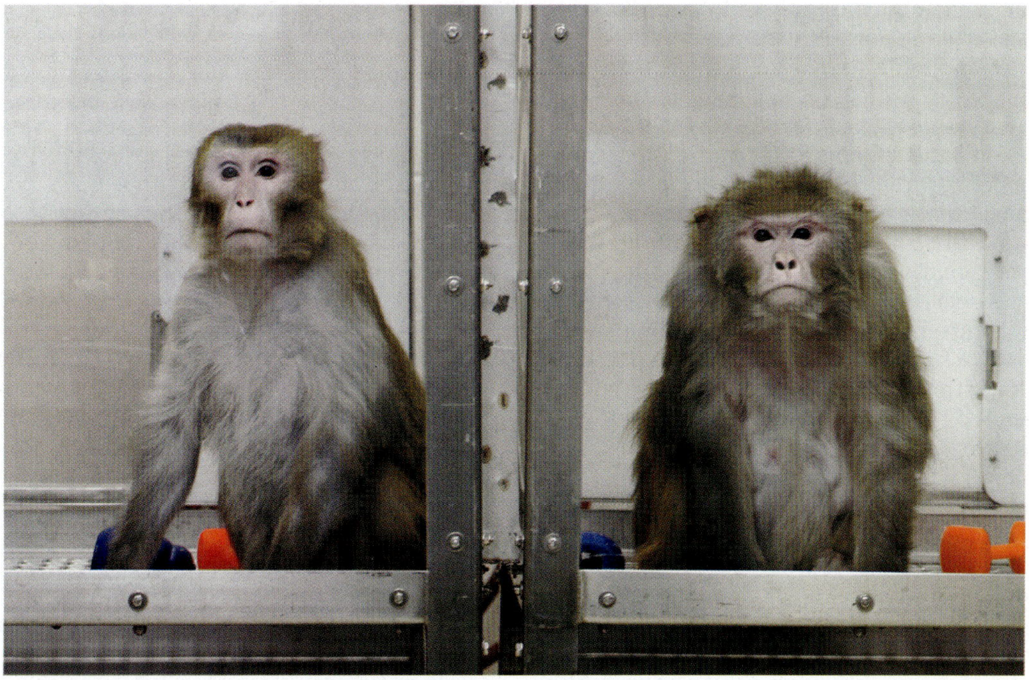

Fig. 19.2 Rhesus monkey Canto (left), on a restricted diet, and Owen (right), a control subject on an unrestricted diet. Both animals are part of long-term, NSF-funded research at the University of Wisconsin–Madison studying the links between diet and aging in monkeys. (Courtesy of Jeff Miller, University of Wisconsin, Madison.)

also focus more on the hormonal effects of estrogen and testosterone on women and men and seek interventions that will enhance these effects in them, respectively.

As facial plastic surgeons, we should be aware of trends and advances in other fields that may impact upon us. For example, there is increasing interest in, but not yet enough research to support, the value of restricting caloric intake by up to 20 to 30% to increase both average and maximal life span.[3] There is some support for this in monkey studies (**Fig. 19.2**). Notwithstanding the current obesity epidemic in North America, would such a trend provide new opportunities for facial rejuvenation and volume restoration in a growing number of people?

Dramatic new cosmetics from the fashion world may also impact thinking about skin care and interventions. For example, at Chanel attempts are being made to apply artificial skin technology to cosmetics.[4] Some say that within a few years, foundations and treatment products will be able to "read" the skin using tiny "enviro" chips to determine the level of moisture, coverage, and texture required. In addition, color cosmetics such as lipsticks and shadows will adapt their hues to complement skin tones in all kinds of lighting, similar to some spectacles today.[5]

◆ Genetic and Tissue Engineering

"Without expectations, there is no future, only an endless present."

—Francois Jacob, Nobel Laureate in Medicine

We would all agree that a greater fundamental knowledge of the intrinsic and extrinsic factors that cause aging would aid us in prevention and management of the aging process. Our current understanding is rudimentary, and we will not see any paradigm shifts in treatments until much more is learned. However, the Genome Project has built the foundation on which we can pursue studies leading to tissue engineering of a variety of tissues, potentially including skin, fat, bone, cartilage, and muscle.

For example, tissue engineering of human septal cartilage has been performed. A small biopsy of septal cartilage can be used to create neocartilage that can be shaped as desired by using an absorbable poly-lactic-*co*-glycolic acid (PLGA) polymer scaffold. This neocartilage has been tested and has essentially the same biomechanical properties as native septal cartilage.[6] Applications would include facial reconstruction and revision rhinoplasty, which could eliminate the need for alloplastic implants, rib grafts, and so forth.

There has been an increasing amount of research being performed on mesenchymal stem cells (MSCs), which are harvested from bone marrow. In one study, the authors were able to differentiate the MSCs into adipose tissue.[7] Currently, we know that fat injections using mature adipocytes are somewhat unpredictable and sometimes temporary. Using preadipocytes is problematic as well. Preadipocytes have a reduced ability to proliferate, unpredictable variability based on anatomic sites, and limited availability. Moreover, with regard to primary preadipocyte cultures, differentiation capacity is clearly donor-dependent and decreases significantly with age. However, the adipocyte-forming capacity of MSCs is similar in both young and old donors; it is possible that MSCs may constitute a better material for soft tissue regeneration than do preadipocytes. The same study also demonstrated that MSCs could be mounted onto PLGA injectable spheres. The adipo-MSCs differentiate into adipocytes on PLGA spheres, and adipo-MSCs on PLGA spheres formed adipose tissue in vivo. For larger defects, the MSCs could also be mounted onto a scaffold to create a three-dimensional soft tissue filler. Furthermore, the same MSCs can be differentiated into osteocytes or chondrocytes if needed.

Gene therapy is also being researched for the treatment of skin cancers. Currently, our primary treatments are anatomic ablative techniques, that is, surgery, cryotherapy, laser therapy, radiation, and topical ointments. Treating genetic problems with anatomically based modalities could become obsolete. In particular, there is extensive research being done on gene therapy for melanoma.[8] It is well recognized that all cancers, including head and neck, reflect complex genetic interventions. How close are we, really, to genetically engineering the cure for those tumors?

Although cloning is possible, having been successfully performed in animals, the ethical issue surrounding human cloning will likely obstruct this development, except by renegade groups. This obviously would pose a substantial ethical dilemma for our profession and for society.

◆ Facial Reconstruction

"As for the future, your task is not to foresee it but to enable it."
—Max Jakobson, Finnish diplomat

Gene therapy provides the hope that, once the causative gene is identified, treatments could be developed to eradicate congenital facial anomalies. As mentioned, with tissue engineering, custom-designed cartilage, bone, fat, muscle, skin, or neurovascular tissues could be uniquely created to reconstruct a given defect. The production of such tissues, or indeed permanent or biodegradable implants, would be enhanced by the use of three-dimensional computed tomography (CT) and magnetic resonance imaging (MRI) for large craniofacial defects. Computer-generated alloplastic patient-matched implants have already been created.[9] Using similar technology, it should be possible to take a three-dimensional CT or MRI scan and use it to design a custom, patient-matched PLGA scaffold. As our understanding of MSCs grows, we would be able to attach the MSCs onto the scaffold and have them differentiate into whatever is needed (i.e., bone, cartilage, soft tissue, etc.). The need for a free flap could be a thing of the past.

It may be possible to have computerized systems that would analyze such a defect, create a program for the appropriate tissue-engineered replacement tissues, plan the operative procedure, and assist the surgeon with the reconstruction. This could all be performed through wireless, voice-activated, interactive computers and robots. It is difficult to perceive a computer-technical interface that could relieve the surgeon of all surgical judgment and the finest technical points of reconstructive surgery—but 100 years from now, who knows?

◆ Soft Tissue Advances

"The future cannot be predicted, but futures can be invented."
—Dennis Gabor, *Inventing the Future*, 1964

There has been tremendous growth in understanding wound healing in the past 15 years. As we begin to figure out how the pieces of this complex puzzle all come together, pharmacotherapies are being developed that will enable us to modulate the wound-healing response.

In 1998, the U.S. Food and Drug Administration (FDA) approved becaplermin (Regranex [Ortho-McNeil Pharmaceuticals, Inc., Titusville, NJ]), a recombinant human platelet-derived growth factor (PDGF) that is used for diabetic neuropathic ulcers to induce granulation, with an off-label use to induce granulation in irradiated wounds.[10–12] Autologous platelet gel has been used to decrease soft tissue bruising, and investigations now are determining if it may also improve wound healing.[13]

In 2004, the growth factor palifermin (rKGF-2; Kepivance [Amgen, Inc., Thousand Oaks, CA]) was approved by the FDA to decrease the severity and duration of oral mucositis in patients undergoing chemoradiation therapy. This agent, when used proactively, appears to decrease wound-healing complications.[14] Research has shown that antifibrogenic factors may decrease scar formation,[15] as may certain herbal remedies.[16]

There continues to be significant interest and research in scar-free healing. More evidence is being accrued that demonstrates that scarless wound repair in gestation is in large part due to the various isoforms of transforming growth factor-β (TGFB) and their receptors.[17] Scientists have experimentally manipulated healing wounds in adult mice, rats, and pigs to mimic the scar-free embryonic profile. These experiments have resulted in scar-free wound healing.[18] It may only be a matter of time until novel pharmaceutical molecules are developed that will prevent scarring during adult wound healing. Scar-improving drugs could have widespread benefits and prevent complications in several tissues; for example, prevention of blindness after scarring due to eye injury, facilitation of neuronal reconnections in the central and peripheral nervous system by the elimination of glial scarring, restitution of normal gut and reproductive function by preventing strictures and adhesions after injury to the gastrointestinal or reproductive systems, and restoration of local motor function by preventing scarring in tendons and ligaments.[19] This means that scarring may no longer be an inevitable consequence of injury or surgery. One might postulate that if we can achieve scar-free healing, will the longer-incisional approaches gain some increasing favor once again with respect to certain endoscopic approaches?

In general, these expected advances in the modulation of wound healing and diminishment of scarring, along with newer biodegradable fixation devices, may portend widened indications for certain endoscopic procedures and/or more traditional approaches. Only time and experience will tell which will prevail. With our current appreciation for maintaining or restoring volume in the soft tissues, as well as lifting ptotic tissues, it is expected in the nearer future that there will continue to be an emphasis on repositioning, tightening, and filling, in contradistinction to aggressive excisional techniques for facial rejuvenation.

The future will come to yield minimally invasive, office-based treatments that will predictably reduce redundant fat pads, thereby making liposuction obsolete. Perhaps these treatments are already upon us, and only fine-tuning of the current technology and techniques is needed. In North America, interest in mesotherapy for body contouring has been growing. Mesotherapy involves injecting various chemicals in the subcutaneous tissue to treat a variety of disorders and ailments. It has been used for years in Europe and South America as a method of "melting fat" for body contouring.[20] At the time of writing, a Medline search from 1950 to the present in the English language did not reveal a single published study on the formulations, dosages, safety, mechanisms of action, or efficacy of mesotherapy. Though there is plenty of anecdotal support that mesotherapy successfully treats cellulite, the scientific support is lacking. In their policy statement,[21] the American Society of Plastic Surgeons "does not endorse the use of injectable treatment (mesotherapy) for any condition at this time."

The future of percutaneous, suture-based lifting procedures is yet to be determined. Early experience would indicate the results are less than hoped for and the complications greater than acceptable for many patients. There is no doubt that the public is always seeking the most for the least, however, and therefore, there will be more research, more products developed, and more ideas presented. It still seems apparent that lifting and recontouring of facial soft tissue requires both appropriate mobilization followed by a period of fixation as wound healing occurs to secure a satisfying long-term outcome.

The advances in tissue engineering to create neotissue will compete with the development of newer and more biocompatible alloplasts that can be custom-molded for a given defect. Biodegradable tissue scaffolding products will improve. All things being equal, cost will be a major factor in the introduction of any newer modality.

With each advance, a more knowledgeable public living in a more connected world will expect higher standards of reconstruction and rejuvenation, placing a higher burden on all professionals providing such care.

◆ Transplantation

"It is the business of the future to be dangerous."
—Alfred North Whitehead, philosopher

Fat transplantation is, once again, receiving increased attention. Progress has been made in harvesting and injecting fat to enhance its viability, but as of yet, there are still no guarantees of consistent and persistent results. There is little doubt the future holds a much greater place for fat transplantation along with fat transposition to recontour the face through fat sculpting as its reliability is improved.

In November 2005, the profession (and indeed the world) was excited to learn of the first partial face transplant (**Fig. 19.3**).[22] The pioneering French team is planning another five transplants in the near future, notwithstanding the controversial nature of the procedure. In the coming years, there will be extensive discussion regarding acquisition of donors for such procedures, selection of recipients, management of immunosuppression, restoration of animation,

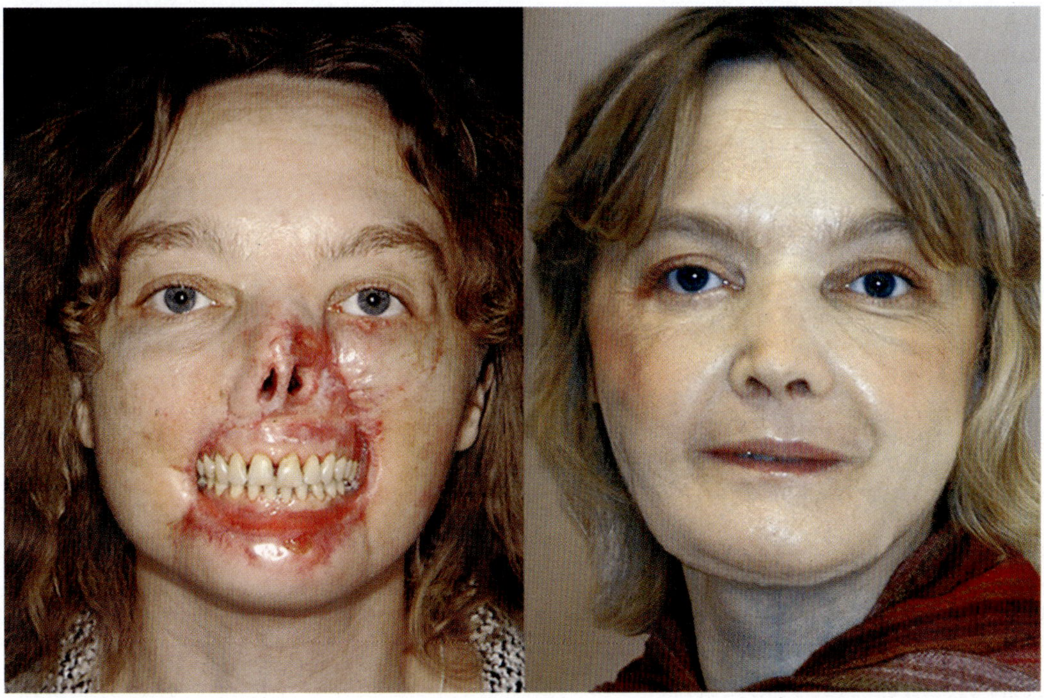

A B

Fig. 19.3 (**A**) Before partial face transplant. (**B**) One year after partial face transplant. (Courtesy of Professor Benoît Lengelé.)

ethical issues, and cost for such procedures. But it is highly likely such procedures will continue to evolve, eventually leading to full face transplantation. There could be a significant increase overall in microvascular transplantation from heterologous donors with advances in immunosuppressive therapy. The next generation of immunosuppressive drugs will have fewer side effects and fewer long-term complications, thereby promoting the use of nonautogenous products. Potential donors sites would include the ear, nose, lips, and eyelids.

Face transplantation will have its polemicists,[23] and those who are pioneering this surgery will have their responses. So it has been with the world's first partial face transplant. In their article "Facing up is an act of dignity: lessons in elegance addressed to the polemicists of the first human face transplant," Drs. Lengelé, Testelin, and Devauchelle responded as follows: "The spirit of excellence is to take care more than others think is wise, to risk more than others think is safe, to dream more than others think is real and to expect more than others think is possible. Elegance is an art of living in the spirit of excellence, seeking to create more passion, grace and beauty than others think is practical."[24]

◆ The Future of Skin Care

> "The trouble with our times is that the future is not what it use to be."
>
> —Paul Valery (1871–1945)

One of the areas of greatest change in the past generation has been skin care. A host of minimally or noninvasive treatments has been developed. These include carbon dioxide laser (CO^2), erbium laser, fractionated laser, radiofrequency (Thermage [Thermage, Inc., Hayward, CA]), phototherapy (e.g., intense pulse light and broadband infrared light), chemotherapy (e.g., glycolic acid), muscle-stimulating systems, and microdermabrasion, among others. The carbon dioxide laser, initially believed to be the answer for skin rejuvenation, has fallen out of its original favor due to its complication rate and long healing time. But many still believe it represents the gold standard for skin rejuvenation in selected patients. New modalities are all seeking to rejuvenate the collagen and elastin in the dermis without traumatizing the epidermis. There have been many promising technologies, and many promises, but nirvana is yet to be reached. The overwhelming consensus is that modalities such as radiofrequency, nonablative lasers, and light technologies are not a replacement for surgery. At the present time, these modalities fill a very defined niche in facial plastic surgery, treating only mild to moderate facial rhytides and skin laxity. There have been a few studies demonstrating greater benefit by combining multiple modalities.[25,26] Because these treatments are all relatively new, long-term results are not yet available. The odyssey, without doubt, will continue. Once reached, the nasty appearance of patients after dermabrasion, chemical peels, and carbon dioxide laser will be a relic of the past.

Novel ways to use energy to resurface and rejuvenate the skin with no down-time are constantly being researched and developed. Injuring skin (thermally, chemically, or mechanically) to stimulate new collagen formation will become obsolete. In ophthalmology, the application of riboflavin and UV-A for cross-linking is being used to treat ectasia and keratoconus. Additional applications are currently undergoing clinical trials.[27] The cross-linking using riboflavin and UV-A is applicable to most collagen types. Long-term effects of this technique have been studied for $\sim$10 years, and the vitamin photosensitizer appears to cause a gentle, biocompatible, nonmutagenic, long-lasting stabilizing effect with some tightening. The degree of tightening can be controlled both by dosing/pulsing the UV-A and varying the riboflavin concentration. According to a senior investigator conducting the clinical trials, this technology should work on skin as well with the proper delivery refinements.[28]

As topical agents such as 5-fluorouracil (5-FU) to treat skin cancers improve in their efficacy, we may see a decrease in the number of radical ablative resections and as much need for Mohs surgery. Other topicals may stimulate the DNA of nascent skin progenitors to generate new skin.

Tremendous advances have been made in the application of botulinum toxin A (Botox; Allergan, Irvine, CA), truly one of the wonder drugs of the new millennium. More than 11 million patients had Botox in 2006. The sculpting of facial musculature is developing into an art form to create a more youthful and relaxed facial dynamic. It is likely there will be increased growth in the indications for the use of this drug, especially as newer botulinum toxins are brought to market.

Injectable fillers have also seen an exponential increase in their use. This is due to the larger number of fillers to choose from and their increasing efficacy. It has been said by some that the perfect filler would last $\sim$2 years, and the current hyaluronic acids (e.g., Juvéderm [Allergan, Irvine, CA] and Restylane [Q-Med, Uppsala, Sweden]) are lasting 6 to 9 months in most people and more than a year in some. With relatively few contraindications, a high safety profile, and satisfying volume replacement effect, they will likely see continued growth in their use. Widespread research in this area will likely see even better products and increased usage. Although the permanent fillers (e.g., ArteFill [Artes Medical Inc., San Diego, CA]) are much improved and often provide excellent results, they are not likely to receive as much favor as the temporary fillers due to their more restricted indications and greater potential for unresolvable complications. As evidenced by one of the earlier, excellent permanent injectables—silicone—misuse, public perception, and government regulation all have the potential to play a significant role in determining the ultimate usage of all of these products. The future is always uncertain in this regard.

◆ Education and Robotics

> "When we have understood the present, it has become the past."
>
> —Andrew Abbott, *Time Matters*

Surgical education will change. Surgical training is frequently compared with pilot training, and yet we are years behind in the development of simulators for surgical training. However, advances are being made. Computer simulators with haptic feedback are being perfected and will become widely available.[29] Currently, they are limited to specific procedures, but these will undoubtedly be expanded in the years to come. It may even be that surgical training will change from being chronology-based to proficiency-based training. This could be more effective and could also be a more accurate determinant of when a given resident is prepared for independent practice. These systems could also be used for surgical rehearsal prior to difficult cases and for research into new procedures.

Surgical robots like the da Vinci are in their infancy (**Fig. 19.4**). Currently, use of surgical robotics is primarily limited to laparoscopic, urologic, and cardiac procedures. An exciting application of surgical robotics is remote telesurgery. There has already been a reported case of a successful lap-cholecystectomy performed on a patient in France by a surgeon in New York.[30] This also has the implication that a given surgeon could potentially create an international practice and never leave home.

It is expected that rhinoplasty will continue to pose one of the greatest challenges to surgeons. Will it be possible through photography, scanning, and computer analysis to generate a planned and quantifiable approach to reduction and augmentation of the nose? And what about the ever-important skin redrapage factor, will it become quantifiable? Could surgical robots perform such a procedure recognizing the variable situations that arise intraoperatively? We are likely still several generations of advances removed from such a scenario, but who knows?

◆ The Profession and the Public

> "The best thing about the future is that it only comes one day at a time."
>
> —Abraham Lincoln

Medicine continues to be the most demanding of professions in its duration of training. We will continue to have the "best of the best" apply to medical school as it is still perceived as the greatest of all of the professions. However, we will lose a proportion of individuals who believe the less regulated world of business, with its potential for greater freedom and higher financial rewards, offers a better future for them. Increased government and regulatory control will be the norm, as will time-limited licensing and recertification procedures. Lifetime learning will be increasingly expected and demanded. Specialization and fractionation of subspecialty groups will continue. The various medical bureaucracies will have a difficult time keeping up with the social changes and public demands confronting them. Physicians will increasingly need to make a career choice—join a

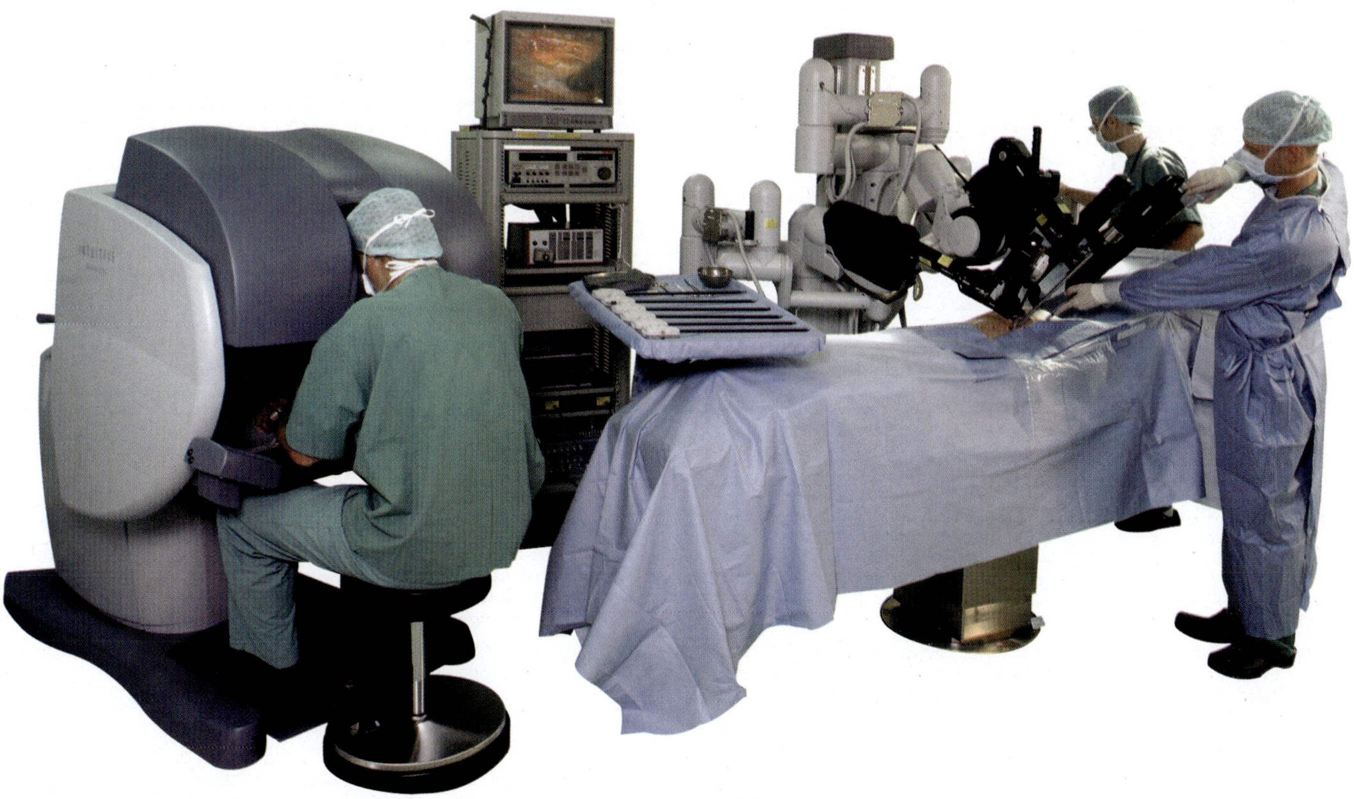

Fig. 19.4 da Vinci Surgical System. (Courtesy of Intuitive Surgical, Inc.)

large group of physicians essentially as an employee or assume the risk of a medical entrepreneur in establishing a practice and business that functions as much as possible outside the realm of bureaucratic control. Professional satisfaction will be difficult to find in the middle.

The public's demand for improved health care standards and accountability of health care providers will increase. The public may even demand physician grading and scoring to be made public. Pay-for-performance initiatives will set standards for procedures that may result in higher-quality care. Health care costs will continue to burgeon, resulting in further pressures on physician payment schedules and hospital budgeting. Some of these costs may be ameliorated by increased cost effectiveness in diagnostic and therapeutic modalities, but this is unlikely. Scrutiny of all of us by government, regulatory bodies, and the public will certainly increase. More surgeons will need to be increasingly involved in their professional organizations, not only for continuing education but also for certification. Fortunately, the state of the American Board of Facial Plastic and Reconstructive Surgery is strong, and its future is bright. "The American Board of Facial Plastic and Reconstructive Surgery has become respected and strong over the past 20 years because a small group of individuals cared enough about education, standards, and dedication to ideals to make this Board and what it represents one of their life's top priorities. Their dedication has infused the specialty with a unique imperative—the more you learn, the more you share with your colleagues. The ripple effect of this imperative will carry facial plastic surgery into the future as expectations to meet and exceed standards are a matter of intense pride among this group of surgeons."[31]

◆ Professional and Ethical Issues

> "I have but one lamp by which my feet are guided, and that is the lamp of experience. I know no way of judging the future but by the past."
>
> —Edward Gibbon

The ultimate goal of all physicians is to relieve suffering and prolong life. As facial plastic surgeons, we are given the added responsibility of treating that part of the body that reflects the person's spirit to the world. As such, we deal with the human psyche as much as with the face itself. Our goal must be to enhance the patient's appearance in a manner that satisfies them and brings to them a sense of comfort that improves their quality of life. As our products, surgical tools, and techniques advance, so will the standards we set for ourselves and those our patients expect from us. We deal daily with the eternal human values, and our appreciation for these will increase. The future will also bring more profound ethical dilemmas, especially related to the use of new and unproved products and transplantation.

Physicians have always had a contractual relationship with their patients, both implied and explicit in the form of the surgical consent. Our profession in general, and in cosmetic surgery in particular, has had its altruistic ideals tested in the face of our capitalistic world. Today, there is a new altruism emanating from the corporate world. Hopefully, it can be merged with the inherent altruistic nature of medicine to the benefit of the many who have not had access to our services. We live increasingly in an interdependent world. To flourish, we will need to look outward as well as inward and be proactive in determining our professional and personal futures. After all, we are each responsible for our own future.

> "The only certain thing about the future is that it will surprise even those who have seen the furthest into it."
>
> —E. J. Hobsbaum, historian

Acknowledgments The authors acknowledge, and express gratitude to, the following individuals who submitted their thoughts on this chapter: Joan Harting Barham, Gary C. Burget, Paul J. Carniol, Jean Carruthers, Stephen C. Duffy, Peter A. Hilger, David B. Hom, Calvin M. Johnson Jr., Theda C. Kontis, Wayne F. Larrabee Jr., Lawrence J. Marentette, Philip J. Miller, R. Stephen Mulholland, Stephen J. Pearlman, Stephen W. Perkins, J. Regan Thomas, G. J. Nolst Trenite, Hade Vuyk, Joseph K. Wong, and Laurie Wirth.

References

1. Polanyi J. [Nobel Laureate in Chemistry] Personal communication, January 2007
2. Adamson PA, Galli SK. Rhinoplasty approaches: current state of the art. Arch Facial Plast Surg 2005;7:32–37
3. Lane MA, Mattison J, Ingram DK, et al. Caloric restriction and aging in primates: relevance to humans and possible CR mimetics. Microsc Res Tech 2002;59:335–338
4. Barham JH. Facing the future. Beauty 2006;Holiday:52–53
5. Barham JH. Facing the future. Beauty 2006;Holiday:52–53
6. Haisch A, Duda GN, Schroeder D, et al. The morphology and biomechanical characteristics of subcutaneously implanted tissue-engineered human septal cartilage. Eur Arch Otorhinolaryngol 2005;262: 993–997
7. Choi YS, Park SN, Suh H. Adipose tissue engineering using mesenchymal stem cells attached to injectable PLGA spheres. Biomaterials 2005;26:5855–5863
8. Schmitz M, Graf C, Gut T, et al. Melanoma cultures show different susceptibility towards E1A-, E1B-19 kDa- and fiber-modified replication-competent adenoviruses. Gene Ther 2006;13:893–905
9. Eppley BL, Kilgo M, Coleman JJ III. Cranial reconstruction with computer-generated hard-tissue replacement patient-matched implants: indications, surgical technique, and long-term follow-up. Plast Reconstr Surg 2002;109:864–871
10. Steed DL, Group DU. Clinical evaluation of recombinant human platelet-derived growth factor for the treatment of lower extremity diabetic ulcers. J Vasc Surg 1995;21:71–81
11. Hom DB, Manivel JC. Promoting healing with recombinant human platelet-derived growth factor–BB in a previously irradiated problem wound. Laryngoscope 2003;113:1566–1571
12. Jakubowicz DM, Smith RV. Use of becaplermin in the closure of pharyngocutaneous fistulas. Head Neck 2005;27:433–438
13. Powell DM, Chang E, Farrior EH. Recovery from deep-plane rhytidectomy following unilateral wound treatment with autologous platelet gel: a pilot study. Arch Facial Plast Surg 2001;3:245–250
14. Spielberger R, Stiff P, Bensinger W, et al. Palifermin for oral mucositis after intensive therapy for hematologic cancers. N Engl J Med 2004; 351:2590–2598

15. Takeuchi M, Tredget EE, Scott PG, et al. The antifibrogenic effects of liposome-encapsulated IFN-alpha2b cream on skin wounds. J Interferon Cytokine Res 1999;19:1413–1419

16. Becic F, Mulabegovi N, Mornjakovi Z, et al. Topical treatment of standardised burns with herbal remedies in model rats. Bosn J Basic Med Sci 2005;5:50–57

17. Chen W, Fu X, Ge S, et al. Ontogeny of expression of transforming growth factor-beta and its receptors and their possible relationship with scarless healing in human fetal skin. Wound Repair Regen 2005; 13:68–75

18. Ferguson MW, O'Kane S. Scar-free healing: from embryonic mechanisms to adult therapeutic intervention. Philos Trans R Soc Lond B Biol Sci 2004;359:839–850

19. Ferguson MW, O'Kane S. Scar-free healing: from embryonic mechanisms to adult therapeutic intervention. Philos Trans R Soc Lond B Biol Sci 2004;359:839–850

20. Matarasso A, Pfeifer TM, and the Plastic Surgery Educational Foundation DATA Committee. Mesotherapy for body contouring. Plast Reconstr Surg 2005;115:1420–1424

21. American Society of Plastic Surgeons. Policy statement—mesotherapy (2005). Available at: http://www.plasticsurgery.org/medical_professionals/health_policy/Policy-Statements.cfm. Accessed January 24, 2007

22. Devauchelle B, Badet L, Lengele B, et al. First human face allograft: early report. Lancet 2006;368:203–209

23. Preminger BA, Fins JJ. Face transplantation: an extraordinary case with lessons for ordinary practice. Plast Reconstr Surg 2006;118: 1073–1074

24. Lengele B, Testelin S, Devauchelle B. Personal communication, January 2007

25. Alexiades-Armenakas M. Rhytides, laxity, and photoaging treated with a combination of radiofrequency, diode laser, and pulsed light and assessed with a comprehensive grading scale. J Drugs Dermatol 2006;5:731–738

26. Sadick NS, Trelles MA. Nonablative wrinkle treatment of the face and neck using a combined diode laser and radiofrequency technology. Dermatol Surg 2005;31:1695–1699

27. Satish H. [Vice President, PriaVision Inc] Personal communication, January 2007

28. Satish H. [Vice President, PriaVision Inc] Personal communication, January 2007

29. Sewell C, Morris D, Blevins N, et al. Quantifying risky behavior in surgical simulation. Stud Health Technol Inform 2005;111: 451–457

30. Challacombe BJ, Kavoussi LR, Dasgupta P. Trans-oceanic telerobotic surgery. BJU Int 2003;92:678–680

31. Wirth L [Executive Director, American Board of Facial Plastic & Reconstructive Surgery]. Personal communication, January 2007

Index

Note: Page numbers followed by *f* and *t* indicate figures and tables, respectively.

D

G

J

K

L

M